FEBS Congress, Part A

Proceedings of the 16th
FEBS CONGRESS

Part A

25–30 June 1984, Moscow, USSR

Edited by
YU. A. OVCHINNIKOV

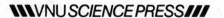 UTRECHT, THE NETHERLANDS

VNU Science Press BV
P.O. Box 2073
3500 GB   Utrecht
The Netherlands

© 1985 VNU Science Press BV

First published 1985

ISBN 90-6764-045-X Part A
ISBN 90-6764-044-1 set of three parts

Printed in Great Britain by J. W. Arrowsmith Ltd, Bristol

PREFACE

The investigation of the chemical nature of cell processes plays a key role in the study of living matter; the present advances in biochemistry, bioorganic chemistry, molecular biology, genetic engineering, etc. are widely known. Practically every day we are witnessing the revelation of new facts, the discovery of new bioregulators and the deciphering of new structures. The new direction in science, which is often called physico-chemical biology, not only strikes our imagination, but also has a considerable influence on the improvement of health care, efficiency in agricultural production and the development of new technologies.

In the summer of 1984, Moscow was the venue of the 16th Meeting of the Federation of European Biochemical Societies (FEBS). More than 4000 participants gathered in Moscow; this included not only Europeans, but also researchers from America, Asia and other parts of the world.

The scientific programme of the 16th FEBS meeting was very wide and covered practically all major aspects of the study of living matter on a molecular level. The lectures and posters presented at the meeting were devoted to the structure and function of biopolymers, the questions of the cell and membrane biology, the pressing problems of immunology, enzymology, neurobiology and modern directions of biotechnology.

The scientific level of all symposia organized within the framework of the meeting was extremely high and has reflected the latest achievments in each particular branch of science.

This three-part publication of the Proceedings of the 16th FEBS Congress includes the lectures that are of particular interest. We unfortunately could not publish all of the contributions—this would be hardly practicable.

On behalf of the organizing committee I should like to express my sincere gratitude to all attendants of the meeting for their active participation in this outstanding biochemical forum. I hope that the spirit of cooperation, mutual understanding and friendship which has marked the Moscow FEBS meeting will contribute to future progress in the study of living matter, to the well being of all nations and to peace and happiness on Earth.

Professor Yu. A. Ovchinnikov
Moscow

ORGANIZING COMMITTEE

CONTENTS

Symposium III
Medical biochemistry

Symposium VII
Evolutionary biochemistry

MECHANISM OF ENZYME ACTION

STRUCTURAL HOMOLOGIES IN ISOENZYMES

F. BOSSA, D. BARRA, L. SCHIRCH° AND S. DOONAN°°
Istituto di Chimica Biologica, Università di Roma;
Centro di Biologia Molecolare del C.N.R., Italy;
° Dept. of Biochemistry, Medical College of Virginia,
Richmond, U.S.A.; °°Dept. of Biochemistry, University
College, Cork, Ireland.

Comparative studies on isoproteins, i.e. proteins which
have similar functions within the same cellular type of a
single organism or of different organisms, or in different
compartments of the same cell, represent a classical but
still valid approach to a detailed description of structure-function relationships in these molecules. Moreover
such studies give ample opportunity for considerations of
(i) the evolutionary history of proteins, (ii) the
mechanisms of their molecular adaptations to the most
varied environments and/or (iii) the structural basis for
their specific intracellular compartmentation.
Our interest in the study of the structural and genetic
relationships between pairs of proteins (or isoenzymes)
which catalyse the same reaction in the cell cytosol and
in the mitochondria originated from work performed on the
determination of the primary structures of both the cytosolic and the mitochondrial isoenzymes of a pyridoxal
phosphate-dependent protein, aspartate aminotransferase
from pig heart.
In this particular case, it was known that both proteins were dimers of similar molecular weight and catalytic properties but with remarkable differences in the
isoelectric points (5.4 and 9.4, respectively for the
cytosolic and the mitochondrial isoenzymes), amino acid
compositions, and N- and C-terminal residues. Thus, the
question was open whether the two proteins were the
result of divergent evolution or arose by a process of
convergent evolution. Determination of the amino acid
sequence of both isoenzymes, accomplished independently
by our groups and by a Russian and a Japanese group ([1]
and references therein) demonstrated that the former was
the correct answer. In fact the 401 residues of the mitochondrial isoenzyme can be aligned along the 11 residue-

Proceedings of the 16th FEBS Congress
Part A, pp. 3–8
© 1985 VNU Science Press

-longer sequence of the cytosolic isoenzyme in such a way that 194 residues (47.1% of the total) occupy identical positions. Moreover, of the non identical residues, 128 substitutions could have occurred by single base changes. It is thus immediately apparent that the two forms arose by divergent evolution from a common ancestral gene, as attested also by the similarity of predicted secondary structure and by the very high degree of similarity in three dimensional structure, appearing from the crystal structure analyses under way in various laboratories on both isoenzymes ([2] and references therein).

A point of particular interest relates to the rates of evolution of the two enzyme forms. Given that the mitochondrial isoenzyme is synthesized in the cytosol and then translocated into the mitochondria it might be expected that there would be extra constraints imposed on its structure compared with the cytosolic form. In fact immunochemical comparisons of isoenzymes from different species [3,4] showed that mitochondrial forms are more closely related immunochemically than are the cytosolic forms. On the other hand, statistical comparisons of amino acid compositions of isoenzymes from various sources suggested a very similar rate of evolution of the two forms [5] and this conclusion is confirmed by direct sequence analysis, which is now complete for the two isoenzymes from chicken heart and for the mitochondrial form from rat liver and almost complete for the two isoenzymes from horse heart and for the mitochondrial form from human and from turkey heart ([6-8] and references therein and unpublished results from our laboratories).

Of particular interest is the comparison of pairs of isoenzymes, such as those from pig, chicken and horse heart; this shows that the percentage identities of sequence of the cytosolic isoenzymes are very similar to those of the mitochondrial forms.

The apparent conflict between results from immunochemical comparisons and from sequence studies can be resolved on the assumption that certain restricted regions of the mitochondrial isoenzymes have been particularly highly conserved during evolution (because of their possible involvement in the mechanism of intracellular compartmentation?) and moreover that some at least of these regions

4

are antigenic. Consistent with this, the three most likely predictable antigenic sites are completely conserved in the mitochondrial isoenzymes, whereas none is conserved in the cytosolic isoenzymes [9].

A structural feature clearly more conserved in the mito chondrial isoenzymes is the sequence of the N-terminal segment; the corresponding segment of cytosolic isoenzymes is not homologous with the mitochondrial forms and shows a relatively low degree of conservation. Another feature which is conserved in the mitochondrial isoenzymes is the reactivity, and hence the environment, of the single accessible sulphydryl group, that of cysteine 166. It is relevant to recall that pieces of evidence are available, which point to a possible role of both the N-terminal segment and cysteine 166 in the uptake of the mitochondrial form by the organelles [10]. Furthermore, Graf-Hausner et al. [6] by comparing the sequences of the pairs of isoenzymes from pig and from chicken identified thirty six residues specifically conserved in the mitochondrial forms, which occur in surface regions of the protein molecule. It is tempting to assume that these highly conserved surface regions are important for the process of selective intramitochondrial import.

Serine hydroxymethyltransferase is another pyridoxal--phosphate dependent enzyme which also exists in eukaryotic cells in two forms, one localized in the cytosol and the other in the mitochondria. The recent availability of sufficient quantities of the mitochondrial isoenzyme allowed a comparison of its structural and functional properties with those of the cytosolic isoenzyme [11]. It was possible to show that the two enzyme forms have similar spectral and functional properties. As far as the structural properties are concerned, the mitochondrial isoenzyme is slightly larger by about 1,000 daltons per subunit, but the amino acid compositions and isoelectric points are essentially identical. Both enzymes have a blocked N-terminal residue, whereas the C-terminus is different. These preliminary data suggested that the two enzyme forms might show a very high degree of homology; in fact one could not rule out the possibility that the slightly larger mitochondrial form differed from the cyto solic one by having an extra piece of about 10 residues

5

attached at either the carboxyl or the amino terminal of the molecule. This would suggest that the two isoenzymes may be encoded by a single gene.

A more detailed comparative investigation of the structural properties of the two enzyme forms has been undertaken, first by isolating the active site peptide from the mitochondrial isoenzyme, which proved indistinguishable from that of the cytosolic one. In contrast, the reactivity of and the sequence around the cysteine residues in the mitochondrial isoenzyme are only in part homologous with those of the cytosolic form. Furthermore, evidence for differences in the structure of the two reactive enzymes was also obtained from the effect of proteases. Incubation of the cytosolic isoenzyme with chymotrypsin results in an increase of catalytic activity, accompanied by the removal of about 25 residues from the amino terminal end of the molecule. In contrast, the mitochondrial isoenzyme is not digested in the native state by protease under the same conditions as the cytosolic form, suggesting that the conformation of this part of the molecule is different [12].

Recently the sequence of the gly A gene of E. coli has been determined and from this an amino acid sequence for the putative serine hydroxymethyltransferase proposed [13]. It was relatively easy to align along the E. coli sequence many tryptic and chymotryptic peptides from the cytosolic mammalian isoenzyme and some of the less numerous peptides from the mitochondrial form, on the basis of obvious homology considerations. In this way 162 residues of the cytosolic isoenzyme appear to have identical positions to residues in the bacterial protein; this corresponds to 39% homology. For the mitochondrial isoenzyme less structural information is at the moment available, but sufficient to demonstrate that the two iso enzymes are homologous proteins and exclude the possibility that they are encoded by a single gene [14].

Lack of space prevents a detailed description of another isoenzyme system which is being studied in our as well as in other laboratories and which is illustrative of a different evolutionary situation, namely the isoenzymes of superoxide dismutase. These enzymes are present in nature as three metalloforms: the first is the copper/zinc form

6

found in the cytosol of eukaryotes, which is completely unrelated to the other two forms, the manganese form of mitochondria and prokaryotes and the iron form of prokaryotes. These latter two forms are in turn strictly correlated [15]; in the case of Propionibacterium shermanii it was possible to obtain evidence that this bacterium can accomodate either iron or manganese on the same protein, depending on the culture conditions. The important point in relation to the present discussion, however, is that there is no sequence homology between the cytosolic and mitochondrial isoenzymes from eukaryotes, which argues for their convergent evolution from unrelated genes.

1. Barra,D., Bossa,F., Doonan,S., Fahmy,H.M.A., Hughes, G.J., Martini,F., Petruzzelli,R. and Wittmann—Liebold, B. (1980). The cytosolic and mitochondrial aspartate aminotransferases from pig heart. Eur.J.Biochem. 108, 405-414.
2. Kirsch,J.F., Eichele,G., Ford,G.C., Vincent,M.G., Jansonius,J.N., Gehring,H. and Christen,P. (1984). Mechanism of action of aspartate aminotransferase proposed on the basis of its spatial structure. J.Mol. Biol. 174, 497-525.
3. Sonderegger,P. and Christen,P. (1978). Comparison of the evolution rates of cytosolic and mitochondrial aspartate aminotransferases. Nature 275, 157-159.
4. Porter,P.B., Doonan,S. and Pearce,F.L. (1981). Interspecies comparisons of aspartate aminotransferases based on immunochemical methods. Comp.Biochem.Physiol. 69B, 761-767.
5. Doonan,S., Barra,D., Bossa,F., Porter,P.B. and Wilkinson,S.M. (1981). Interspecies comparison of aspartate aminotransferases based on amino acid compositions. Comp.Biochem.Physiol. 69B, 747-752.
6. Graf—Hausner,U., Wilson,K.J. and Christen,P. (1983). The covalent structure of mitochondrial aspartate aminotransferase from chicken. J.Biol.Chem. 258, 8813-8826.
7. Christen,P., Graf-Hausner,U., Bossa,F. and Doonan,S. (1984). Comparison of covalent structures of the isoenzymes of aspartate aminotransferases. In: Transaminases, P. Christen and D.E. Metzler (eds.) John Wiley,

New York, in press.

8. Martini,F., Angelaccio,S., Barra,D., Doonan,S. and Bossa,F. (1984). Partial amino-acid sequence and cysteine reactivities of cytosolic aspartate amino-transferase from horse heart. Biochim.Biophys.Acta, in press.

9. Doonan,S., Doonan,H.J., Barra,D.and Bossa,F. (1982). Prediction of antigenic determinants of aspartate aminotransferase isoenzymes from amino acid sequences. Biochem.Soc.Trans. 10, 106-107.

10. Passarella,S., Marra,E., Doonan,S., Saccone,C. and Quagliarello,E. (1984). Trasport of mature proteins into isolated mitochondria: a model system to investigate mitochondrial biogenesis. Biochem.Soc.Trans. 12, 381-384.

11. Schirch,L. and Peterson,D. (1980). Purification and properties of mitochondrial serine hydroxymethyl-transferase. J.Biol.Chem. 255, 7801-7806.

12. Schirch,L., Gavilanes,F., Peterson,D., Bullis,B., Barra,D. and Bossa,F. (1984). Structural studies on rabbit liver cytosolic and mitochondrial isozymes of serine hydroxymethyltransferase. In: Chemical and bio logical aspects of Vitamin B_6 catalysis, A.E. Evange-lopoulos (ed.). Alan R. Liss, New York, pp.301-308.

13. Plamann,M.D., Stauffer,L.T., Urbanovski,M.L. and Stauffer,G.V. (1983). Complete nucleotide sequence of the E. coli gly A gene. Nucleic Acids Res. 11, 2065-2075.

14. Barra,D., Martini,F., Angelaccio,S., Bossa,F., Gavilanes,F., Peterson,D., Bullis,B. and Schirch,L. (1983). Sequence homology between prokaryotic and eukaryotic forms of serine hydroxymethyltransferase. Biochem.Biophys.Res.Commun. 116, 1007-1012.

15. Parker,M.W., Schininà,M.E., Bossa,F. and Bannister, J.V. (1984). Chemical aspects of the structure, function and evolution of superoxide dismutases. Inorganica Chimica Acta 91, 307-317.

8

THE ROLE OF MULTIELECTRON AND SYNCHRONIOUS PROCESSES IN ENZYME CATALYSIS

Likhtenstein G.I.
Institute of Chemical Physics of Academy of
Science Chernogolovka, Moscow Region 142432
USSR

The conception of synchronious concert mechanisms has been accepted by biochemists for
explanation of outstanding catalytic behaviour
of enzymes for a long time. Ideas about multielectron mechanisms appeared resently in
connection with the convertion of small chemically inert molecules such as N_2 fixation and
water photooxidation in mild condition (1-4).
These reaction remain the chellenging problems
as processes of enormous biological importance
as well as attractive objects for solution of
general problems of enzyme catalysis. In this
paper some theoretical and experimental aspects of concert and multielectron mechanisms
will be discussed and the criteria for its
realization will be formulated.

GENERAL PRINCIPLES

According to modern concepts, the occurrence
of an elementary step of chemical processes,
including catalytic reactions, proceeds at a
sufficient rate characteristic for enzymic
catalysis ($K = 10^1 + 10^7 s^{-1}$), provided the following factors are operating in concert: (1).
Thermodynamic feasibility of the step (2).
Positive overlap of electron and nuclear wave
functions in the final and initial states (3).
The matching of the nuclear environment and
the electron configuration. The latter is
achieved upon synchronization of nuclei as a
result of the rapid vibrational relaxation

Proceedings of the 16th FEBS Congress
Part A, pp. 9–15
© 1985 VNU Science Press

during the time comparable to the duration of
an elementary step of an adiabatic chemical
reaction (10^{-13}s) (3-6). The efficiency of the
fit is sharply diminished during this time
with increasing the number of nuclei participating in the process. According to the theory
developed by Aleksandrov (6) the value of synchronization probability ($\measuredangle$) is given by the
formula

$$\measuredangle = \frac{n}{2^{n-1}} \left(\frac{nKT}{\pi E_{(n)}} \right)^{n-1/2} \qquad (1)$$

where n is the number of vibrational degrees
of freedom of the nuclei participating in the
concerted transition, $E(n)$ is the activation
energy.

Concerted and multielectron mechanisms are
energy preferable, but less probable owing to
participation of a considerable number of nuclei. This allows formulation of the principls
of "optimal motion" (3-5). According to this
principle, the number of nuclei whose configuration is changed in the elementary act of a
chemical reaction must be sufficiently large
to provide the favourable energetic of the
step and at the same time, sufficiently small
for the high value of the nuclear synchronization probability to be maintained during motion along the path to reaction products.

Let us consider as an example the possible
four-electron mechanisms. Evidently, the direct transport of four electrons from the filled orbitals of a metal to the substrate in a
binuclear complex is absolutely ruled out for
energetic and relaxation reasons. Such a transport increases sharply the electrostatic
energy of the system and obviously requires a
substantial rearrangement of the nuclear configuration of the environment. The interaction
in a transition-metal complex with substrates
(N_2, for example) occurs through transfer of 4

electrons from the orbitals of a metal to the antibonding π*-orbitals of the substrates and a simultaneous transfer from the bonding orbitals of the substrate to the vacant d-orbitals of the metal atom. Such an electron transport may cause significant changes in the electron structure of the substrate, without changing substantially the total energy of the system.

REDUCTIVE FIXATION OF N_2

The central enzyme of biological fixation of N_2 catalyzes coupled reactions: (1) reduction of N_2 to NH_3, and (2) hydrolysis of ATP to ADP and inorganic phosphate. The active form of the enzyme nitrogenase is formed by a combined action of two components: an iron-containing protein (FeP) and an iron-molybdenum protein (FeMoP). In 1970 Likhtenstein and Shilov (1) showed that the formation of N_2H and N_2H_2 derivatives as intermediate products in the N_2 ase reaction is energetically unfourable even when an account is taken of the additional consumption of the energy released in the ATP-hydrolysis. On the other hand, the hydrolysis of ATP can provide an increase in the reduction potential of the system up to-600 to-700mv, which is quite sufficient for the formation of a hydrazine derivative.

The predictions of thermodynamic consideration have been in principle confirmed experimentally in biological and model systems (2-4, 7). Some data on the structure and function of the active center of nitrogenase are summerized in Fig.1. The nitrogenase active center consists of a whole ensemble of iron-sulphur clusters (Fe_4S_4-clusters, presumably), as well as of a FeMo-containing clusters (so-called FeMo cofactor). All clusters are disposed in close proximity to each other and to the ATP center. These distances are suitable for tunneling of electrons between the clusters and for direct chemical interaction between Fe_4S_4 clusters and ATP. The electrons run one by one from Fe- to FeMo-proteins and owing to coupled hydrolysis of ATP a superreduced state of FeMo cofactor is formed:

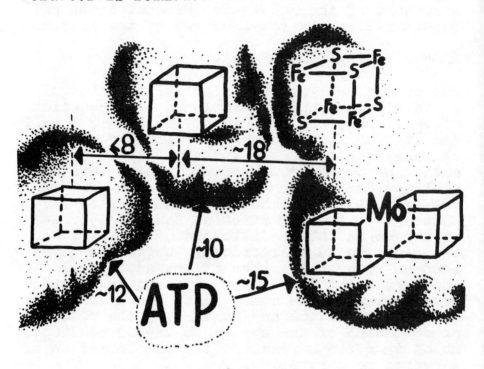

a.

b.

FIGURE 1. Proposed model of the N_2ase active center (a) and coupled reaction ATP hydrolysis and electron transfer (b). (r in Å)

When 4 electrons are collected, the four-electron mechanism of N_2 reduction is realized. The hydrazine derivative has been indeed revealed in the nitrogenase reduction.

The most optimal mechanism is presumably a four-electron one, which involves two Mo atoms of two molecules of the FeMo cofactor. The presence of iron-clusters with a great electron capacity in the immediate vicinity of Mo atoms allows reducing the rearrangement of the nuclear environment to a minimum upon electron transfer from molybdenum to N_2.

WATER OXIDATION

In biological photosynthesis, the decomposition of water with evolution of oxygen occurs under the action of a relatively mild oxidant: the cation-radical of chlorophyll which is the product of one-electron photooxidation with $E_0 = 0.9-1.1$ eV. The potentials of the water oxidation by one-, two- and four-electron mechanisms are equal, respectively, to 2.7 eV (the hydroxyl radical), 1.36 eV (hydrogen peroxide) and 0.81 eV (molecular oxygen). It is evident that the smoothest thermodynamic profile of the reaction is provided by the four-electron mechanism (2-4). This mechanism can be realized in photosystem II in tetra or binuclear manganese containing complex. The cluster nature of the manganese complex has been convincingly demonstrated in (8).

The evolution of dioxygen from water may be described as a sequence of elementary steps: four one-electron steps of oxidation of the manganese complex by the chlorophyll cation-radical and one four-electron step of O_2 evolution. Each one-electron step is accompanied by elimination of a proton, which contributes to the preservation of the total charge of the complex and considerably simplifies the last decisive step of the process. One of the possible mechanisms of water oxidation is given by the scheme:

$$\begin{bmatrix} H_2O & \\ H_2O & Mn_4 \end{bmatrix}^{n+} \xrightarrow[-4\bar{e},4H^+]{4h\nu} \begin{bmatrix} O^- & \\ O^- & Mn_4 \end{bmatrix}^{n+1} \xrightarrow{O_2} \begin{bmatrix} Mn_4 \end{bmatrix}^{n+}$$

HYDROLYTIC ENZYME REACTION. LYSOZYME.

The tipical example of concert hydrolytic reaction is hydrolysis of glucoside bond in the lysozyme active center. The reaction is affected presumably by synchronious attack of two carboxyle groupes (one protonated and one deprotonated) and water molecules. This implicates milty-orbital overlapping (virtually multielectron mechanism) and synchronious replacement not less then 12 nuclea of catalytic and substrate groups.

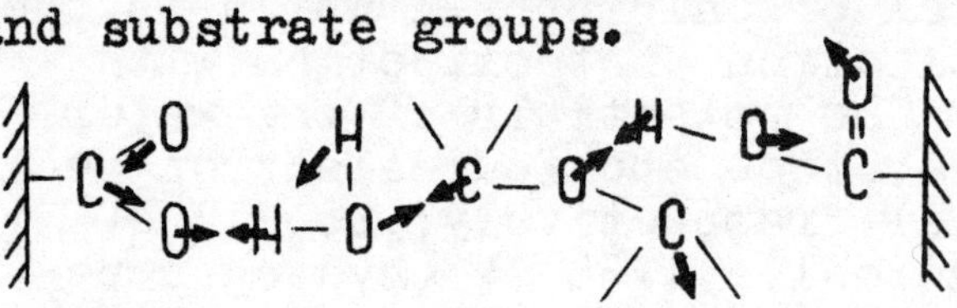

FIGURE 2. Lysozyme reaction.

In such a case the value of synchronization factor is to be very low ($\alpha \approx 10^{-10}$–10^{-12}). That why such a concert mechanism seems to be questionable.

CONCLUSION

The following general requirements for realization of synchronious and multielectron mechanisms can be formulated: (1). Thermodynamic feasibility. (2) Effective overlapping of orbitals involved in the reaction:"orbital symmerty conservation selection rule".(3) Large value of synchronization factor. New "selection rule on synchronization" has to be put into practice to examine possibilities of chemical and biochemical reactions.

The optimum combination of these factors provided good conditions for multielectron and limited concert reactions and may be generalized as principal of optimum motions at elementary act.

REFERENCES

1. Likhtenstein, G.I., Shilov, A.E. (1970). On the thermodynamic fixation of molecular nitrogen. Zhur. Fiz. Khim. 44, 849-856.
2. Semenov, N.N., Shilov, A.E. and Likhtenstein, G.I. (1975). Multi-electron redox processes in chemistry and biology. Dokl. Akad. Nauk SSSR, 221, 1374-1378.
3. Likhtenstein, G.I. (1979). Polynuclear Redox Metalloenzymes. Nauka. Moscow.
4. Likhtenstein, G.I. (1984). Chemical Physics of Redox Metallo-Enzyme Catalysis. Springer Verlag. Heidelberg. Berlin.
5. Likhtenstein, G.I. (1977). On the principles of "optimal motion" in elementary acts of chemical and biological processes. Kinetika i Kataliz. 28, 878-885.
6. Aleksandrov, I.V. (1976). Dependence of the rate of concerted chemical reaction on the number of degrees of freedom involved in the transition. Teor.Eksp. Khim. 12,299-305.
7. Shilov, A.E. (1978). N_2 fixation in proton media in mild condition. In:Atreatise of dinitrogen fixation, R.W.F. Hardy, F.Bottomley, R.C.Burns (eds). Wiley Interscience, New York, pp.518-537.
8. Kulikov, A.V., Bogatirenko, V.R., Likhtenstein, G.I., Allakhverdiev, S.I., Klimov, V.V., Shuvalov, V.A. and Krasnovsky, A.A. (1983). Magnetic interaction of manganese in the reaction centers of photosystem II. Biofizika, 28, 3, 357-363.

DIFFERENCES IN THE CATALYTIC MECHANISMS OF SERINE AND CYSTEINE PROTEINASES

POLGÁR, L. & ASBÓTH, B.

Institute of Enzymology, Biological Research
Center, Hungarian Academy of Sciences,
Budapest, Hungary

The basic features of the mechanism of action of
serine proteinases, like chymotrypsin and subtilisin, are illustrated in the scheme below. It

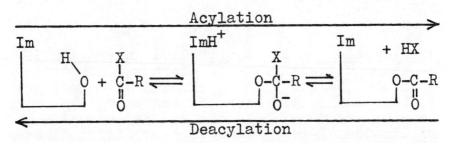

is seen that the nucleophilic attack by the serine hydroxyl group on the carbonyl carbon atom
of the substrate is catalyzed by a histidine residue as a general base. This leads to the formation of a tetrahedral intermediate and an imi-
dazolium ion. The intermediate breaks down by
general acid catalysis to an acyl-enzyme, an
imidazole base and alcohol or amine. The acyl-
-enzyme is hydrolyzed through the reverse reaction pathway of acylation.

Lack of general base-catalysis in the acylation step of cysteine proteinase catalysis

It was originally suggested that cysteine proteinases, whose protagonist is papain, operate

Proceedings of the 16th FEBS Congress
Part A, pp. 17–22
© 1985 VNU Science Press

via the same mechanism but instead of serine a
cysteine residue is the nucleophile. However,
we have pointed out that the nucleophilic attack
by the cysteine is not assisted by general base-
-catalysis. This difference arises from the formation of a thiolate-imidazolium ion-pair in
the free cysteine enzyme, which implies that
the proton is already on the imidazole when the
thiolate ion attacks the substrate. The arguments supporting ion-pair formation were the
lack of D_2O effect in acylation (1) and spectroscopic detection of a thiolate ion-like form of
Cys-25 (2). Proton NMR studies have also shown
that histidine-159 is in the protonated form
below pH 8, where the ion-pair was proposed to
exist (3).

Stabilization of the tetrahedral intermediate
The other difference to be discussed concerns
the stabilization of the tetrahedral adduct generated in the formation and decomposition of
the acyl-enzyme of both the serine and cysteine
proteinases. X-ray diffraction studies indicated
that the negative oxyanion of the tetrahedral
adduct can interact with backbone -NH- or side
chain amide groups in both serine proteinases
(4) and papain (5). To test this possibility, we
synthesized thiono ester substrates which contain a sulphur atom in place of the carbonyl
oxygen atom. As the reactivities of the oxo and
thiono ester bonds are similar in alkaline hydrolysis (6), a considerable difference with the
thiono substrate relative to the corresponding
oxo ester should give information about the role
of the oxyanion binding site in catalysis.

Reaction of oxo and thiono esters with serine
proteinases. The second-order rate constants
for acylation of chymotrypsin and subtilisin

Table 1.

Second-Order Rate Constants ($M^{-1}s^{-1}$) for Acylation of Serine Proteinases by Oxo and Thiono Esters

	Methyl N-benzoylglycinates		Ethyl N-acetylphenylalaninates	
	k_O	k_S	k_O	k_S
Chymotrypsin	31	<1	15 000	<1
Subtilisin	18	<0.6	25 000	<2

are shown in Table 1 (for experimental details see ref. 6). It is seen that the thiono esters are not hydrolyzed by either serine proteinase at a measurable rate (the data represent upper limits). Particularly in the case of the better substrate (the phenylalanine derivative), the differences in the rate constants for the oxo and thiono compounds are considerable, more than 4 orders of magnitude with both chymotrypsin and subtilisin. Since the acylation rate constant ($k = k_2/K_s = k_{cat}/K_m$) is a complex constant which involves binding, the binding constants (K_s or K_i) were also determined. The values showed that binding was not significantly affected by the oxygen to sulphur change (6). Accordingly, the substantial difference in the acylation rate constants may be attributed to poor catalysis with thiono esters rather than to the impediment of the formation of the enzyme-substrate complex. This implies that substrate binding in the oxyanion binding site is critical in the transition state (tetrahedral adduct) while it is less important in the ground state (Michaelis complex) of the reaction.

Hydrolysis of oxo and thiono esters by cysteine
proteinases. Table 2 shows that cysteine proteinases are less reactive towards the thiono derivative of a specific substrate than towards

Table 2.

Kinetic Parameters of the Reactions of Cysteine
Proteinases with the Oxo and Thiono Ethyl Esters
of N-Benzyloxycarbonyl-Phenylalanylglycine

	k_{cat}/K_m $(M^{-1}s^{-1})$	k_{cat} (s^{-1})
Papain		
Oxo ester	430 000	9.1
Thiono ester	240 000	0.77
Oxo/Thiono	1.8	12
Chymopapain		
Oxo ester	10 000	0.75
Thiono ester	4400	0.05
Oxo/Thiono	2.3	15
Papaya peptidase A		
Oxo ester	320 000	16
Thiono ester	100 000	1
Oxo/Thiono	3.2	16

the corresponding oxo ester, but the difference
is much less than in the case of the specific
substrates of serine proteinases (1.8-3.2 as
compared with more than 10 000).

Table 2 also shows the k_{cat} values, which were
found to be practically equal to the first-or-
der deacylation rate constants by the added nucleophile method (7). The 12-16-fold difference

between the rate constants for the oxo and thio-no substrates shows that replacement of sulphur for the oxygen atom does not seriously affect deacylation either.

Conclusion
Owing to the lack of general base-catalysis in acylation and the less stringent geometry in transition state stabilization, cysteine protei-nases have a simpler mechanism as compared with the more sophisticated mechanism of action of serine proteinases. This may be worth conside-ring when designing relatively simple catalysts with enzymic activity which is one of the grea-test challenges to the present day organic che-mists. Furthermore, as a relatively simple me-chanism is expected to be realized readily du-ring evolution, cysteine proteinases, as com-pared with serine proteinases, might represent a more ancient family of enzymes.

Reference list

1. Polgár, L. (1973). On the mode of activation of the catalytically essential sulfhydryl group of papain. Eur. J. Biochem. 33, 104-109.
2. Polgár, L. (1974). Mercaptide-imidazolium ion-pair: the reactive nucleophile in papain catalysis. FEBS Lett. 47, 15-18.
3. Lewis, S.D., Johnson, F.A. and Shafer, J.A. (1981). Effect of cysteine-25 on the ioniza-tion of histidine-159 in papain as deter-mined by proton nuclear magnetic resonance spectroscopy. Evidence for a His-159-Cys-25 ion pair and its possible role in catalysis. Biochemistry 20, 48-51.
4. Kraut, J. (1977). Serine proteases: structure and mechanism of catalysis. Ann. Rev. Biochem. 46, 331-358.

5. Drenth, J., Kalk, K.H. and Swen, H.M. (1976). Binding of chloromethyl ketone substrate analogues to crystalline papain. Biochemistry 15, 3731-3738.
6. Asbóth, B. and Polgár, L. (1983). Transition-state stabilization at the oxyanion binding sites of serine and thiol proteinases: hydrolyses of thiono and oxygen esters. Biochemistry 22, 117-122.
7. Bender, M.L., Clement, G.E., Gunter, C.P. and Kézdy, F.J. (1964). The Kinetics of α-Chymotrypsin Reactions in the Presence of Added Nucleophiles. J. Am. Chem. Soc. 86, 3697-3703.

A NEW CONFORMATIONAL MODEL FOR SUBSTRATES OF COLLAGEN PROLYL HYDROXYLASE

V.S. ANANTHANARAYANAN

Department of Biochemistry, Memorial University of Newfoundland, St. John's, Nfld., Canada A1B 3X9

Prolylhydroxylase catalyses the conversion of selected proline (Pro) residues into 4-hydroxyproline (Hyp). Only those Pro residues which occur in position 3 of the typical collagen triplet, $-Gly-R_2-R_3-$, are hydroxylated by the enzyme and the extent of hydroxylation is apparently governed by the nature of the residues adjoining the -Pro-Gly- segment (1). Since the unhydroxylated collagen molecule is found to be structurally and functionally defective (1), the understanding of the conformational aspects of Hyp incorporation in collagen is very important.

EARLIER DATA AND THE β-TURN HYPOTHESIS

We have been interested in the conformational aspects of proline hydroxylation. Our earlier studies led us to propose (2) that the structural feature that distinguishes the Pro residues that are hydroxylated by prolyl hydroxylase is the β-turn conformation at the -Pro-Gly- segments of the nascent (unhydroxylated) poly-peptide chains. Our proposal was based mainly on theoretical and experimental studies on the conformation of -Pro-Gly- segments in synthetic peptides and globular proteins which revealed the high propensity of this sequence for the β-turn (3,5). In contrast, the -Gly-Pro- sequence, which is unsuitable for hydroxylation, shows a preference for a relatively extended conformation similar to the polyproline-II (PP-II) helix (5). We attributed the variations in the extent of proline hydroxylation in different parts of

Proceedings of the 16th FEBS Congress
Part A, pp. 23–30
© 1985 VNU Science Press

the collagen molecule to the influence of the residues adjoining the -Pro-Gly- segments on the stability of the β-turn (2). This suggestion was based on the experimental data on the tripeptides: N-acetyl-Pro-Gly-X (X = Gly, Ala, Leu, Ile or Phe) and on theoretical analysis of tetrapeptide sequences in proteins (4). In a later study (6), we synthesized a variety of peptides which, from spectroscopic data, were found to favour the β-turn conformation, although the exact β-turn type depended on the amino acid sequence. The interaction of these peptides with purified prolyl hydroxylase was then examined (6,7). All the peptides were found to act as inhibitors of the hydroxylation of the synthetic substrate (Pro-Pro-Gly)$_5$, thus lending support to our earlier β-turn hypothesis.

NEED FOR A MODIFIED THEORY

Our previous studies (6,7) showed that β-turn tri-peptides (eg. tBoc-Pro-Gly-Val-OH) acted only as inhibitors of the synthetic substrate but not as substrates themselves, while the pentapeptide, tBoc-Gly-Val-Pro-Gly-Val-OH was both an inhibitor and a substrate. This indicates that the minimal peptide sequence for a β-turn is necessary but not sufficient for proline hydroxylation. Further, it is known that polyproline in the PP-II conformation and native triple-helix collagen are effective inhibitors of prolyl hydroxylase although neither of them contained the β-turn. There were also no data available to show that (Pro-Pro-Gly)$_n$, in the "denatured" form in which it is hydroxylated, would contain β-turn segments at the -Pro-Gly- junctions.

ADDITIONAL EXPERIMENTAL DATA

To clarify the above points, we carried out the synthesis of several additional peptides and studied their interactions with prolyl hydroxylase as in the earlier study (6). To our surprise (and intial dismay), we found that not only the β-turn tripepides (eg. tBoc-Pro-Gly-Ala-OH) but several dipeptides viz.- tBoc-Pro-Gly-OH, tBoc-Pro-DAla-OH and tBoc-Gly-Pro-OH, which obviously cannot sustain the β-turn conformation, also acted as inhibitors of the synthetic substrate (Table I). None of these peptides, however, was hydroxylated by the enzyme. These results seemed to indicate that prolyl hydroxylase recognized non-β-turn conformation as well. We then synthesized a series of peptides which had additional residues besides those minimally needed to form the β-turn. Interestingly, all these peptides were found to undergo significant hydroxylation, albeit to varying extents (Table II). This is marked in contrast to the data on peptides having the minimal β-turn sequence or less (Table I).

NEW MODEL FOR SUBSTRATE CONFORMATION

An insight into the exact conformational requirement for proline hydroxylation was obtained by a careful analysis of the ocnformation of the inhibitors and substrates. The tripeptides tBoc-Pro-Gly-Ala-OH, tBoc-Pro-Gly-Val-OH and tBoc-Pro-DAla-Ala-OH shown in Table I and also several other tripeptides used in our earlier study (6,7) had, as mentioned before, the β-turn conformation. In comparison, the dipeptides shown in Table I were found to have either a 'bent' or a 'rigid' structure. X-ray crystallographic data on tBoc-Pro-Gly-OH (8) and tBoc-Pro-DAla-OH (9) show that the conformational angles for the Pro residues are close to those observed for the 2nd residue in type I or type II β-turn ($\Phi \cong -60°$ and $\psi \cong 150-175°$), while those for the Gly and DAla residues are such that they would cause a 'bend' similar to the one made by the 3rd residue in type I or type II β-turn, respectively. In other words, these peptides have a 'partial β-turn' structure. In marked contrast, the crystal structure data on tBoc-Gly-Pro-OH (10) reveal an extended structure where, in particular, the Φ, ψ values for the Gly residue are high ($\cong 180°$).

Table I. Inhibition of Hydroxylation by Synthetic Peptides

Peptide[a]	Inhibition(%)[a]	Conformation (Reference)
tBoc-Pro-Gly-Ala-OH	90	β-turn (6)
tBoc-Pro-Gly-Val-OH	80	β-turn (6)
tBoc-Pro-DAla-Ala-OH	70	β-turn (6,9)
tBoc-Pro-Gly-OH	40	'bent structure'(8)
tBoc-Pro-DAla-OH	50	'bent structure'(9)
tBoc-Gly-Pro-OH	35	'rigid' structure (10)

[a]Expressed with respect to $(Pro-Pro-Gly)_5 \cdot 4H_2O$ as substrate. Error limits + 5 to + 10%. The inhibitor concentration was 10 mM for tripeptides and 20 mM for dipeptides. See ref. 6 for details.

Table II. Hydroxylation of Synthetic Peptides by Prolyl Hydroxylase.

Peptide[a]	Hydroxylation(%)[b]	Conformation[c] (Reference)
t-Boc-Pro-Gly-NHCH$_3$	3	PP-II+β-turn (11)
N-Ac-Pro-Pro-Gly-Pro-OH	6	PP-II+β-turn (13)
tBoc-Pro-Pro-Gly-Pro-NHCH$_3$	7	n.a.
tBoc-Val-Pro-Gly-Val-OH	14	PP-II+β-turn (12)
tBoc-Gly-Val-Pro-Gly-Val-OH	40	n.a.

[a]Peptide concentration used was 20 mM; conditions same as in ref. 6.
[b]Expressed with respect to $(Pro-Pro-Gly)_5 \cdot 4H_2O$ as reference (100%).
[c]n.a.: not available.

Turning now to the conformation of the oligopeptide substrates of prolyl hydroxylase, the data on the crystal structures of tBoc-Pro-Pro-Gly-NHCH$_3$ (11) and tBoc-Val-Pro-Gly-Val-OH (12) and the minimum energy conformation of N-acetyl-Pro-Pro-Gly-OH and (Pro-Pro-Gly)$_n$ in its 'denatured' state (13), reveal that the N-terminal Pro-Pro or X-Pro part of these peptides adopts a PP-II-like conformation while the Pro-Gly segment assumes the β-turn. We may reasonably expect a similar conformation in the other peptides listed in Table II because of their analogous sequences. We therefore conclude that the structural requirement for the enzymic proline hydroxylation is the PP-II + β-turn conformation. We further propose that the PP-II structure is required at the binding site while the β-turn is necessary at the catalytic site of the active site of prolyl hydroxylase. Thus peptides that have structures resembling either the PP-II or β-turn would serve as inhibitors. This then would account for the inhibition data presented in Table I as well as the available data on several other peptides and polypeptides including polyproline and native collagen.

A schematic representation of our new model for proline hydroxylation is shown in Figure 1, which depicts the polyproline-II 'arm' of the substrate at the binding site and the β-turn at the catalytic site. Further studies are now in progress to understand the effect of chain length and the influence of neighbouring residues on the stability of the PP-II + β-turn structure and therefore on the extent of proline hydroxylation.

ACKNOWLEDGEMENT

I thank my colleagues Dr. S. Attah-Poku and Ms. Prabha Mukkamala for the experimental data on the peptides. This work was supported by the Canadian Heart Foundation.

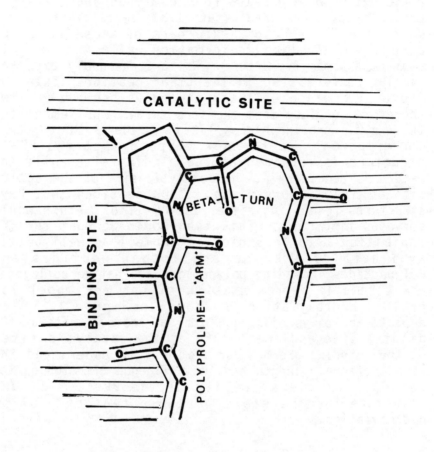

Figure 1.   Model of the active site of prolyl hydroxylase. Arrow indicates the position of hydroxylation.

REFERENCES

Bornstein, P. and Traub, W. (1979). The Chemistry and
Biology of Collagen. In: The Proteins, H. Neurath and
R.L. Hill (eds). Academic Press, New York, Vol. IV,
pp. 412-632.
Brahmachari, S.K. and Ananthanarayanan, V.S. (1979).
β-turns in nascent procollagen are sites of post-
translational enzymatic hydroxylation of proline.
Proc. Natl. Acad. Sci. (USA) 76, 5119-5123.
Zimmerman, S.S. and Scheraga, H.A. (1977). Influence of
local interactions on protein structure. I.
Conformational energy studies of N-acetyl-N'-methyl-
amines of Pro-X and X-Pro dipeptides. Biopolymers 16,
811-843.
Brahmachari, S.K. (1978). Ph.D. Dissertation (Indian
Institute of Science, Bangalore, India).
Stimson, E.R., Zimmerman, S.S. and Scheraga, H.A.
(1977). Conformational studies of oligopeptides
containing proline and glycine. Macromolecules 10,
1049-1060.
Chopra, R.K. and Ananthanarayanan, V.S. (1982).
Conformational implications of enzymatic proline
hydroxylation in collagen. Proc. Natl. Acad. Sci.
(USA) 79, 7180-7184.
Ananthanarayanan, V.S. (1983). Conformational critera
for, and consequence of proline hydroxylation in
collagen. In: Conformation in Biology, R. Srinivasan
and R.H. Sarma (eds). Academic Press, New York, pp.
99-111.
Benedetti, E., Pavone, V., Toniolo, C., Bonora, G.M.
and Palumbo, M. (1977). Solid state and solution
conformation of N-tert-butyloxycarbonyl-L-prolyl-
glycine. Macromolecules 6, 1350-1356.
Cameron, T.S. and Ananthanarayanan, V.S., to be
published.
Tanaka, I., Kozima, T., Ashida, T., Tanaka, N. and
Kakudo, M. (1977). Benzyloxycarbonylglycyl-L-proline.
Acta Cryst. B33, 116-119.
Tanaka, I., Ashida, T., Shimonishi, Y. and Kakudo, M.
(1977). The crystal and molecular structure of the

tert-butyloxy-carbonyl-L-prolyl-L-prolylglycinamide".
Acta Cyrst. 35, 110-114.

Yagi, Y., Tanaka, I., Yamane, T. and Ashida, T. (1983).
Crystal structures of repeating peptides of elastin.
3. N-(tert-butyloxycarbonyl)-L-valyl-L-prolylglycyl-L-
valine and its monohydrate crystal. J. Amer. Chem.
Soc. 105, 1242-1246.

Lee, E., Nemethy, G., Scheraga, H.A. and
Ananthanarayanan, V.S. (1984). β-bend conformation of
CH_3CO-Pro-Pro-Gly-$NHCH_3$. Implications for
posttranslational proline hydroxylation in collagen.
Biopolymers 23, 1193-1206.

FUNCTIONAL DYNAMICS OF PROTEOLYSIS

V.K. ANTONOV
Shemyakin Institute of Bioorganic Chemistry, USSR
Academy of Sciences, Moscow, USSR

Proteolysis, like other enzyme-catalyzed reactions, is
a multistep process, each step involving functionally
important changes of reacting substances. The term
"functional dynamics" summarizes these changes. Numerous data available nowadays that the formation of the
productive enzyme-substrate complex is not an instan-
taneous process (1). The rapid, usually diffusion-
-controlled step of the enzyme-substrate interaction
is followed by the relatively slow step of the isomerization of the complex formed:

$$E + S \; \underset{}{\overset{K_s}{\rightleftharpoons}} \; E_oS \; \underset{k_{-2}}{\overset{k_2}{\rightleftharpoons}} \; E_pS \; \overset{k_3}{\longrightarrow} \tag{1}$$

What is the difference between these two complexes?
We lack precise information but it is reasonable to
suppose that the first, "external" complex (E_oS) is
formed due to longrange, isotropic forces. In case of
peptide substrates some kind of "anchoring" of the
substrate by the group defining the primary specificity
of the enzyme may occur. At the next stage secondary
interactions are realized and the right orientation of
the entire substrate and enzyme is achieved. Thus the
experimentally available kinetic constants $K_{m(app)}$ and
k_{cat} may depend on the equilibrium position between
the "external" and "internal" complexes (Table 1).
For a series of substrates with identical or similar
primary specificity, that is with similar K_s values,
and different secondary interactions, K_p increasing
changes k_{cat} without affecting $K_{m(app)}$, but when
K_p exceeds a unity k_{cat} reaches its maximum value and

Proceedings of the 16th FEBS Congress
Part A, pp. 31–40
© 1985 VNU Science Press

$K_{m(app)}$ decreases. Fig. 1 shows that this is the case
for substrates of some proteases, especially pepsin,
where the systematic change of A and B peptide moieties
causes the k_{cat} increase followed by the decrease in
$K_{m(app)}$ values.

Table 1. Meaning of the experimental kinetic constants[*]

K_p	k_3	k_{cat}	$K_{m(app)}$
$\ll 1$	$\ll k_{-2}$	$k_2 k_3/k_{-2}$	K_s
$\ll 1$	$\gg k_{-2}$	k_2	K_s
$\gg 1$	$\ll k_{-2}$	k_3	$K_s k_{-2}/k_2$
$\gg 1$	$\gg k_{-2}$	k_3	$K_s k_3/k_2$

[*]
$$K_p = \frac{k_2}{k_{-2}+k_3} \quad ; \quad K_s = \frac{k_{-1}}{k_1} \qquad (Eq.\ 1)$$

The question arises what are the structural features
of the "internal" enzyme-substrate complex which are
essential for the high rate of the amide bond hydrolysis? To answer the question it is necessary, first
of all, to point out the types of nucleophilic groups
of the enzyme. Recently our laboratory has developed
the methods for differentiation between covalent (Eg. 2)
and general base (Eq. 3) modes of proteolysis. They
are based on the investigation of ^{18}O incorporation
from heavy-oxygen water into the substrates, acyl-
-transfer (or transpeptidation) products and products
of hydrolysis. The results of these studies (7 - 10)
evidence that amide hydrolysis by serine and thiol
proteases proceeds by the covalent mechanism with formation of an intermediate acyl-enzyme, but in case
of carboxylic and metal-dependent proteases water
participates as a nucleophile and no acyl-enzymes are
formed.
  Recently most of the investigators (cf. e.g. (11))

32

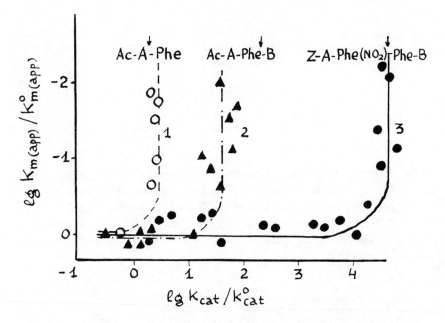

Fig. 1. Plots of log K_m (relative) vs. log k_{cat} (relative) for series of substrates of carboxypeptidase A (1), chymotrypsin (2) and pepsin (3). Kinetic data are taken from (2 - 6).

$$
E-X^- \quad \underset{NHR_2}{\overset{R_1}{C}}=O \rightleftharpoons E-X-\underset{NHR_2}{\overset{R_1}{C}}-O^- \rightleftharpoons E-X-\overset{R_1}{C}=O \underset{H_2O}{\rightleftharpoons} E-X-\underset{OH}{\overset{R_1}{C}}-O^- \rightleftharpoons E-X^- + \underset{OH}{\overset{R_1}{C}}=O
$$

$$
\underset{R_3NH_2}{\quad} \quad E-X-\underset{NHR_3}{\overset{R_1}{C}}-O^- \rightleftharpoons E-X^- + \underset{NHR_3}{\overset{R_1}{C}}=O
$$

(2)

have come to the conclusion that such an attractive hypothesis as "charge relay system" does not hold in case of serine proteases. Consequently, nucleophilicity of catalytic groups of most proteases is very low. To understand the high velocity of proteolysis one needs to fing out another reason rather than the state

33

of the enzyme catalytic groups.

$$E-X^- \quad H-\bullet \quad \overset{\underset{|}{R_1}}{\underset{NHR_2}{C}}=O \rightleftarrows E-XH \cdot H\bullet-\overset{\underset{|}{R_1}}{\underset{NHR_2}{C}}-O^- \rightleftarrows E-X^- \cdot \overset{\underset{|}{R_1}}{\underset{OH}{C}}=\bullet \rightleftarrows E-X^- + \overset{\underset{|}{R_1}}{\underset{OH}{C}}=\bullet$$

$$\updownarrow$$

$$R_3NH_2$$

$$E-XH \cdot \ ^-\bullet-\overset{\underset{|}{R_1}}{\underset{OH}{C}}-NHR_3 \rightleftarrows E-X^- + \overset{\underset{|}{R_1}}{\underset{NHR_3}{C}}=\bullet \qquad (3)$$

The main factor stabilizing amides is the resonance in a planar amide group. Two ways exist to decrease the resonance stabilization of amides - the twisting (A) and bending (or pyramidalyzation) (B). The degree of pyramidalyzation depends on the distance between a carbonyl carbon

and nucleophile as well as on the basicity of the nucleophilic group. As follows from quantum-chemical calculations, some degree of pyramidalyzation may exist even at the van der Waals distance between reacting groups (Fig. 2). Fluctuation may shorten this distance and result in increasing pyramidalyzation which, in turn, enhances the electrophilicity of the amide carbonyl carbon. Pyramydalyzation corresponds to the change of the amide bond structure during the nucleophilic addition. Is the enzyme capable of decreasing the resonance stabilization of the amide bond in substrates? Some crystallographic data show that this may be the case. Table 2 demonstrates that in some enzyme-quasisubstrate complexes the potentially susceptible amide bond has substantial degree of pyramidalyzation.

The nucleophilic attack develops simultaneously up

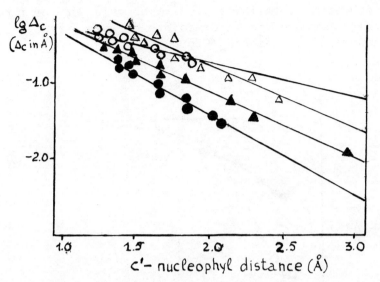

Fig. 2. Dependence of the degree of pyramidalyzation of the amide bon of the distance between the carbonyl carbon of the substrate (MeCONHMe) and the nucleophyl for CH_3OH (1), CH_3O^- (2), CH_3S^- (3) and $H_2O-HCOO^-$ system (4). Calculated by CNDO/2 method.

Table 2. Pyramidalyzation of the amide bond[x]

Enzyme	Ligand	Bond	Δ_c, Å (FLA B)
Chymotrypsin	BPTI	$Lys^{15}-Ala^{16}$	0.38
Trypsin	BPTI	$Lys^{15}-Ala^{16}$	0.28
--	BPTI (free)	$Lys^{15}-Ala^{16}$	0.008
Ealastase	$CF_3COLysAlaNHC_6H_4CF_3$	CF_3CONH	0.042
Carboxy-peptidase A	GlyTyr	CONH	0.012
Thermolysin	$C_6H_5(CH_2)_2COPheOH$	CONH	0.06

[x] Calculated from the atomic coordinates of the complexes. Source (12 - 17).

up to the equilibrium state when started with appropriate degree of pyramidalysation. The structure of the equilibrium compound is intermediate between planar amide and real tetrahedron (Fig. 3).

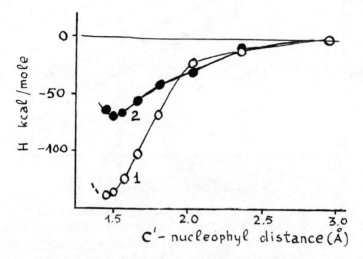

Fig. 3. Change of the energy at the nucleophilic attack of MeCONHMe by MeOH (1) and MeO⁻ (2). The initial state of the CONH corresponds to that shown in Fig. 2 for 3A distance. Calculated by CNDO/2 method, programme GEOMO.

Formation of the tetrahedral intermediate terminates when the proton abstraction takes place or, in case of sufficiently basic leaving group, reaction may proceed without formation of the tetrahedral intermediate (18).

Thus it is reasonable to suppose that in the productive enzyme-substrate complex the amide bond to be broken is not planar but pyramidal to a certain degree, that decreases its resonance stabilization and inceases the electrophilicity of the amide carbonyl carbon.

Many enzymes which do not form the acylenzyme intermediate nevertheless are capable of catalizing the acyl transfer or transpeptidation reactions. In these cases the properties of the enzyme-product complex resulted from the substrate hydrolysis must differ from those

formed upon simple and product interactions. Stability
of the latter does not correspond to the experimentally
observed initial rates of transpeptidation (19). It
seems that dissociation of the products must also be
a stepwise process (20). For pepsin it was experimentally proved by J. Fruton et al. (21).

In conclusion, I would like to emphasize that the
concept presented here explains the efficiency of proteolysis in terms of resonance destabilization of the
amide bond in the ground state of the reaction, thus
diminishing the barrier of the elementary step of its
chemical transformation. The enzyme stabilizes this
highly reactive but energetically unfavourable form of
the substrate (S_a) (Fig. 4). The activation barrier

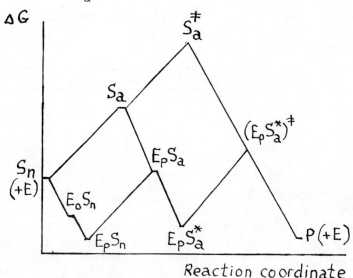

Fig. 4. Diagram of changes in free energy along the
reaction coordinate (22).

of the elementary step of chemical transformation for
an enzymic reaction may be the same as the transformation barrier of this active form of the substrate
in solution just due to the similar structures of the
ground states for both processes. In model reaction
we have to select the non-planar (S_a) rather than

37

planar (S_n) amide as a ground state. In this case the efficiency of catalysis is equal to the inverse equilibrium constant between planar and non-planar amide in solution or proportional to the free energy of active substrate stabilization by the enzyme (22). The concept does not require any strain or transition state stabilization.

I believe that experimental verification of these ideas will be a step forward in establishing a general theory of enzymic hydrolysis of carboxylic acid derivatives.

REFERENCES

1. Antonov, V. K. (1980). Specificity and mechanism of proteolytic enzymes. Bioorgan. Khimiya. 6, 805-839.
2. Klyosov, A. A. and Vallee, B. L. (1977). Substrate specificity and kinetics of carboxy-peptidase A action: Role of a metal of the active center in specificity of binding and catalysis. Bioorgan. Khimiya. 3, 806-815.
3. Bauer, C-A., Thompson, R. C. and Blout, E. R. (1976). The active centers of Streptomyces griseus protease 3 and ∝-Chymotrypsin: Enzyme-Substrate Interactions Remote from the Scissile Bond. Biochemistry 15, 1291-1295.
4. Bauer, C-A., Thompson, R. C. and Blout, E. R. (1976). The active centers of Streptomyces griseus protease 3, ∝-Chymotrypsin and Elastase: Enzyme--Substrate Interactions close to the Scissile Bond. Biochemistry 15, 1296-1299.
5. Zinchenko, A. A., Rumsh, L. D. and Antonov, V. K. (1977). Kinetic and thermodynamic analysis of pepsin specificity. Bioorgan. Khimiya 3, 1663-1670.
6. Medzihradszky, K., Voynick, I. M., Medzihradszky--Schweiger, H. and Fruton, J. S. (1970). Effect of Secondary Enzyme-Substrate Interactions on the Cleavage of Synthetic Peptides by Pepsin. Biochemistry 9, 1154-1162.
7. Antonov, V. K., Ginodman, L. M., Kapitannikov, Yu. V.,

Barshevskaya, T. N., Gurova, A. G. and Rumsh, L. D.
(1978). Mechanism of pepsin catalysis. General
base catalysis by the active site carboxylate ion.
FEBS Lett. 88, 87-90.

8. Antonov, V. K., Yavashev, L. P., Volkova, L. I.,
Sadovskaya, V. A. and Ginodman, L. M. (1979).
Catalytic mechanism of leucine aminopeptidase.
Bioorgan. Khimiya 5, 1427-1429.

9. Antonov, V. K., Ginodman, L. M., Rumsh, L. D.,
Kapitannikov, Yu. V., Barshevskaya, T. N., Yavashev,
L. P., Gurova, A. G. and Volkova, L. I. (1980).
How to distinguish the covalent and general base
mechanisms of enzymic hydrolysis? Bioorgan.
Khimiya 6, 436-446.

10. Antonov, V. K., Ginodman, L. M., Rumsh, L. D.,
Kapitannikov, Yu. V., Barshevskaya, T. N., Yavashev,
L. P., Gurova, A. G. and Volkova, L. I. (1981).
Studies of the mechanisms of action of proteolytic
enzymes using heavy oxygen exchange. Eur. J.
Biochem. 117, 195-200.

11. Kossiakoff, A. A. and Spencer, C. A. (1981).
Direct Determination of the Protonation States of
Aspartic acid-102 and Histidine-57 in the Tetra-
hedral Intermediate of the Serine Proteases:
Neutron Structure of Trypsin. Biochemistry 20,
6462-6474.

12. Blow, D. Personal communication.

13. Huber, R., Kukla, D., Bode, W., Schwager, P.,
Bartels, K., Deisenhofer, J. and Steigemann, W.
(1974). Structure of the complex formed by bovine
trypsin and bovine pancreatic trypsin inhibitor.
II. Crystallographic refinement at 1.9 Å resolution.
J. Mol. Biol. 89, 73-101.

14. Huber, R. Personal communication.

15. Hughes, D. L., Sieker, L. C., Bieth, J. and Dimi-
coli, J. L. (1982). Crystallographic study of the
binding of a trifluoroacetyl dipeptide anilide
inhibitor with elastase. J. Mol. Biol. 162, 645-658.

16. Quicho, F. A. and Lipcomb, W. N. (1971). Carboxy-
peptidase A: A protein and an enzyme. Adv. Prot.
Chem. 25, 1-78.

17. Kester, W. R. and Matthews, B. W. (1977). Crystal-
    lographic study of the binding of dipeptide inhi-
    bitors to thermolysin. Implications for the mecha-
    nism of catalysis. Biochemistry 16, 2506-2516.
18. Komiyama, M. and Bender, M. L. (1979). Do cleavages
    of amides by serine proteases occur through a
    stepwise pathway involving tetrahedral intermediates?
    Proc. Nat. Acad. Sci. USA 76, 557-560.
19. Antonov, V. K., Rumsh, L. D. and Tichodeeva, A. G.
    (1974). Kinetics of pepsin-catalysed transpeptida-
    tion: Evidence for the "amino-enzyme" intermediate.
    FEBS Lett. 46, 29-33.
20. Antonov, V. K. (1981). Non-covalent intermediates
    in catalysis by proteolytic enzymes. In: Proteinases
    and their inhibitors. V. Turk and Lj. Vitale (Eds).
    Mladinska Khimiya/Pergamon Press, Ljubljana,
    Oxford, pp. 141-150.
21. Sachdev, G. P. and Fruton, J. S. (1976). Kinetic
    of Action of Pepsin on Fluorescent Peptide Sub-
    strates. Proc. Nat. Acad. Sci. USA 72, 3424-3427.
22. Karpeiskii, M. Ya., Yakovlev, G. I. and Antonov,
    V. K. (1980). Does the enzyme decrease the acti-
    vation energy of the elementary step of chemical
    transformation of a substrate? Bioorgan. Khimiya 6,
    645-654.

PROTEIN CONFORMATIONAL RELAXATION IN ENZYME CATALYSIS

L. A. BLUMENFELD
Institute of chemical physics, USSR Academy of Sciences,
Kosygin Str. 4, moscow, 117977, USSR

In the course of chemical reactions of proteins one
can expect the formation of specific long-living
conformationally nonequilibrium states. A fast local
chemical change is accompanied by the vibrational
relaxation of the active center and its immediate sur-
roundings and takes place with the structure of the
whole protein globule remaining practically unchanged.
The transition to a new conformational state is of
relaxational nature, requires coordinated disruption
and formation of a multitude of secondary bonds and
can last for microseconds, milliseconds, and even
seconds. In this way there appears a long-living
specific nonequilibrium state: active center is already changed, but the structure of the main volume
of protein globule remains the same. A structural
strain between the relaxed and unchanged regions is
slowly lifted in the course of protein relaxation.

  Two basic ideas of the proposed approach can be
formulated as follows (1-3): 1) Conformational relaxation of proteins and their complexes must be regarded
as motion along a specific mechanical degree of freedom.
2) This relaxation is an elementary act of many enzyme
processes and of the energy coupling of intracellular
chemical reactions. The rate of substrate - product
transformation is determined by the rate of conformational relaxation of the substrate - enzyme complex.
This relaxation includes not only the changes in the
system of protein secondary bonds, but also the chemical
changes necessary to ensure the substrate - product
transition. Relaxation proceeds under the action of
a force that pushes a system directionally along the
reaction coordinate. Such a mechanism which includes
irreversible stages, can, naturally, be realized only
far from the state thermodynamic equilibrium substrate

Proceedings of the 16th FEBS Congress
Part A, pp. 41–47
© 1985 VNU Science Press

- product, and the probability of its realization
increases with the increase of the system free energy
change in the course of the catalized reaction (4).
Similar ideas have been applied to muscle contraction
(5, 6) and to oxidative phosphorylation (7).

We have studied the appearance of the protein conformationally nonequilibrium states in the course of
ATP synthesis energetically ensured by the electron
transfer through electron transport chains (ETC) in the
inner mitochondrial membrane (Fig. 1). In the first

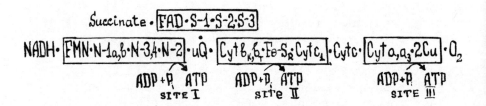

Figure 1. A scheme of mitochondrial ETC

complex carrier-transformer is non-heme-iron protein
of ferredoxin type designated usually as N-2 (8).
Energy liberated during electron transfer through N-2
is utilized for ATP synthesis. The active centers of
these proteins are iron-sulfur centers (ISC). The
technique of low-temperature EPR spectroscopy was
firstly applied to the ISC study in 1971 (9, 10). We
have shown that this method can detect mitochondrial
ISC in conformationally nonequilibrium states. Spin-
-lattice magnetic relaxation of these centers is determined by two-phonon Orbach' process (11, 12). In this
case spin-lattice relaxation time, T_1, is determined

by energy gap, $\Delta = 3|j|$, between ground (S=1/2) and
first excited (S=3/2) spin states: $1/T_1 \frown \exp(-3|j|/kT)$.

T_1 is extremely sensitive to the value of exchange
integral j, which in its turn, depends exponentially
on iron-iron distance. The method of "temperature
curves", I(T), permits to detect small changes in ISC

42

structure. Temperature dependence of differential
intensity of on of EPR signal components is recorded
at constant microwave power. Fig. 2 shows typical EPR
spectrum of mitochondria. Fig. 3 shows I(T) curve for
N-2 center. Within certain temperature interval Curie
law holds true (II). The decay of I at higher temperatures (III) is due to the signal broadening caused by
T_1 decrease. At low temperature I value passes through
a maximum and decreases due to power saturation (I).
Analysis of I(T) curve allows to estimate j and make
conclusions concerning the changes of iron-iron distance
in ISC.

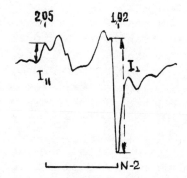

Figure 2. Part of the EPR spectrum of mitochondria at
20K. Arrows indicate the measured intensities of the
$g_{||}$ and $g_{\perp}$ components of the N-2 center EPR signal

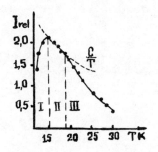

Figure 3. Typical I(T) curve. P=50mw. $g_{||}$ component
of EPR signal of reduced equilibrium N-2 center in rat
liver mitochondria

Ohnishi (13) suggested that there exist low- and
high-potential forms of N-2 center localized at two
sides of mitochondrial first coupling site. In our
laboratory the existence of these two forms has been
proven experimentally and shown that they represent
different conformational states of one and the same
center (14-17). Low-potential form is conformationally
nonequilibrium (N-2n), and high-potential - equilibrium
(N-2e) state of this center. N-2n has lower T_1 value
and increased iron-iron distance as compared with N-2e.
In a state 4 (18) mitochondria (lack of ADP, slow
electron transport) practically all reduced N-2 centers
are recorded in the mechanically strained state N-2n.
Addition of surplus ADP transforms mitochondria into
state 3 (fast electron transport) and practically all
N-2 centers - into N-2e state. These data, as well as
results obtained with uncoupled mitochondria and under
conditions of reversed electron transfer imply the
following scheme of N-2 transformations in the course
of electron transfer (Fig. 4). An electron from pre-
ceeding carrier is transferred to the N-2 lowest unoccupied orbital. N-2 is now in a long-living N-2n
state, relaxation of which in coupled mitochondria
is accompanied by ATP synthesis. During relaxation
the energy of the highest occupied orbital of the reduced N-2 center decreases to the level of the lowest
unoccupied orbital of the next ETC carrier, electron
can be transferred farther, and N-2 is again in the
oxidized state. During conformational relaxation las-
ting scores of milliseconds (19) the energy transduction

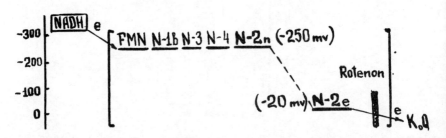

Figure 4. A scheme of N-2 changes during electron transfer

is realized. At low ADP content the frequency of relaxation acts is low, and they are the rate-limiting stages of the overall process. Therfore, at any given time moment only small part of N-2 centers exists in the reduced N-2e state. Under conditions of ADP surplus the after relaxation electron transfer becomes rate--limiting stage, and EPR method regusters N-2e.

The possibility of ATP synthesis in coupled and uncoupled mitochondria was also minutely studied in our laboratory (20, 21). The interpretation of obtained data can be briefly formulated as follows. A jump-like increase of the pH value leads to ionization of certain acid groups of ETC proteins (and/or of ATP-synthetase) with pK 8.1-8.3, and to the formation of protein conformationally nonequilibrium states (22) in the course of whose relaxation free ATP is formed. The immediate energy source is in this case a reaction of the type:

$$AH + OH^- \longrightarrow A^- + H_2O$$

REFERENCES

1. Blumenfeld, L. A. (1981). Problems of Biological Physics. Springer-Verlag, Heidelberg.
2. Blumenfeld, L. A. and Koltover, V. K. (1972). Energy Transformation and Conformational Transitions in Membranes as Relaxational Processes. Mol. Biol. 6, 161-166.
3. Blumenfeld, L. A. (1972). On elementary act of enzyme catalysis. Biofizika 17, 954-958.
4. Blumenfeld, L. A. (1983). Physics of Bioenergetic Processes. Springer-Verlag, Heidelberg, 109-110.
5. Gray, B. F. and Gonda, I. (1977). The Sliding Filament Model of Muscle Contraction. 1. J. Theor. Biol. 69, pp. 167-185.
6. Gray, B. F. and Gonda, I. (1977). The Sliding Filament Model of Muscle Contraction. 2. J. Theor. Biol. 69, pp. 187-230.
7. Cartling, B. and Ehrenberg, A. (1978). A Molecular Mechanism of the Energetic Coupling of Sequence of Electron Transfer Reactions to Endergonic Processes. Biophys. J. 23, 451-461.

8. DeVault, D. (1976). Theory of Iron-sulfur Center
   N-2 Oxidation and Reduction by ATP. J. Theor.
   Biol. 62, 1115-1139.
9. Orme-Johnson, N. R., Orme-Johnson, W. R., Hansen,
   R. F., Beinert, H. and Hatefi, J. (1971).
   EPR Detectable Electron Acceptors in Submitochon-
   drial Particles with Special References to the
   Iron-sulfur Compound of DPNH-Ubiquinon Reductase.
   BBRC 44, 446-457.
10. Ohnishi, T., Asakura, T., Jonetani, T. and
    Chance, B. (1971). Spin-lattice Relaxation and
    Exchange Interaction in 2-Iron, 2-Sulfur Proteins.
    J. Biol. Chem. 246, 5960-5974.
11. Gayda, J. P., Gibson, J. F., Cammach, R., Hall,
    D. O. and Mullinger, R. (1976). EPR studies at
    Temparature Below 77K on Iron-Sulfur Proteins
    of Yeast and Bovine Heart Submitochondrial Parti-
    cles. BBA 434, 154-163.
12. Burbaev, D. Sh. and Lebanidze, A. V. (1979).
    Estimation of Exchange Integral between Iron atoms
    in Ferredoxin Active Center. Biofizika 24, 392-395.
13. Ohnishi, T. (1976). Studies on the Mechanism of
    the Site 1 Energy Conservation. Europ. J. Biochem.
    64, 91-103.
14. Burbaev, D. Sh. (1979). Two forms of N-2 Center
    in mitochondria. Biofizika 24, 1099.
15. Blumenfeld, L. A., Burbaev, D. Sh. and Lebanidze,
    A. V. (1977). Nonequilibrium state of N-2 center
    in mitochondria and tissues. In: Magnetic Resonance
    in Biology and Medicine, N. M. Emanuel (ed).
    Nauka, Moscow, 82.
16. Blumenfeld, L. A., Burbaev, D. Sh., Lebanidze,
    A. V. and Vanin, A. F. (1977). EPR study of non-
    equilibrium states of iron-sulfur centers of
    soluble pea ferredoxin, membrane-bound ferredoxin,
    and N-2 center in mitochondria.
    Stud. Biophys. 63, 143-148.
17. Blumenfeld, L. A. (1978). The physical aspects
    of energy transduction in biological systems.
    Quart. Rev. Biophys. 11, 251-308.
18. Chance, B. and Williams, G. R. (1956). The respi-
    ratory chain and oxidative phosphorylation.

Adv. Enzymol. 17, 65-134.

19. Blumenfeld, L. A. and Davidov, R. M. (1979).
    Chemical reactivity of metalloproteins in confor-
    mationally out-of-equilibrium states. BBA 549,
    225-240.

20. Malenkova, I. V., Kuprin, S. P. Davidov, R. M.,
    and Blumenfeld, L. A. (1980). ATP synthesis in
    mitochondria induced by fast pH increase.
    DAN SSSR 252, 743-746.

21. Malenkova, I. V., Kuprin, S. P., Davidov, R. M.
    and Blumenfeld, L. A. (1982). pH-jump-induced
    ADP phosphorylation in mitochondria. BBA 682,
    179-183.

22. Blumenfeld, L. a., Greschner, S., Genkin, M. V.,
    Davidov, R. M. and Roldugina, N. M. (1976).
    Kinetic study of conformational changes in ferri-
    cytochrome C induced by pH change.
    Stud. Biophys. 57, 110.

STRUCTURAL DYNAMICS IN ENZYME ACTIVITY AND MODULATION

P. DOUZOU, T.E. BARMAN, F. TRAVERS AND C. BALNY
INSERM U 128, CNRS, B.P. 5051, 34033 Montpellier Cedex,
et I.B.P.C., 13 rue P. et M. Curie, 75005 PARIS, France.

A way of studying the sequential stereochemical changes
accompanying the interconversion of enzyme-substrate
intermediates as revealed by transient kinetic is to
slow them down by lowering the temperature (1). Such
"temporal resolution" has been achieved with a number
of different classes of enzymes ; with the aid of the
differences in the energies of activation of the rate
constants of the reaction pathway, one can map the struc--
tures of kinetically significant transient species (2).
Further, the antifreezes used (usually organic solvents
at high concentrations, cryosolvents) may themselves
selectively affect certain rate constants and thus
facilitate the thermal resolution of elementary steps.
At room temperatures cryosolvents may contribute to
"break" the sequential pathway, i.e. making the time
of transformation of one intermediate to another long
enough for the measurement of the rate-constant
concerned. Here, it is possible to investigate the effect
of biological solutes on partial processes and thus
any eventual modulation of the pace of an enzyme
reaction.

Working at subzero temperatures and high pressures
permits one to gain information about the "activation
volume" ($\Delta V^{\neq}$) of single interconversions of intermediates, and then to detect stereochemical changes. Doing
the same in the presence of biological solutes might
permit to obtain further structural and energetic features of activation processes stepping the reaction
pathway, under the influence of ligands and solutes
influencing the pace of reactions.

Here we deal with this "baro-cryoenzymic" approach
which can provide information about the dynamics of regulatory enzymes and a new understanding in the most
subtle mechanisms of enzyme reactions.

Proceedings of the 16th FEBS Congress
Part A, pp. 49–56
© 1985 VNU Science Press

In this laboratory, several model systems have been used for new cryoenzymic and baro-cryoenzymic approaches as tools to analyze the fine regulatory mechanisms of enzyme systems.

Our favorite model is myosin ATPase which is involved in muscle contraction. Detailed knowledge of myosin ATPase is a prerequisite for the understanding of muscle contraction, but in spite of the fact that it has received much attention, the intimate mechanism of the conversion of the chemical energy of ATP to the mechanical energy required for the sliding of the myosin and actin filaments remains uncertain. Most authors agree that the mechanism can be narrowed down to one asking about the stereochemical changes of the enzyme intermediates of the acto-myosin system during the course of ATP hydrolysis. But because of the rapidity of certain of the key steps of the ATPase reaction pathway, such changes are difficult to study at the molecular level.

The first four steps of the seven step Bagshaw-Trentham scheme (3) are (Scheme 1) :

$$M + T \underset{k_{-2}}{\overset{K_1}{\rightleftharpoons}} M.T \underset{k_{-2}}{\overset{k_2}{\rightleftharpoons}} M^*.T \underset{k_{-3}}{\overset{k_3}{\rightleftharpoons}} M.D.Pi \overset{k_4}{\longrightarrow} M+D+Pi$$

where M = myosin, T = ATP, D = ADP.

The main technique used to investigate this pathway is the rapid-flow quench method ; here enzyme and ATP are mixed in a suitable device, the reaction mixture allowed to age and then quenched by the addition of a quencher (6). The mixture is then assayed by a suitable analytical technique. Changes in the time scale, the nature of the quencher and the ratio of enzyme to substrate permit to obtain the constants of the reaction pathway (Table I).

In Scheme 1, the initial "binding" steps 1 and 2 can be studied in isolation by the ATP chase technique (4). By studying the dependence of the rate of binding of ATP to myosin on the ATP concentration, one can show the mechanism involved : an hyperbolic relationship indicates a two step and a linear one a one step binding process. The results obtained with myosin are shown in Fig. 1 ; this illustrates the usefulness of 40 % ethylene glycol in obtaining elementary kinetic constants by decreasing an equilibrium constant (K_1) and a rate constant k_2.

Method (quencher)	Time scale	Constant obtained
ATP chase (ATP)	$1/k_2$	K_1, k_2
Pi burst (acid)	$1/(k_3+k_{-3})$	k_3+k_{-3}
Pi burst (acid)	$1/k_4$	$k_4.K_3/(1+K_3)$ or k_6 (depending on temperature)
Pi burst single turn over (acid)	$1/k_4$	K_3, k_4

Table I - Methods for obtaining kinetic constants of myosin ATPase (Scheme 1). From (4) and (7).

In water these constants could not be obtained. But the usefulness of 40 % ethylene glycol does not end here : it is an antifreeze allowing for work down to - 20 °C (5,7).

K_1 is presumably the equilibrium constant for the formation of the collision complex M.ATP. k_2 is the rate constant of the first conformational change of myosin leading to a second enzyme substrate complex, $M^{\ddagger}$.ATP by an induced fit (8). This is a key intermediate of myosin where the ATP is close to a conformation leading to its cleavage. The M.ATP $\rightarrow$ $M^{\ast}$.ATP isomerization is essentially irreversible (3) and from a thermodynamic view the properties of $M^{\ast}$ are of great interest. $M^{\ast}$ATP can be stabilized at subzero temperatures. At 0 °C, its concentration can reach 80 %, and its half lifetime is 12 min at - 15 ° C. (Table II).

Temperature (°C)	K_3	k_o	$M^{\ast}$ATP fraction of Mo in steady state	to,5
+ 15	1	0.06	0.5	12 s
+ 5	0.4	0.02	0.7	35 s
- 5	0.16	0.006	0.85	2 mn
- 15	0.06	0.0001	0.95	12 mn

Table II - Accumulation of a key intermediate of myosin

ATPase, M*ATP, with decrease in temperature. $k_O = k_4 K_3/(1+K_3)$; from (7).

Thus, M*ATP, which was "virtual" in aqueous solution, becomes stable in mixed solvents at subzero temperatures.

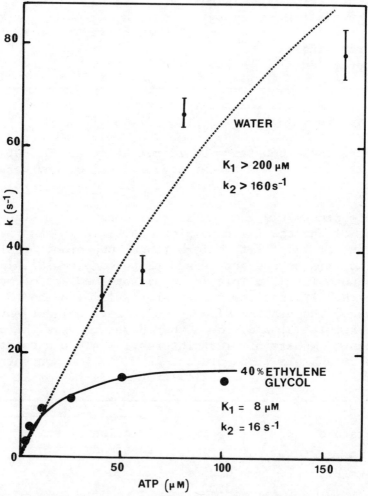

Fig. 1 - Dependence of rate of binding of ATP to myosin on [ATP] in 5 mM KCl, pH 8, 15 °C. The solvent was water or 40 % ethylene glycol. K_1 and k_2 were estimated by assuming an hyperbolic law (4).

It could be analyzed by the available spectroscopic techniques, e.g. NMR. It can also, as we will see, be produced under increasing pressure, in various conditions of medium, or yet be used as a starting, "precharged" system for the study of further steps.

An intrinsic fluorescence signal can be used as a probe of the conversion M.ATP $\xrightarrow{k+2}$ M*.ATP, and the kinetics of this conversion can be recorded at subzero temperatures under increasing pressure (1 to 1000 bars) to measure the "activation volume" ($\Delta V^{\neq}$) of the conversion. This volume is the volume change occuring when M.ATP is activated to the transition state, and $\Delta V^{\neq}$ equals the volume of the system containing the activated complex ($V_{ES}{\neq}$) minus the volume of the system containing the ground state complex (V_{ES}).

The dependency of the rate constant k, for a reaction can in simple cases be expressed as $k = k_0.\exp(-\Delta V^{\neq}/RT)$ (eqn. 1) where k_0 includes the thermodynamic parameters $\Delta H^{\neq}$ and $\Delta S^{\neq}$.

$\Delta V^{\neq}$ can be estimated from the slope of a plot of the logarithm of k versus the pressure. This procedure is formally analogous to the Arrhenius plot technique for determining activation energies (9), and $\Delta V^{\neq}$ is derived from the equation : $\Delta V^{\neq} = -RT. \Delta(\ln k)/\Delta P$. Estimates of $\Delta V^{\neq}$ involved in the interconversion of enzyme-substrate intermediates, and here during the conversion M ATP $\rightarrow$ M*ATP, are obtained with a special device combining rapid mixing of reactants, subzero temperatures (down to -20°C) and increasing pressure (1 to 1500 bars). Preliminary results are very encouraging and baro-cryoenzymic studies should be a useful approach to detect conformational changes during catalysis and, in the case of myosin, to demonstrate the postulated "induced-fit" process.

One of the most important implications of the anti-freeze effect on the binding steps of myosin ATPase activity is the finding that the rate constant k_{+2} is very sensitive to changes in the medium (Table III).

It can be seen that k_{+2} varies by a factor 5 between pH 6.4 and 8.0 and by 3 between 5 and 150 mM KCl. These variations could be recorded as a function of pressure to determine both k_{+2} and $\Delta V^{\neq}$ variations under the influence of the pH and of the ionic strength, namely

of weak and strong electrolytes these being pacemakers
of the reaction pathway.

pH	KCl (mM)	Ethylene glycol (% v/v)	K_1 (µM)	$k_2 (s^{-1})$
8	5	0	$\geqslant 200$	$\geqslant 160$
8	5	40	8	16
8	150	40	110	45
6.4	150	40	27	8

Table III - Variation of K_1 and k_2 of myosin ATPase with
experimental conditions at 15 °C (4).

We plan to undertake such investigation so as to compare
the effect of solvent and solutes (e.g. KCl, above) on
k_{+2} and $\Delta V^{\neq}$. From such a study it should be possible to
determine whether a change in k_{+2} is due to a change in
$\Delta V^{\neq}$ or $\Delta H^{\neq}$ and $\Delta S^{\neq}$ which can be studied independently
as a function of the temperature (eqn. 1). This postula-
ted energy change should be linked to the fact that
strong electrolytes probably influence the degree to
which water can organize around the amino-acid side
chains and peptide linkages transfered during the confor-
mational event, and modify both the $\Delta V^{\neq}$ and the $\Delta G^{\neq}$ (k_{+2})
values of the interconversion. By influencing the degree
to which water organizes around transfered enzyme groups,
electrolytes and presumably other solutes and ligands,
as well as cryosolvents at selected concentration may
act on the time course of a reaction pathway.
　Electrolytes and cosolvents have in common the property
of changing the structure of water and therefore the
solvation of exposed protein groups, and then of chan-
ging favorably or unfavorably the $\Delta V^{\neq}$ and $\Delta G^{\neq}$ of the
interconversion of intermediates, depending on their
concentration. Cosolvents used at concentrations at
which they are reversible inhibitors of rate processes
and "breakers" of the reaction pathway open the way to
baro-cryoenzymic studies focusing on transient steps and
species that are not considered in the steady-state kinetic treatment based on recordings of the rate-limiting
step.

The quantitative breakdown of reactions into a series
of simple one step processes is thus a prerequisite for
carrying out these dynamic studies where the intermediates are at once controlled, perturbed and converted. We
have seen that k_{+2} is very sensitive to the environment
thus changing the pace of the reaction. K_1 and k_{+3} are
also perturbed, but k_{+4}, which is the rate-limiting constant, is practically unaffected by solutes and antifreeze
(7). Thus, the overall constant k_{cat} is insensitive to
the experimental conditions, while steps 1, 2 and 3 are
sensitive and therefore able to respond to changes in
environment in vitro and in vivo . On the other hand,
lowering the temperature may increase or decrease the
steady-state concentrations of the various intermediates,
providing means for their detection or effacement.

The results reported here show the advantages brought-
about by the use of solvent and temperature perturbations
: a magnification of the subtle and pacesetting effects
of biological solutes, followed by the perturbation of
the reaction pathway which offers new analytical possibilities. Many other enzyme-systems could be investigated
in this way to reveal the possible effects of biological
solutes (electrolytes, ligands, modulators) on their
transient intermediates and therefore on the time-course
of their reaction pathway.

The finding that the induced-fit accompanying the binding of ATP to myosin represents a large part of the
free energy of the overall hydrolytic process and may
present different lifetimes depending on environmental
conditions, suggests further study and understanding of
the coupling between chemical and mechanical energy on
the acto-myosin system. Storage and release of energy
by transient species and structures as well as their
expressions at the molecular level become experimentally
accessible.

These results are also a reminder of the fact that
most enzymes are not mere catalysts : they are involved
in regulatory process, in which the pace of the reaction
pathway is as essential as the velocity for handling
properly the energy required, released or converted during their functionning.

In sum, perturbations of a reaction pathway by

cryoenzymology is an invaluable tool for gaining access
to the most subtle, dynamic mechanisms involving protein
structures, while their pressure-dependence may reveal
some of their specific energetic features.

References

(1) Douzou, P. (1977). Cryobiochemistry : an introduction
    Academic Press, New York.
(2) Douzou, P. & Petsko, G.A. (1984). Proteins at work :
    "stop-action" pictures at subzero temperatures.
    Adv. Prot. Chem. 36, 345-361.
(3) Trentham, D.R., Eccleston, J.F. & Bagshaw, C.R. (19
    76). Kinetic analysis of ATPase mechanisms. Q. Rev.
    Biophys. 9, 217-281.
(4) Barman, T.E., Hillaire, D. & Travers, F. (1983).
    Evidence for the two-step binding of ATP to myosin
    subfragment-1 by the rapid-flow-quench method.
    Biochem. J. 209, 617-626.
(5) Biosca, J.A., Travers, F. & Barman, T.E. (1983). A
    Jump in an Arrhenius plot can be the consequence
    of a phase transition. The binding of ATP to myo-
    sin subfragment-1. FEBS Letters 153, 217-220.
(6) Barman, T.E. & Travers, F. (1985). The rapid flow
    quench method in the study of fast reactions in
    biochemistry. Extension to subzero conditions.
    Meth. Biochem. Anal., in press.
(7) Biosca, J.A., Travers, F., Hillaire, D. & Barman, T.
    E. (1984). Cryoenzymic studies on myosin subfrag-
    ment-1 : perturbation of an enzyme reaction by
    temperature and solvent. Biochemistry 23, 1947-
    1955.
(8) Koshland, D.E. (1958). Application of a theory of
    enzyme specificity to protein synthesis. Proc.
    Natl. Acad. Sci. USA. 44, 98-101.
(9) Laidler, K.S. (1951). The influence of pressure on
    the rates of biological reactions. Arch. Biochem.
    Biophys. 30, 226-236.

PROTEIN MOTION AND ENZYME ACTION

ROBERT J.P. WILLIAMS
Inorganic Chemistry Laboratory, University of Oxford,
South Parks Road, Oxford OX1 3QR, U.K.

In about 1974 three NMR research groups(1)(2)(3) discovered that side chains of certain residues inside proteins had high mobility. Subsequently similar mobility
has been uncovered in a wide range of proteins. These
observations forced a reappraisal of crystallographic
data concerning proteins and have generated much theoretical analysis. The practical consequences of the new
knowledge have not been well analysed. It is one purpose of this paper to look at enzyme action in the light
of mobile structures. The mobility is now known to
extend to segments of proteins. We believe it to be
very important in protein/protein binding and in protein
antigenicity.

At about the same time NMR measurements showed that
the binding of inhibitors to the groove of lysozyme
caused small changes in structure all over the protein
(4). These changes are in addition to the changes which
were recognised by crystallography, i.e. the closing of
the gap between the faces of the groove. Since that
time we have shown that similar long range effects are
observable even on binding an electron at the iron of
cytochrome c (5) or more markedly on binding calcium
ions to calcium binding proteins (6). Many of the observations have been confirmed by crystallographic
studies. This second group of facts again forces a reappraisal of the nature of enzyme action since they
imply that a protein is a cooperative body when its properties can not be described in terms of isolated functional groups. All groups have an interactive energy
with the whole protein. All proteins therefore have a
allosteric capability but in some it has been developed
functionally. It is in part this cooperativity in pro-

Proceedings of the 16th FEBS Congress
Part A, pp. 57–70
© 1985 VNU Science Press

teins which has allowed evolution to search so effectively for the best solutions to structure/mobility/
function relationships and to build intercommunicating
protein/protein machinery.

In order to demonstrate these points I turn to a description of a protein, cytochrome c, which has been
investigated in extreme detail by both X-ray crystallography and NMR studies in solution.

CYTOCHROME C: CRYSTAL AND SOLUTION STRUCTURE STUDIES

Elsewhere we analyse several accurate crystal structure
studies (7). Here we shall summarise the findings.
(a) The surface and hydration sphere of cytochrome c are
not definable by a structure. They are too mobile. The
reported surface structures differ widely from one
crystal structure to another in the same oxidation
state, from one molecule to another in the same crystal,
from one oxidation state to another. The surface groups
have very high temperature factors i.e. mobility.
(b) The regions of contact between molecules in crystals
distort the structure locally, Fig.1.
(c) The structures change quite noticeably on change of
charge at the haem even at a long distance from the
haem.
(d) Substitution of amino-acids from horse to tuna to
rice cytochrome c cause only small main chain movements
but considerable side-chain alterations.

We have extended these observations by very detailed
studies of cytochrome c structure in solution (7).
While the fold of the backbone must be very similar to
that in crystals there are some clear local differences
between the Fe(III) form of say tuna cytochrome c in
solution and either of the two Fe(III) structures in its
crystal and between the Fe(II) structure in solution and
in its crystal. These differences are readily analysed
by NOE and coupling constant studies and are found to
involve positional changes of greater than 1Å of some
hydrophobic residues, and centre on two regions of the
polypeptide chain and the surface.

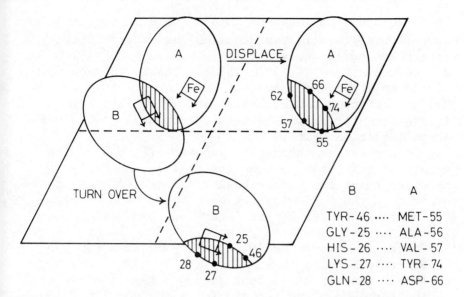

Fig.1 Rice cytochrome c molecules in crystals. Diagram
shows the packing top-left and top-right. Bottom right
describes the area (distorted) where molecules contact.

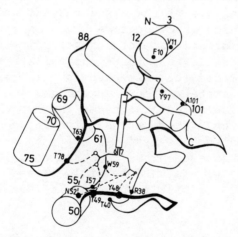

Fig.2 The black dots on the structure of cytochrome c
show groups whose residues change relative position on
going from the Fe(III) to the Fe(II) protein. The haem
propionates are shown and their binding indicated by
dashes.

(1) The chain from Thr40 to Thr63. This region includes the relatively mobile residue Ile57 and the relatively rigid residues 46 and 48, see Fig.3.
(2) The chain from Ile75 to Thr78. These residues form a relatively rigid 3_{10} bend.
(3) The surface residues, Val111 and Ile81 also have different conformations between the crystal and solution in one oxidation state.

We have observed changes in the same regions of the protein on switching between the Fe(III) and Fe(II) states in solution. Additional redox-linked changes are observed in the following regions, Fig.2.
(4) The residues around the C-terminus and its contact with the protein surface.
(5) The region around Phe10 including small motions of the N-terminal helix.
This shows that there is long range cooperative trans-mission throughout the protein for a change of but one electron.

The changed interaction between haem propionates and the iron charge, Fig.2, has been proposed as the source of the redox conformation change.

Finally an analysis of the pseudocontact shifts of the assigned resonances of cytochrome c has indicated the presence of conformational heterogeneity in the region around Thr9, Phe82, Ile85, Leu94 and thioether-2 to the left of the haem crevice, although in this case it is not possible to state whether the changes occur between the crystal and solution or between the two oxidation states in solution. There is no point in an analysis of surface residues such as lysines.

We conclude that cytochrome c has to be described as a cooperative body with a variety of localised mobilities. Yet relatively speaking it is a very rigid protein.

Amino-acid Substitution and Modification
We have studied many different mitochondrial cytochromes c. These include proteins from different biological species, proteins changed by semi-synthesis and proteins changed by selective chemical modification. We have

observed that in one case a change, from a serine to a
threonine, had no effect on the structure but that in
all other cases changes were observed not only at the
sites of chemical change but also elsewhere, sometimes
at considerable distances away. Again the protein
behaves as a cooperative unit. The region of the
protein around Ile57, which is a relatively mobile
region, is particularly sensitive to chemical change,
and indeed to all changes of conditions. These studies
imply that the interpretation of site-specific
mutagenesis experiments (which are exactly the same as
the above) may be extremely difficult. Is there really
site-specific mutagenesis?

Mobility of the Structure (4)

We have studied the mobility of many aliphatic and
aromatic groups in cytochrome c.   Figure 3 gives a
mobility map. It is particularly interesting that some
regions of the protein are almost rigid e.g. around
Tyr67, Trp59, Phe10, Phe48 while other regions are much
more mobile e.g. around Trp33, Ile57, Tyr74, Phe82 and
the C-terminus. The group mobilities and the
distortions of structure again suggest that a domain of
the structure from 38-57 can move relative to the rest
of the protein although the centre part of this domain
around 46-48 is more firmly held. In the structure this
domain is to the Met-80 side of the haem and rests
against the 70-80 part of the structure see Fig.2. This
could be important for our understanding of the folding
pattern, the chemical reactivity at the iron and the
antigenic properties of the protein. We have pointed
out that the relaxation of the solvent cage around the
iron is essential part of electron transfer (5) and
indeed of any other reaction in an enzyme groove. The
long-range changes, see Fig.2, in structure and mobility
are indications of energy partition into the protein for
bound intermediates, here the bound electron.

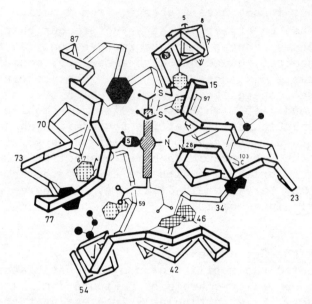

Fig.3 The mobility map of cytochrome c. The hatched residues are relatively rigid, filled residues are mobile.

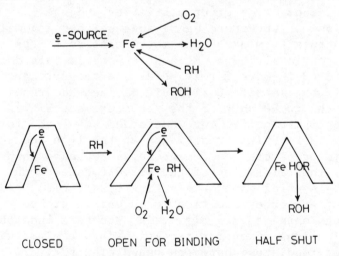

Fig.4 The proposed opening and shutting of P-450. The enzyme is not cross-linked and is helical. Reaction occurs in the half-shut state and via a further open state when product is lost.

FURTHER PROTEIN STRUCTURES IN SOLUTION BY NMR

From the NMR and structural studies of cytochromes $\underline{c}$,
lysozymes, and the calcium binding proteins, which are
groups of proteins of decreasing structural rigidity
from very rigid to highly mobile ("melting points"
~100° C to 40° C) we conclude that
(1) Most side-chains of proteins especially on surfaces
and surfaces of grooves will be highly mobile. Some of
this mobility can go undetected by X-ray crystal
studies. This mobility includes many rotational and
librational states. There is little significance to be
attached to the structures of exposed surfaces as seen
in crystals. Internal side-chains e.g. of aromatic
groups usually have quite high flip rates but they are
very idiosynchratic and their motion can not be detected
in crystals.
(2) Segmental motions are small but not uncommon. Parts
of many proteins open up relatively easily.
(3) On change of binding partner, e.g. oxidation state,
inhibitor, metal ion etc. a protein behaves as a cooperative unit. The cooperativity has a smaller structural
effect the tighter the protein fold. In calcium binding
proteins it is large, in cytochrome $\underline{c}$ it is small.
Cross- linking, as in cytochrome $\underline{c}$ and lysozyme but not
calmodulin, restricts change.
(4) It follows from the combination of mobility (which
reflects ease of adjustment of structure) and cooperativity (which reflects the long-range nature of forces
inside proteins) that the energetics of these proteins
are global not local. We suspect that this is true for
all proteins. The consequences of these facts for the
discussion of enzyme activity will now be pursued but we
must look first to see if enzymes are a limited group of
proteins by examining sequences and structures.

Sequences and Mobility (8)
It is usual to discuss sequence: structure: function
relationships. I believe this to be incorrect. The
connectivity pattern is sequence:structure: mobility:

function. Sequences which give rise to cooperative units such as β-sheets and α-helices are of low chain mobility internal to these units. The interaction between strands in a sheet is more powerful than the interactions between helices or between sheets and helices. A protein made from a sheet, e.g. a β-barrel, is then likely to be very rigid, e.g. superoxide dismutase. A protein made from only α-helices is likely to be segmentally deformable. The deformations will be limited by -S-S-, porphyrin, or metal ion cross-links. Finally loops connecting the two main elements of secondary structure are likely to be deformable. Sometimes such loops are not even visible in the electron density maps and are drawn into X-ray "structures". We may then suppose that those sequences which give helix-loop-helix units are not very suitable for the construction of enzymic active sites where selectivity of activity is essential. Too much mobility is disadvantageous. It is better to use β-sheets. On the other hand control-proteins which respond to triggers should be helical. The extreme deformability of a protein would be a type of pre-melting glass transformation. If we wish to transmit messages through a protein structure we require that the deformability is relatively great and we surmise that the "melting point" will be low. Table I illustrates these connections between protein classes and secondary structure.

ACTIVITY OF ENZYMES

It is generally recognised that the activities of enzymes require a structure in one state at least plus knowledge of structural changes and mobilities to define the geometry of the reaction path and of energy states to describe the energetics (9). The case of cytochrome c is the simplest possible since the substrate is the electron and the reaction is electron transfer. There are two states and we have shown that they differ in geometry. We know a great deal about the mobility and the energy states of the system. The change of unit

64

TABLE I. SINGLE DOMAIN PROTEINS OF DIFFERING STRUCTURE

Helical (α)	Mixed α/β	Sheet (β)
Myoglobins	Lysozyme (S-S)	Neurotoxin (S-S)
Cytochrome c' (S-C)	Cytochrome c (S-C)	Protease inhibitor (S-S)
Haemerythrin	Carboxypeptidase	Superoxide dismutase
Parvalbumin	Subtilisin	Prealbumin
Calcium binding proteins	Papain (S-S)	Ribonuclease (S-S)
Haemoglobins	Cytochrome b_5 (Fe)	Immunoglobin (S-S)
Cro repressor	Thermolysin (Ca)	Rubredoxin (Fe-S)
protein or	Flavodoxin	Carbonate
bacteriophage λ	Triose phosphate	dehydratase
Insulin (S-S)	isomerase	Trypsin (S-S)
Cytochrome b_{562}	Phospholipase A_2 (S-S)	Acid protease
Peptide of F_0		

TABLE II. COMPARISON BETWEEN ZINC AND NON-ZINC ENZYMES

Reaction	Zinc-dependent Enzyme Substrate	Metal-independent Enzyme Substrate
Hydration	CO_2,Levalinic Acid	None
Protein Hydrolysis	Carboxy-terminal,	Endopeptide
Phosphate Ester	Amino terminal	None(?)
Hydrolysis	Di-peptides	
	Terminal phosphate	Phosphate transfer
RNA/DNA Hydrolysis	Non-specified Nucleotides	Ribonucleotides
RNA Polymerase	No specific bases	None
β-lactamase	Penicillins	Penicillins
Aldolase	Several aldols	Several aldols
Phospholipase	(C) Lipid esters	(A) Lipid Esters

charge is a cooperative event which alters the melting
point of the protein by 40°. Accessibility to the iron
atom is very greatly changed. The surface of the protein in different oxidation states is differentially
recognised by chromatographic materials and antibodies.
Moreover we know that certain regions are deformable
and are deformed in crystals. It turns out that the
most adjustable parts of the surface are the strongest
antigenic sites. Now this is a very rigid protein. If
this description of cytochrome c is accepted then the
description of other enzymes which are more loosely
folded must be more complicated in terms of mobility,
especially their activities, which involve large substrates and many states.

Cytochrome c gives further cause for thought in that
some of the ring flip rates have activation energies of
100kJoules. Now these rings, and groups such as valine,
leucine and isoleucine which could also flip, are effectively the medium in which the enzyme reaction occurs.
The solvent of any enzyme reaction (the protein side
chains which are not attacking groups) could be
described as a viscous liquid of highly anisotropic
motion locally. Given the above activation energy,
100kJoules, for the temperature dependence of the visco-
sity of this solvent it could be that many activation
energies derived from studies of enzyme catalysis do not
refer to chemical steps but to physical "solvent" visco-
sity i.e. movements of protein side-chains.

The Use of Metal Ions in Enzymes

The fact that the reactions of small substrates are
often catalysed by metal ions e.g. the reactions of CO_2,
urea, ethanol, glycol, and small phosphate esters,
whilst larger substrates such proteins, polysaccharides,
and polynucleotides do not require metal ions strongly
suggests that the activation of the two classes of substrate may be different, Table II. Metal
ions can break bonds by direct Lewis acid attack and
their attacking power is readily enhanced by binding
(entatic-state)[9] but the organic side-chains of proteins
such as RSH, ROH and so on are very poor attacking

66

groups. It is probable, following Pauling and Jencks, that the enzyme action involves the use of binding energy to strain the bonds under attack – a mechanism well suited to the attack on large substrates but not on small substrates. The selectivity for large substrates can then be by selective binding but that for small substrates just by selective exclusion. The idea of studying enzymes in order to understand attacking groups is then false for organic attacking groups. The protein works as a cooperative unit folding around the large substrate so as make optimal the strain on the selected bond to be broken as is seen in lysozyme. Here we know that the protein binding groove, the attacking groups and the interactions deep in the protein change on binding inhibitors.

The mobility can be put to many other uses for example in kinases where a hinge motion has been proposed. The same model can be applied to cytochrome P-450 and is well illustrated by reference again to the properties of cytochrome c, e.g. in the reaction with cyanide ions.

Enzymes Requiring Large Motion

Proteins, enzymes, are very vulnerable catalysts. They are unstable to hydrolysis and must not activate water randomly. They are also vulnerable to oxidation and must not activate oxygen randomly. Despite this they must use the reagents water and oxygen as substrates in many reactions. Now it is not only the proteins which must be preserved from attack but a large number of small molecules inside cells are vulnerable to the same reagents, water and oxygen. Such reagents are ATP, phenols etc. The interior of a cell must be very low in free zinc or copper both of which are quite good catalysts per se. Notwithstanding these problems the catalysts of the cell must use ATP and must use oxidation by oxygen with selectivity of attack on quite large substrates. How is it done? The answer seems to be that the catalytic site is created by the binding of the substrate which is selected for attack. Such attack requires preferred order of reaction based upon the schemes.

(1) Selected substrate bound, enzyme conformation change, then attacking group, O_2, introduced. Example: cytochrome P-450, see Fig.4.
(2) Two selected substrates bound, enzyme conformation change, then reaction occurs. Example: kinases.
The details of the changes and the energetics of these changes in the protein concern us here. They require mobility and cooperativity within structure.

It is obvious that P-450 only activates oxygen after the substrate, sterol, has been bound and that the sterol literally protects the enzyme during reaction. It is obvious too that the kinase protein protects ATP from hydrolysis, aided by Mg^{2+} ions (as is the case for free ATP) until the second substrate is bound when the enzyme moves so as to bring substrates together and possibly to move the protection from the βγ bond by moving the Mg^{2+} ion. Now inspection of such protein movement either directly in kinases or indirectly for P-450 by studying the binding of CN^- to cytochrome c or of O_2 to hemoglobin shows that the protein is involved in a global sense but this requires many mobile groups and segments. We can not understand the energetics unless we understand the mobility and cooperativity of the protein. With this understanding it will be possible to conect the reactions of P-450 itself to its required electron-transfer network and then on to such reactions as that of cytochrome oxidase. It will also be possible to connect the reaction of kinases to calmodulin control and then on to ATP-synthetases via calcium pumps. Proton pumps and ATP-synthesis may be visualised in a similar manner.

CONCLUSION

This essay, and it is more of an essay than a scientific article, has as its theme the central point that a protein which is an enzyme is a mobile cooperative unit. The demonstrations by NMR are clear. The extension of the ideas to the function of enzymes implies that there is always flow of energy between the whole enzyme and

the substrate during the reaction cycle. It is easy to
see then why it proves difficult (impossible?) to understand enzymes from static structures or from the point
of view of attacking group reactivity. Equally in-
triguing is the thought that it is possible to see how
in evolution trial and error changes can search for
solutions since the idea of essential conserved aminoacids and non-essential amino acids in a sequence should
be changed for the most part to a discussion of degrees
of usefulness of all the amino-acids in a sequence
through their mobilities and cooperative interactions.
There are many ways, using compensating changes of
several amino acids, of producing a very functional
cytochrome c̲. It may be too strong to say that every
amino acid in a sequence is involved in an enzyme's
activity, but it is a better basis for analysis of the
way enzymes work than a blind adherence to the idea of a
local active site. Such is the lesson from NMR studies
of proteins.

REFERENCES
1. Snyder, G.H., Rowan, R., Karplus, S., Sykes, B.D.
      (1976) Tyrosine Assignments of a Trypsin
      Inhibitor, Biochemistry 14,3765-3774
2. Wagner, G., De Marco, A., Wuthrich,K. (1976)
      Dynamics of Amico-acid Residues, Biophys Structure
      Mech.2,139-184
3. Campbell, I.D., Dobson, C.M., Williams, R.J.P.
      (1975) PMR Studies of Tyrosine Residues in
      Lysozyme, Proc.Roy.Soc.London A345,23-31
4. Campbell, I.D., Dobson, C.M., and Williams R.J.P.
      (1978) Structures and Energetics of Proteins, Adv.
      Chem.Phys.39,55-80
5. Moore, G.R., Huang, Z-X., Eley, C.G.S., Barker,
      H.A., Williams, G., Robinson, M.N., Williams,
      R.J.P.(1982) Electron Transfer in Biology:
      Cytochrome c̲, Faraday Soc Disc Chem Soc (London)
      74,311-329

6. Levine, B.A., Dalgarno, D.C., Esnouf, M.P., Klevit, R.E., Scott, G.M.M., Williams, R.J.P. (1983) The Mobility of Calcium Trigger Proteins, Ciba Foundation Symposium No.93 on Mobility and Function in Proteins and Nucleic Acids, Pitman London p72-95
7. Moore, G.R., Williams, G., Williams, R.J.P. J.Molec. Biol. The Structure of Cytochrome c in Solution submitted
8. Williams, R.J.P. (1980) On First Looking into Nature's Chemistry, Chem.Soc.Reviews (London) 9,281 324,325-370
9. Vallee, B.L., Williams, R.J.P. (1968) Metallo-proteins: The Entatic Nature of their Active Sites, Proc.Natl.Acad.Sci.US 59,498-503

MICROENVIRONMENTAL PROPERTIES AND CONFORMATIONAL CHANGES IN GLYCOGEN PHOSPHORYLASE. DENATURATION PROFILES OF SURFACE AND BURIED SPIN-LABELLED SITES

C.T. CAZIANIS, T.G. SOTIROUDIS AND A.E. EVANGELOPOULOS
The National Hellenic Research Foundation, 48 Vassileos
Constantinou Avenue, Athens 116 35, Greece.

The denaturation profile of Glycogen Phosphorylase
(EC 2.4.1.1) by urea and/or propylurea has been studied
earlier (1-4). In these studies, where several techniques including ESR spectroscopy were used, denaturation
of this enzyme was examined as a total phenomenon of the
macromolecule. Phosphorylase b, however, provides the
possibility to be specifically spin labelled at sites
with entirely different microenvironments and catalytic
action (5).
The intent of this work was to study phosphorylase denaturation and monitor quantitatively the local unfolding
of a critical regulatory enzyme at different regions by
different kinds of denaturants. For this purpose, phosphorylase b spin labelled at a) a surface and not essential for activity -SH group and b) a buried -NH$_2$ group
critical for the catalytic activity, have been used to
monitor the denaturation processes by ESR spectroscopy.

MATERIALS AND METHODS

All chemicals used in this work were of the highest grade
commercially available. Phosphorylase b and the paramagnetic analogue of FDNB as well as the corresponding spin
labelled enzyme (0.75 labels per monomer) were prepared
as described previously (5). Spin labelled phosphorylase
b with the iodoacetamide derivative (0.7 labels per monomer) was prepared as described by Campbell et al. (6).
Denaturation was performed by adding an appropriate volume of a concentrated solution of the corresponding denaturant to a volume of spin labelled enzyme stock solution
to attain the desired final denaturant concentration.
The ESR spectra were recorded immediately on a Varian E4

Proceedings of the 16th FEBS Congress
Part A, pp. 71–78
© 1985 VNU Science Press

spectrometer operating at X-band. Sedimentation velocity experiments were carried out as reported previously (5).

RESULTS AND DISCUSSION

The effect of four types of denaturants on the structure of phosphorylase b was examined: 1) Detergents (anionic, cationic and non ionic, 2) urea, 3) guanidine hydrochloride and 4) an aliphatic alcohol. The pH used for these studies was slightly alkaline (pH 8.0), because preliminary experiments had shown that at neutral pH many denaturants caused precipitation of the spin labelled enzyme even at low concentrations. To follow the denaturation, we used the ratio β/α (Fig. 1). This parameter is used as a means quantitatively monitoring structural changes of macromoleculecules which are reflected in changes in the motional freedom of the protein bound spin label with respect to its environment. This ratio is expected to decrease as denaturation loosens (or unfolds) the tertiary structure surrounding the label.

Detergents represent a special group of protein denaturants because they are able to produce a drastic conformational change at remarkably low reagent concentrations. SDS causes dramatic changes on the tertiary and quarternary structure of phosphorylase molecule. These changes include dissociation to subunits, unfolding of the polypeptide chains and breakdown of the schiff base which unites pyridoxal phosphate with the apoenzyme (4).

As shown in Fig. 1A, the spectroscopic titration of FDNB spin labelled phosphorylase b with SDS, revealed two basic steps in the denaturation process. Thus, in the presence of the anionic detergent, the mobility of the label originally decreases and then increases as the concentration of SDS in the system is raised. In contrast, the IA-spin labelled enzyme (Fig. 1B) presents a continuous increase of the mobility of the label in the whole titration range, suggesting a continuous unfolding of phosphorylase b domain near the IA-spin labelled sites.

The first step of the denaturation profile of the FDNB spin labelled enzyme is probably due to a conformation change leading to an immobilization of the label.

The possibility that the first step of the above dena-

72

turation profile is due to the formation of tetra-
mers or polydispersed aggregates of phosphorylase b was
excluded since the sedimentation pattern of the enzyme
examined under similar denaturation conditions, showed
no aggregated material. Of course the possibility of a

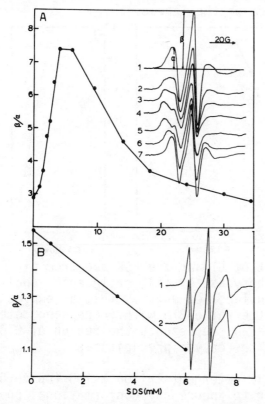

Fig. 1. Effect of SDS on the ESR spectrum of spin labelled phosphorylase b. A, FDNB spin labelled enzyme; B,
IA-spin labelled enzyme. The quantity β/α was plotted
against SDS concentration. Insets: A, ESR spectra of
FDNB spin labelled enzyme recorded at 1, 0; 2, 1.5; 3, 2;
4, 4; 5, 9.5; 6, 14 and 7, 18.2 mM SDS. B, ESR spectra
of IA spin labelled enzyme recorded at 1,0 and 2, 3.3 mM
SDS.

direct interaction of the ligand with the spin label or
a direct hindering of the motion of the label cannot be
completely excluded.

The cationic detergent cetyl trimethylammonium bromide was found to precipitate phosphorylase b up to about 10mM of denaturant with concomitant decrease of the mobility of both spin labels (Fig. 2). Further increase of the detergent concentration results in gradual increase of the motional freedom of the labels.

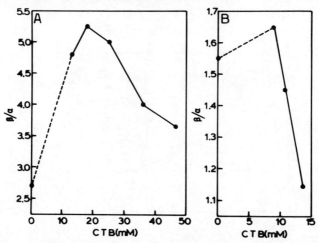

Fig. 2. Effect of CTB on the ESR spectrum of FDNB spin labelled phosphorylase b, (A), or IA spin labelled enzyme, (A), or IA spin labelled enzyme, (B), as expressed by the ESR change of the ratio β/α with increasing detergent concentration. (---), represents the region of CTB concentrations where the enzyme precipitates.

The non ionic detergent Triton X-100 (up to 5% v/v) does not appear to induce any conformational change to both spin labelled conjugates.

The above surfactants tested were of type A amphiphiles, i.e. they display lyotropic mesomorphism (7). As far as the activity of phosphorylase b is concerned, type A surfactants were found to act as inhibitors (8). In contrast, some surfactants of type B, like sodium cholate were found to act as allosteric activators of the enzyme (8). In this respect it must be added that ESR measurements demonstrated that while the mobility of the FDNB spin label bound to phosphorylase b decreases cooperatively with increasing bile salt concentration, the mobility of the IA spin label is unaffected even at high bile salt concentrations (8).

The environmental conformational changes of spin label-led phosphorylase b during denaturation with urea were found similar to those with SDS. That is, the denatura-tion profile of FDNB spin labelled enzyme is biphasic (Fig. 3A), while the mobility of the IA spin label increa-ses constantly as phosphorylase b is unfolded in presence of urea (Fig. 3B).

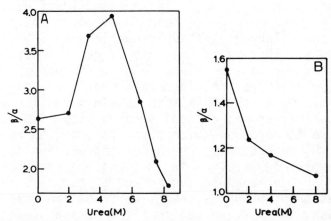

Fig. 3. Effect of urea on the ESR spectrum of FDNB spin labelled phosphorylase b, (A), or IA spin labelled enzyme, (B), as expressed by the ESR change of the ratio β/α with increasing denaturant concentration.

The denaturation of reduced muscle phosphorylase b by urea has been also studied by Chignell et al. (1), using fluorescence and circular dichroism techniques. They found two intermediates in the denaturation profile, the first of which is stable near 4M urea. This intermediate is perhaps similar with the transition of the FDNB spin labelled enzyme, observed also near 4M urea. Jones and Cowgill (2), studying the effect of urea on the fluores-cence intensity and fluorescence polarization of the co-enzyme of reduced phosphorylase b, found a plateau region between 1.2 and 2.0 M and a second plateau at 3.6 M urea. These results are in accordance with those of Fig. 3A, while the IA spin label is unable to detect any transi-tion states.

Most proteins with an ordered native structure undergo

a marked transition upon the addition of guanidine hydrochloride, which is usually completed at a concentration
of from 6 to 8M guanidine (9).

In the case of phosphorylase b we found that the mobility of both spin labels increases with increasing concentration of guanidine hydrochloride. Thus, while in
general the enzyme precipitates up to 2.7M of the denaturant, for the FDNB spin labelled phosphorylase b the ratio β/α was found 1.18 and 1.15 at 3 and 4M of guanidine
respectively and for the IA spin labelled enzyme, denatu-
ation at the sulphydryl sites is complete by 3.5M guanidine (β/α=1). That is in the case of guanidine denaturation of phosphorylase b, the unfolding process of the enzyme molecule at the protein domain near the buried NH_2
groups modified by the FDNB spin label is similar to that
at the domain near the exposed sulphydryls. The above
results are in agreement with those reported by Price and
Stevens (10) according to which phosphorylase b is rapidly and completely unfolded in 3M guanidine hydrochloride.

All of the denaturants considered so far have led to
the formation of products that seem to be randomly coiled.
In contrast, it is known (9) that the action of some organic substances such as aliphatic alcohols falls into a
different category: the denatured product possesses an ordered conformation, which however, is usually quite different from the native structure. Fig. 4 shows the titra-

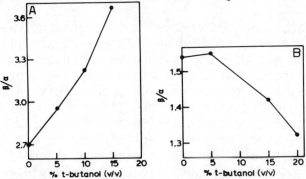

Fig. 4. Effect of t-butanol on the ESR spectrum of FDNB
spin labelled phosphorylase b, (A), or IA spin labelled
enzyme, (B), as expressed by the ESR change of the ratio
β/α with increasing alcohol concentration.

tion of the ESR spectra of FDNB and IA spin labelled conjugates of phosphorylase b by t-butanol, an aliphatic alcohol which in addition is known to activate the enzyme in absence of AMP (at low concentrations) (11). As we can see, while the mobility of the IA spin label increases with increasing alcohol concentration, the motional freedom of the FDNB spin label decreases, suggesting that the region of the enzyme molecule in the vicinity of the fast SH groups is most readily denatured.

ABREVIATIONS

FDNB, 1-fluoro-2,4-dinitrobenzene; IA, Iodoacetamide.

REFERENCES

1. Chignell, D.A., Azhir, A. and Gratzer, W.B. (1972). The Denaturation of Muscle Phosphorylase b by Urea. Eur. J. Biochem. 26, 37-42.
2. Jones, D.C. and Cowgill, R.W. (1971). Evidence for the Binding of Pyridoxal 5´-Phosphate in a Hydrophobic Region of Glycogen Phosphorylase b Dimer. Biochemistry 10, 4276-4282.
3. Bhat, R.K., Smith, T., Greer, L. and Steiner, R.F. (1978). Properties of Monomeric Phosphorylase b Formed by the Action of. Propylurea. Arc. Biochem. Biophys. 190, 677-686.
4. Oikonomakos, N.G., Sotiroudis, T.G. and Evangelopoulos, A.E. (1977). Probing of Protein Microenviroment by Fluorescein Derivatives: A Study with Glycogen Phosphorylase b. In: Bioenergetics of Membranes, L. Packer, G.C. Papageorgiou and A. Trebst (eds). Elsevier/North Holland Biomedical Press, Amsterdam, pp. 27-38.
5. Cazianis, C.T., Sotiroudis, T.G. and Evangelopoulos, A.E. (1980). Spin-Labelling of Phosphorylase b Using a Paramagnetic 1-Fluoro-2,4-Dinitrobenzene Derivative. Biochim. Biophys. Acta 621, 117-129.
6. Campbell, I.D., Dwek, R.A., Price, N.C. and Radda, G.K. (1972). Studies on the Interaction of Ligands with Phosphorylase b Using a Spin-Label Probe. Eur. J. Biochem. 30, 339-347.

7. Helenius, A. and Simons K. (1975). Solubilization of Membranes by Detergents. Biochim. Biophys. Acta 415, 29-79.
8. Sotiroudis, T.G., Cazianis, C.T., Oikonomakos, N.G. and Evangelopoulos, A.E. (1983). Effect of Sodium Cholate on the Catalytic and Structural Properties of Phosphorylase b. Eur. J. Biochem. 131, 625-631
9. Tanford, C. (1968). Protein Denaturation. Adv. Prot. Chem. 23, 121-282.
10.Price, N.C. and Stevens, E. (1983). The Denaturation of Rabbit Muscle Phosphorylase b by guanidinium Chloride Biochem. J. 213, 595-602.
11.Dreyfus, M., Vandenbunder, B. and Buc, H. (1978). Stabilization of a Phosphorylase b Active Conformation by Hydrophobic Solvents. FEBS Lett. 95, 185-189.

THE COENZYME PQQ AND QUINOPROTEINS, A NOVEL CLASS OF OXIDOREDUCTASE ENZYMES.

J.A. DUINE, J. FRANK,JZN. AND J.A. JONGEJAN.

Laboratory of Biochemistry, Julianalaan 67,
2628 BC Delft, The Netherlands.

INTRODUCTION.

From biochemical textbooks we know that there are two
groups of coenzymes involved in catalysis by oxidoreductases:
1)Flavins (FAD, FMN) and related compounds such as the
pteridins (THF, biopterin, methanopterin, etc.) and
deazaflavins (factor $F420$).
2)Nicotinamide nucleotides (NAD, NADP).
  Based on this, dehydrogenases are subdivided in two
classes: the NAD/NADP-dependent group, which are generally
cytoplasmic enzymes and the flavoprotein dehydrogenases,
which are dye-linked, respiratory chain bound enzymes.
However, during the past years it has become clear that
there exists a third class of oxidoreductases. In the
following, this recently discovered group of so-called
quinoproteins and their coenzyme PQQ will be described.

DISCOVERY OF THE COENZYME PQQ.

In Nature there exist bacteria (methylotrophs) which are
specialized in degrading C_1-compounds such as methane,
methanol, formaldehyde, methylamine, etc. The enzyme
involved in the conversion of methanol into formaldehyde
is called "methanol dehydrogenase" (1). However, it shows
several curious properties:

Proceedings of the 16th FEBS Congress
Part A, pp. 79–88
© 1985 VNU Science Press

-Although it is dye-linked and coupled to the respiratory chain, its absorption spectrum is quite different from that of a flavoprotein.
-Furthermore, its absorption spectrum does not change on addition of the substrate methanol.
-Since on denaturation of the enzyme a low molecular weight fluorescent compound appears in the supernatant, having properties resembling those of a pteridin, it was thought for many years that this enzyme was a "pterido-protein".

The fact that the absorption spectrum of the enzyme does not change on addition of substrate was very disturbing as it gave doubts about a correlation between the expected presence of a coenzyme, the absorbance above 300 nm, and the appearance of a fluorescing compound on denaturation of the enzyme. Hence the possibility existed that an "un-coloured compound" was the coenzyme, e.g. a metal ion. In attempts to discover the presence of paramagnetic metal ions by ESR, it was found by accident that the enzyme showed a signal originating from an organic free radical with a g-value of 2.0045 and a very small top to top width of about 6 Gauss when the signal was measured in the derivative mode (2,3). These data indicated that the free radical was neither a flavin nor a pteridin but a quinone.

Denaturation of the enzyme under anaerobic conditions gave further information, since it was possible to measure the hyperfine ESR spectrum of the detached free radical. Furthermore, an identical free radical could be induced in the fluorescing compound by reduction. In this way we could prove that the fluorescing compound was indeed the coenzyme Mathematical analysis of the hyperfine spectrum revealed that it was a hydrophilic o-quinone with 2 N's and 3 H's, one of which was exchangeable (3). Now well-known quinones like e.g. ubiquinones, are lipophilic compounds and they do not contain nitrogen. So at that moment it was realized that the fluorescing compound obtained from methanol dehydrogenase was a novel coenzyme. Based on this finding, two important questions could be formulated. First, what is its structure. Second, are there other enzymes which use this coenzyme or is its function restricted to methanol dehydrogenase. To answer the first question, after we

learned to purify the coenzyme and established its chromatographic properties, it was isolated in reasonable amount
from whole cells (4). For this purpose, about one ton of
single cell protein consisting of bacteria grown on methanol (kindly provided in the form of "Pruteen" by ICI, Agri
cultural Division, U.K.) was extracted.

In this context it is perhaps illustrative to mention it
was found afterwards that this is a very poor source. On
the other hand, substantial amounts of PQQ can be very
easily isolated by ion exchange chromatography from the
culture medium of bacteria grown on alcohols (Table 1).

Table 1

PQQ IN THE CULTURE MEDIUM

Organism	Growth Substrate	PQQ (nM)
A. *calcoaceticus* LMD 79.41	ethanol	100
A. *calcoaceticus*	p-hydroxybenzoic acid	65
Ps. *aeruginosa* LMD 80.53	succinate	0
Ps. *aeruginosa*	ethanol	2800
Ps. *aeruginosa*	glucose	580
Pseudomonas *putida* LMD 72.6	ethanol	1850
Hyphomicrobium X	methanol	4400

By usual techniques like NMR and MS we elucidated the
structure. As said already it is an o-quinone with a
quinoline- and a pyrrole-ring. The three carboxylic acid
groups in the structure make this compound very hydrophilic. In view of this properties it has been given the semi-
systematic name "pyrrolo-quinoline quinone", abbreviated
to PQQ (5). Enzymes having PQQ as prosthetic group are
called "quinoproteins", in analogy with names like flavoproteins, hemoproteins etc. Independently, orther workers
(6) had isolated an acetone adduct from methylotrophic
bacteria. The structure was determined by X-ray diffraction and the compound named "methoxatin".

PROPERTIES OF PQQ.

Reduction of PQQ.

Reduction of PQQ with one electron steps (Fig.1) leads to
the semi-quinone form (PQQH·) and subsequently to the
quinol form (PQQH$_2$)(7). All redox forms have been found in
methanol dehydrogenase.
For some unknown reason,
methanol dehydrogenase
as it is isolated has
the coenzyme in its semi-
quinone form, possibly
explaining why the ab-

PQQ
pyrrolo-quinoline
quinone

PQQH·
pyrrolo-quinoline
semiquinone

PQQH$_2$
pyrrolo-quinoline
quinol

sorption spectrum of the enzyme does not change on addition of substrate. Apparently, the semi-quinone cannot acom-
modate the two electrons derived from the substrate. Although the existence of a three-electron reduced form of
PQQ in the enzyme has been claimed (8), the evidence given
could be refuted (9). On the other hand, the four-electron
reduced form of PQQ (PQQH$_4$) can be obtained by reduction
with NaBH$_4$ under aerobic conditions. However, this compounds seems biologically irrelevant as it has not been
observed so far in biological systems.

Addition compounds.
As mentioned already, a PQQ solution shows fluorescence.
When, however, the excitation spectrum is compared with
the absorption spectrum, large differences are observed.
Since the PQQ used in these measurements was chromatogra-
phically pure, it was very unlikely that the fluorescence
originated from an accompanying impurity. Surprisingly,
on cooling the solution the differences between the spectra diminished. Mathematical analysis of the absorption
spectrum at different temperatures showed that the spectrum consisted of two species. One of these was identical
to the excitation spectrum. NMR measurements under the
same conditions revealed that PQQ in a solution at room
temperature is for a large part (40%) hydrated at the C$_5$-
position (10). Covalent addition of aldehydes, ketones,
urea, amines and ammonia to PQQ has also been observed
(10). Especially the latter compound is interesting as

82

ammonia is an activator for methanol dehydrogenase. In this
context it may be relevant to mention that a reaction takes
place between methanol and PQQ only when NH_3 is present in
the model system. Adducts with amines may play a role in
the catalytic cycle of methylamine dehydrogenase and plasma amine oxidases (see below).

Chromatographic analysis.
The property to form addition compounds is also obvious
from HPLC chromatogramms of PQQ on a reversed phase column
as the peak of PQQ is unusually broad, probably resulting
from addition of H_2O and/or methanol from the solvent. Although the analysis of PQQ can be improved by transforming
it into a stable adduct, e.g. with acetone, still a more
sensitive test was developed. This was based on the observation that periodate oxidation of $PQQH_4$ yields a very in-
tensively fluorescing compound. Using this procedure, low
amounts of PQQ could be determined, even in an untreated
culture medium (11).

QUINOPROTEINS.

Occurrence.
To answer the question whether PQQ is restricted to methanol dehydrogenase or not, several enzymes from which it
was apparent from the literature that they had properties
incompatible with the enzyme groups in the classification
system, were investigated. Some examples are given in
Table 2.

QUINOPROTEINS

Enzyme	EC number	Organism
methanol deh.	1.1.99.8	methylotrophic bacteria
glucose deh.	1.1.99.16	*Gluconobacters, Acinetobacters,* *E.coli, Ps. aeruginosa*
methylamine deh.	1.4.99.3	*Thiobacillus* A_2, *Ps.* spec.
alcohol deh.	1.1.99.8	*Acetobacters,* alkane-degr.bact.
amine oxidase	1.4.3.6	bovine plasma

Enzymology.

In view of the limited space, it is impossible to discuss
the enzymes in full detail. No common trait can be indicated except that all the enzymes show a very broad substrate specificity, although this may be a coincidence.
Methanol- and alcohol dehydrogenase, both are isolated with
PQQ in a semi-quinone form. Glucose dehydrogenase, however,
contains PQQ (12). There is good reason to believe that
the free radical in the first two enzymes is an artifact,
somehow related with the need for an activator of these
enzymes in the assay (13). Thus, although the mechanism in
vitro consists of a hydride transfer from the substrate to
the enzyme and reoxidation of the enzyme via one-electron
steps in the presence of activator (9), the mechanism in
vivo may be different. Finally it should be mentioned that
apoenzymes have been obtained from the quinoprotein enzymes in which PQQ is non-covalently bound. Besides providing an opportunity to study the recombination process
between apoenzyme and PQQ or a modified compound, this
finding has been exploited to develop a biological assay
for PQQ (11).

Bioenergetical aspects.

Methanol dehydrogenase is bound to the respiratory chain
at the level of cytochrome c (13). The same applies to
methylamine dehydrogenase (14), although in this case a
copper-containing protein is situated between the enzymes.
This conclusion about the coupling site is supported by
the results of proton translocation and growth yield
experiments (1) and is explainable from the relatively
high redox potential of the couple $PQQ/PQQH_2$ (+ 90 mV)(7).
In contradiction with this is the recent finding of a
NAD-linked, PQQ-containing methanol dehydrogenase which
exists in a complex with NADH dehydrogenase (15). Furthermore, glucose dehydrogenase in *Acinetobacter calcoaceticus*
is coupled to cytochrome b. These examples show that a
large variation exists in the nature of the natural electron acceptors for quinoproteins.

The way of coupling to the respiratory chain is closely
connected to the question how these enzymes are localized
in the cell. All the available evidence for the bacterial

84

quinoproteins indicates that they are periplasmic enzymes
(16). It is perhaps not fortuitous that quinoprotein enzymes are found (12,17) in bacterial species which have to
maintain very steep gradients(for instance Acetic acid
bacteria have to withstand concentrations of acetic acid
as high as 2.5 M). A complicating factor is, however, the
fact that other enzymes converting the same substrate are
simultaneously present. *Pseudomonas aeruginosa* grown on
ethanol contains a quinoprotein- as well as an NAD-dependent alcohol dehydrogenase. Since cyclopropane-derivatives
appeared to be excellent suicide substrates in vitro (Fig.
2)(18), these compounds were tested for the selective inactivation of quinoprotein alcohol dehydrogenases in the
cell.

Quinoprotein
PQQ   PQQ adduct

R = H, OH, OC$_2$H$_5$

The results demonstrated (19) that these compounds are very
promishing as tools for selectively inactivating the quinoprotein alcohol dehydrogenases in vivo. It is anticipated
that these suicide substrates may be very helpful in the
study of unresolved questions in the bioenergetics of
methane oxidation and related problems.

THE ROLE OF PQQ IN MAMMALIAN SYSTEMS.

Copper-containing amine oxidase (EC 1.4.3.6), also known
as diamine oxidase or plasma amine oxidase has been
studied for many years (20).Although it was known that this
enzyme also contains an organic prosthetic group (covalently bound to the protein), much confusion exists on the
nature of this. Originally, it has been suggested that it

85

could be pyridoxal phosphate since the enzyme becomes inactivated by adding carbonyl-group reagents such as hydrazines. However, this view contradicts the results from mechanistic studies, although the difficulties can be circumvented by assuming a special interaction between pyridoxal phosphate and the copper ion. Another suggestion has been that the prosthetic group is a ring-opened flavin derivative. In view of the properties of the enzyme we reasoned that PQQ could also be a good candidate since it has carbonyl-groups and shows redox behaviour. As mentioned already, PQQ reacts with amines and model studies of PQQ and basic amino acids showed the formation of many degradation products. Therefore, it was decided to derivative the prosthetic group in the enzyme. From the compounds tested, 2,4-dinitrophenylhydrazine looked very promising as it produced a stable model compound and reacted with the prosthetic group in the enzyme. Proteolytic degradation of the derivatized enzyme revealed that the enzyme has covalently bound PQQ as prosthetic group (21).

The finding of the first mammalian quinoprotein raises several important questions. For instance, is PQQ synthesized by the organism itself, or is it provided by the food or by bacteria in the digestive tract? The latter possibility is not unlikely, since normal laboratory strains of *Escherichia coli* synthesize the apo-enzyme of glucose dehydrogenase but not PQQ. The functionality of this enzyme could be demonstrated by using a mutant blocked in the uptake of glucose via the phosphotransferase system. The experiments showed that this mutant could grow on glucose, only in the presence of PQQ (22). The existence of quinoprotein apoenzymes in many bacterial strains may be explained by assuming that in the natural environment PQQ is provided by other organisms. The examples in Table 1 show indeed that there exist several bacteria which excrete PQQ into their culture medium. Also the second possibility is not unrealistic. Substantial amounts of PQQ (2 mg/ml) are found in tabel vinegar. In view of the important role of copper-containing amine oxidases in the regulation of cell growth, studies on the biosynthesis of PQQ and its role as a vitamin seem very important.

REFERENCE LIST.
1) Anthony, C. (1982). The Biochemistry of Methylotrophs. Academic Press, New York.
2) Duine, J.A., Frank,Jzn. J. and Westerling, J. (1978). Purification and properties of methanol dehydrogenase from *Hyphomicrobium* X. Biochim.Biophys.Acta 524, 277-287.
3) Westerling, J., Frank,Jzn. J. and Duine, J.A. (1979). The prosthetic group of methanol dehydrogenase from *Hyphomicrobium* X: electron spin resonance evidence for a quinone structure. Biochem.Biophys.Res.Commun. 87, 719-724.
4) Duine, J.A. and Frank,Jzn. J. (1980). The prosthetic group of methanol dehydrogenase. Purification and some of its properties. Biochem.J. 187, 221-226.
5) Duine, J.A., Frank,Jzn. J. and Verwiel P.E.J. (1980). Structure and activity of the prosthetic group of methanol dehydrogenase. Eur.J.Biochem. 108, 187-192.
6) Salisbury, S.A., Forrest, H.S., Cruse, W.B.T. and Kennard, O. (1979). Nature 280, 843-844.
7) Duine, J.A., Frank,Jzn. J. and Verwiel, P.E.J. (1981). Characterization of the second prosthetic group in methanol dehydrogenase from *Hyphomicrobium* X. Eur.J.Biochem. 118, 395-399.
8) Mincey, T., Bell, J.A., Mildvan, A.S. and Abeles, R.H. (1981). Mechanism of action of methoxatin-dependent alcohol dehydrogenase. Biochemistry 20, 7502-7509.
9) De Beer, R., Duine, J.A., Frank,Jzn. J. and Westerling, J. (1983). The role of pyrrolo-quinoline semiquinone in the mechanism of action of methanol dehydrogenase. Eur.J.Biochem. 130, 105-109.
10) Dekker, R.H., Duine, J.A., Frank,Jzn. J., Verwiel, P.E.J. and Westerling, J. (1982). Covalent addition of H_2O, enzyme substrates and activators to pyrrolo-quinoline quinone, the coenzyme of quinoproteins. Eur.J.Biochem. 125, 69-73.
11) Duine, J.A., Frank,Jzn. J. and Jongejan, J.A. (1983). Detection and determination of pyrrolo-quinoline quinone, the coenzyme of quinoproteins. Anal.Biochem. 133, 239-243.
12) Duine, J.A., Frank,Jzn. J. and Van Zeeland, J.K. (1979). Glucose dehydrogenase from *Acinetobacter*

calcoaceticus: a quinoprotein. FEBS Lett. 108, 443-446.

13) Duine, J.A., Frank,Jzn. J. and De Ruiter, L.G. (1979). Isolation of a methanol dehydrogenase with a functional coupling to cytochrome c. J.Gen.Microbiol. 115, 523-526.

14) Tobari, J. and Harada, Y. (1981). Amicyanin: an electron acceptor of methylamine dehydrogenase. Biochem. Biophys.Res.Commun. 101, 502-508.

15) Duine, J.A., Frank,Jzn. J. and Berkhout, M.P.J. (1984). NAD-dependent, PQQ-containing methanol dehydrogenase: a bacterial dehydrogenase in a multienzyme complex. FEBS Lett. 168, 217-221.

16) Alefounder, P.R. and Ferguson, S.J. (1981). A periplasmic location for methanol dehydrogenase from Paracoccus denitrificans: implications for proton pumping by cytochrome aa_3. Biochem.Biophys.Res. Commun. 98, 778-784.

17) Ameyama, M., Matsushita, K., Ohno, Y., Shinagawa, E. and Adachi, O. (1981). Existence of a novel prosthetic group, PQQ, in membrane-bound, electron transport chain-linked, primary dehydrogenases of oxidative bacteria. FEBS Lett. 130, 179-183.

18) Dijkstra, M., Frank,Jzn. J. Jongejan, J.A. and Duine, J.A. (1984). Inactivation of quinoprotein alcoholdehydrogenases with cyclopropane-derived suicide substrates. Eur.J.Biochem. 140, 369-373.

19) Groeneveld, A., Dijkstra, M. and Duine, J.A. (1984). Cyclopropanol in the exploration of bacterial alcohol oxidation. FEMS Microbiol.Lett. (in press).

20) Yasunobu, K.T., Ishizaki, H. and Minamiura, N. (1976). The molecular, mechanistic and immunological properties of amine oxidases. Mol.Cell.Biochem. 13, 3-29.

21) Lobenstein-Verbeek, C.L., Jongejan, J.A., Frank,Jzn., J. and Duine, J.A. (1984). Bovine serum amine oxidase: a mammalian enzyme having covalently bound PQQ as prothetic group. FEBS Lett. 170, 305-309.

22) Hommes, R.W.J., Postma, P.W., Neijssel, O.M., Tempest, D.W., Dokter, P. and Duine, J.A. (1984). Evidence of a quinoprotein glucose dehydrogenase apoenzyme in several strains of *Escherichia coli*. FEMS Microbiol. Lett. 24, 329-333.

ESR MEASUREMENTS WITH THE PYRUVATE DEHYDROGENASE COMPLEX FROM ESCHERICHIA COLI

DIETER F. SCHRENK AND HANS BISSWANGER
Physiologisch-chemisches Institut, University of Tübingen
Hoppe-Seyler-Str. 1, D-7400 Tübingen, FRG

The pyruvate dehydrogenase complex is the most highly organized enzyme of the cell, consisting of three different components, each catalyzing a partial step of the whole reaction sequence. In the enzyme complex from E. coli each of these three components is present as 24 identical subunits (1). The pyruvate dehydrogenase complex connects the glycolytic pathway with the citric acid cycle and, thus, with the energy metabolism of the cell. This role as a key enzyme of the cell metabolism is confirmed by various regulatory influences the enzyme complex is subject to. Intermediates of glycolysis exert an activating effect and citric acid intermediates inhibit the activity of the enzyme (2,3). Furthermore the energy pool of the cell has a regulatory effect, where AMP is an activator and GTP and ATP are inhibitors (2,4,5). Acetyl CoA is a strong feedback inhibitor of the enzyme complex (4,6) and a positive cooperative effect of pyruvate on the reaction rate has been reported (6). All these effects are thought to occur through mediation of the pyruvate dehydrogenase (E1) component of the enzyme complex. The E1 component which catalyses the initial step of the overall reaction seems to play the role of a regulatory subunit of the enzyme complex.

Up to now the allosteric binding site of the feedback inhibitor acetyl CoA, though postulated by different groups to be located on the E1 component of the pyruvate dehydrogenase complex (4,6,7) is not yet unequivocally proven. The inhibitory effect of acetyl CoA on the partial reaction of the E1 component differs markedly from that effect the cofactor exerts on the overall reaction of the

Proceedings of the 16th FEBS Congress
Part A, pp. 89–94

enzyme complex (6). The dihydrolipoamide acetyltransferase (E2) component possesses a product binding site for acetyl CoA and product inhibition should occur at this site.

With the aid of a spin-labelled analogue of acetyl-CoA, 3-carboxy-2,2,5,5-tetrametylpyrrolidine-1-oxyl- CoA- thio-ester (CoA-SL) synthetized according to the method of Weidman et al. (8), we tried to investigate this complica-te situation in more detail. The chemical structure of this compound in comparison to acetyl CoA is shown in Fig. 1. It can be seen that the acetyl group of acetyl CoA is substituted by a more bulky residue. At first it should be shown whether the spin-label is able to substitude for the physiological feedback inhibitor.

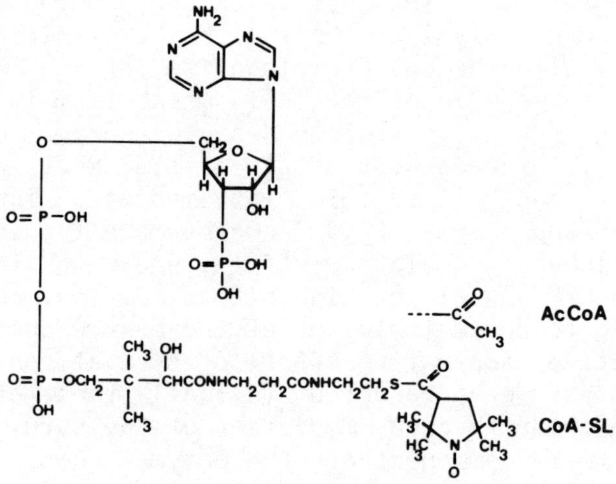

Fig. 1. Structural formula of CoA-SL and of acetyl CoA.

The kinetic experiment presented in Fig. 2 shows that CoA-SL is an inhibitor of the catalytic reaction of the E1 component with nearly the same efficiency (K_i = 20 μM) as acetyl CoA itself (K_i = 15 μM). Furthermore, this diagram shows that a competition exists between both inhibitors, thus is seems plausible to assume that both compounds act on the same site of the enzyme.

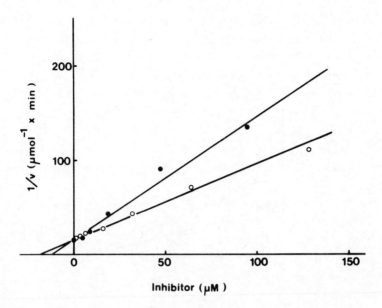

Fig. 2. Inhibiton of the activity of the El component by acetyl CoA (●) and by CoA-SL (○), measured at 25°C. Conditions for the enzyme tests are the same as described in (6).

CoA-SL shows typical ESR spectra with three sharp peaks. Addition of a twofold molar surplus of the El component to CoA-SL results in a considerable decrease of the peak amplitudes, which is an indication for an immobilization of the spin-label. This decrease can be used to measure the binding of CoA-SL to the enzyme.

Increasing amounts of the spin-label were added to the El component and binding was obtained from the relative decrease of the high-field peak amplitude of ESR spectra. As can be seen from the Scatchard plot in Fig. 3 normal hyperbolic binding of the spin-label reveals and from the straight line one binding site per El monomer and a dissociation constant of $\underline{K}_d = 15.9$ µM in the order of magnitude

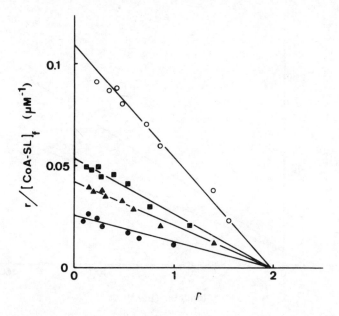

Fig. 3. Binding of CoA-SL to the El component in the absence ($\bigcirc$) and in the presence of 47 μM acetyl CoA ($\bullet$), 0.2 mM fructose-1,6-bisphosphate ($\blacksquare$), and 0.2 mM AMP ($\blacktriangle$), respectively. $[\text{CoA-SL}]_f$ is free CoA-SL, r is the amount of CoA-SL bound divided by the total El concentration.

of the inhibition constant ($\underline{K_i}$ = 20 μM) can be extrapolated. When the same experiment was done in the presence of acetyl CoA a clear competition reveals. The same is true also for AMP and for fructose-1,6,-bisphosphate, which were both reported to be activators of the pyruvate dehydrogenase complex (2,4,5). No influence on the binding of the spin-label could be detected with the inhibitors ATP and GTP, with CoA, with pyruvate and with thiamine diphosphate. From these results follows that the inhibition site for acetyl-CoA must be separate from the catalytic center and, actually, is a real allosteric site. The inhibitors ATP and GTP must possess an additional binding site, while the binding site of the activators AMP and fructose-1,6-bisphosphate overlaps with the acetyl CoA binding site. The main effect of the activators may consist in a reversion of the feedback inhibition. From Fig. 3 it can be seen, that CoA-SL is able to dislodge both activators completely from their binding sites on the E1 component, but the reverse is not true. As can be seen from Fig. 4 only an incomplete competition occurs, when the E1 component was incubated with a constant amount of the spin--label in the presence of varying amounts of AMP and of fructose-1,6-bisphosphate respectively, while acetyl CoA removes CoA-SL completely from its binding site. It may be concluded that acetyl CoA covers the whole allosteric site, while the activators are only able to bind to part of this site.

As is the case with the E1 component binding of CoA-SL to the E2 component of the pyruvate dehydrogenase complex results in a decrease of the peak amplitudes in the ESR

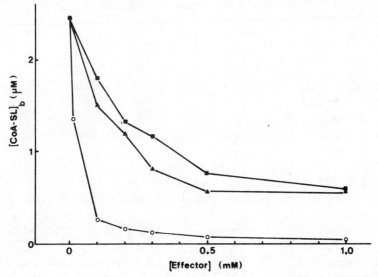

Fig. 4. Binding of acetyl CoA (○), AMP (▲), and fructose-1,6-bisphosphate (■) to the E1 component in the presence of 7.8 μM CoA-SL. The decrease of the fraction of CoA-SL bound to the enzyme ($[CoA-SL]_b$) was obtained from the relative peak amplitudes in ESR spectra.

spectra and normal hyperbolic binding is found. In contrast to the behaviour of the allosteric site, binding of the spin-label to the E2 component can be completely reversed by acetyl CoA as well as by CoA. It is obviously the product binding site of the E2 component which is found in this experiment and two binding sites for the spin-label per polypeptide chain were found. This is in contrast to the data obtained with the amino acid sequence analysis, where three highly homologous domains per E2 polypeptide chain revealed (9). Acetylation experiments with the lipoyl residues of this enzyme component, however, claim for only two active sites (10,11) in accordance with our results.

To sum up with CoA-SL as an analogue for acetyl CoA we were able to distinguish between the product binding site on the E2 component and the regulatory allosteric site on the E1 component. This gives additional evidence that the pyruvate dehydrogenase complex from E. coli is the greatest allosteric enzyme described up to now (12).

REFERENCES

1. Reed, L.J. (1974) Acc.Chem.Res. 7, 40-46.
2. Shen, L.C. & Atkinson, D.E. (1970) J.Biol.Chem. 245, 5974 -5978.
3. Bisswanger, H. (1972) Ph.D. Thesis, Tübingen.
4. Schwartz, E.R. & Reed, L.J. (1970) Biochemistry 9, 1434-1439.
5. Shen, L.C., Fall, L., Walton, G.M. & Atkinson, D. (1968) Biochemistry 7, 4041-4045.
6. Bisswanger, H. & Henning, U.(1971) Eur.J.Biochem. 24, 376-384.
7. Shepherd, G.B. & Hammes, G.G. (1976) Biochemistry 15, 311-317.
8. Weidman, S.W., Drysdale, G.R. & Mildvan, A.S. (1973) Biochemistry 12, 1874-1883.
9. Stephens, P.E., Darlison, M.G., Lewis, H.M. & Guest, J.R. (1983) Eur.J.Biochem. 133, 481-489.
10. Danson,M.J.& Perham,R.N.(1976) Biochem.J.159,677-682.
11. Hale,G. & Perham, R.N.(1979) FEBS Lett. 105, 263-266.
12. Bisswanger, H. (1984) J.Biol.Chem. 259, 2457-2465.

QUANTUM CHEMICAL APPROACH TO OXIDOREDUCTION OF FLAVINS
IN FLAVOPROTEINS

KUNIO YAGI AND KICHISUKE NISHIMOTO*
Institute of Applied Biochemistry, Yagi Memorial Park,
Mitake, Gifu 505-01, and *Department of Chemistry,
Faculty of Science, Osaka City University, Osaka 558,
Japan

INTRODUCTION

The role of the coenzyme, flavin adenine dinucleotide
or flavin mononucleotide, in oxidoreduction catalysed by
flavoproteins is to mediate electron transfer from a
donor to an acceptor. Therefore, the reactivity of
flavins in flavoproteins depends upon their electron-
accepting and electron-donating ability.

Obviously, the situation of flavins in flavoproteins
is different from that in their aqueous solution. The
most characteristic difference is due to the fact that
hydrogen bonding occurs at definite hetero atoms of the
isoalloxazine nucleus in the former, whereas all hetero
atoms are involved in the latter. We proposed the occurrence of hydrogen bonding at definite hetero atoms
from the data of model experiments [1,2], and from the
electronic structures of hydrogen-bonded flavins obtained by calculation [3]. This was actually shown with
flavoproteins by X-ray crystallography [4,5].

Hydrogen bonding can be described by a resonance
hybrid of the following structures:

$$X - H -- Y \ (I) \quad (X - H)^- -- Y^+ \ (II) \quad X^- -- (H - Y)^+ \ (III)$$

where structures (II) and (III) represent the charge
transfer interaction in hydrogen bonding. Accordingly,
hydrogen bonding formation brings about a charge transfer from a proton acceptor (electron donor) to a proton
donor (electron acceptor), which induces electronic polarization in the isoalloxazine nucleus and influences
the reactivity of flavin. The present communication
summarizes the data obtained by ab initio molecular

Proceedings of the 16th FEBS Congress
Part A, pp. 95–100
© 1985 VNU Science Press

orbital (MO) calculations on model systems, oxidized and
reduced lumiflavin-water complexes.

ELECTRON ACCEPTABILITY OF OXIDIZED FLAVIN

It had been found by MO calculation using the P-P-P
method that in oxidized flavin N(5) has the largest size
of frontier orbital in the isoalloxazine nucleus [3].
This was confirmed by ab initio MO calculations [6].
The lowest unoccupied MO (LUMO) coefficients are illustrated in Fig. 1. It is obvious that N(5) can best
accomodate the incoming electrons or nucleophiles.
    To study the effect of hydrogen bonding at hetero
atoms on the electron acceptability of flavin, ab initio
MO calculations were made on oxidized lumiflavin-water
complexes (Fig. 2). The calculated data are summarized
in Table 1. According to the frontier electron theory,
the electron acceptability of a given atom is proportional to the square of the atomic orbital (AO) coefficient of its LUMO. Therefore, the magnitude of the
effect of hydrogen bonding on the electron acceptability
of N(5) is in the order of N(5) > O(14) > N(1) > O(12) >
N(3)H. Since LUMO is an electron-accepting orbital, a
decrease in LUMO energy means an increase in electron
acceptability of a whole molecule. It is noted in this

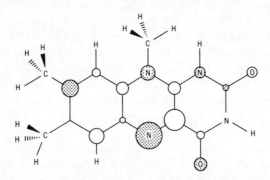

Fig. 1. Schematic illustration of LUMO of oxidized
lumiflavin. The radius of the circle is proportional to
the absolute value of the AO coefficient of the corresponding atom. ⊙ and ○ represent the values of coefficients which are positive and negative, respectively.

case that the order of the effect of hydrogen bonding on electron acceptability of the whole flavin molecule coincides with that of its N(5).

ELECTRON-DONATING ABILITY OF REDUCED FLAVIN

It had been found by MO calculation using the P-P-P method that N(5) and C(4a) are the most susceptible atoms for attack by electrophiles [3]. This is consistent with nuclear magnetic resonance data which indicate that upon reduction the changes in the chemical shifts of N(5) and C(4a) are much larger than those of the other atoms [7]. However, which atom, N(5) or C(4a),

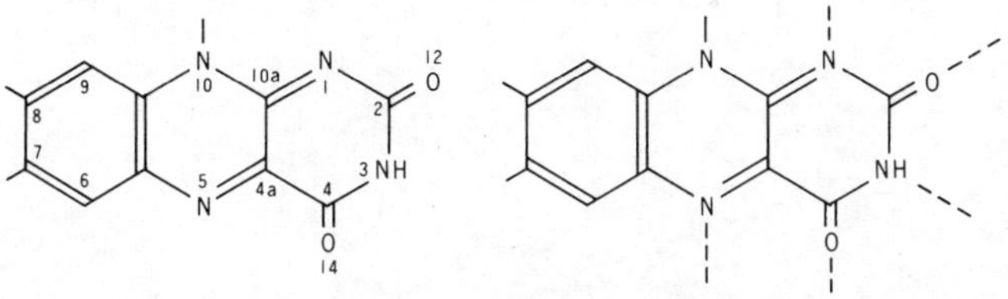

No hydrogen bonding   N(1), O(12), N(3)H, O(14),
                          N(5)-hydrogen bonding

Fig. 2. Hydrogen bonding at hetero atoms of the iso-alloxazine nucleus of flavin.

Table 1. Effect of Hydrogen Bonding on Oxidized Lumi-flavin.

Hydrogen bonding	No	N(1)	N(5)	N(3)H	O(12)	O(14)
ΔQ	–	-0.021	-0.026	0.074	-0.038	-0.046
ΔE	–	5.64	5.78	7.81	6.25	5.51
LUMO energy	0.135	0.127	0.124	0.148	0.128	0.126
Coefficient of LUMO at N(5)	0.543	0.548	0.552	0.532	0.545	0.550

ΔQ: calculated charge migration, ΔQ = Q(H-bonded oxidized lumiflavin) - Q(free oxidized lumiflavin).
ΔE: hydrogen bonding energy (kcal/mol).

is more favorable for reaction with an electron acceptor
has not yet been determined. To elucidate this problem,
we have recently carried out ab initio MO calculation on
reduced lumiflavin [8]. The highest occupied MO (HOMO)
coefficients are illustrated in Fig. 3. The energy of
HOMO is a measure of the electron-donating ability of
a molecule, and atoms having larger HOMO coefficients
are more liable to be attacked by electrophiles. As can

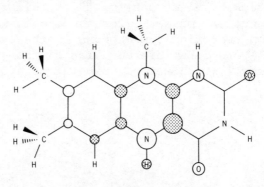

Fig. 3. Schematic illustration of HOMO of reduced lumiflavin. The radius of the circle is proportional to the
absolute value of the AO coefficient of the corresponding atom. ⊙ and ○ represent the values of coefficients
which are positive and negative, respectively.

Table 2. Effect of Hydrogen Bonding on Reduced Lumiflavin.

Hydrogen bonding	No	N(1)H	N(5)H	N(3)H	O(12)	O(14)
ΔQ	–	0.028	0.025	0.026	−0.035	−0.035
ΔE	–	7.07	4.63	6.22	4.89	4.79
HOMO energy	−0.184	−0.175	−0.170	−0.177	−0.190	−0.192
Coefficient of HOMO at C(4a)	0.407	0.424	0.396	0.416	0.397	0.399

ΔQ: calculated charge migration, $\Delta Q = Q$(H-bonded reduced
 lumiflavin) − Q(free reduced lumiflavin).
ΔE: hydrogen bonding energy (kcal/mol).

be seen from the figure, N(5) and C(4a) are the most active among the reactive sites, and their magnitudes are almost the same. However, the net charge of N(5) is negative (-0.335), but that of C(4a) is slightly positive (+0.018) [8]. Therefore, neutral electrophiles such as O_2 would easily attack C(4a), but scarcely N(5), due to the repulsion of the electron cloud.

Effects of hydrogen bonding at hetero atoms of reduced flavin on its reactivity are summarized in Table 2. Hydrogen bonding at N(5)H, N(1)H and N(3)H increases the HOMO energy, while that at O(12) and O(14) decreases it. The coefficient of HOMO energy at C(4a) is increased by hydrogen bonding at N(1)H and N(3)H, while it is decreased by that at N(5)H, O(12) and O(14).

CONCLUSION

Ab initio MO calculations on oxidized and reduced lumi-flavin indicate that the most liable electron-accepting site is N(5) and the best electron-donating site is C(4a) in the isoalloxazine nucleus. The calculations made on oxidized and reduced lumiflavin-water complexes revealed that hydrogen bonding at definite hetero atoms increases the reactivity of flavin, while that at the other atoms decreases it. For instance, a reduced lumiflavin complex possessing hydrogen bonding at N(1)H and N(3)H has the highest reactivity at C(4a), while that possessing hydrogen bonding at all hetero atoms has lower reactivity than that without hydrogen bonding. To realize the occurrence of hydrogen bonding at definite hetero atoms, the environment of flavin should prefera-bly be hydrophobic. In fact, the flavin coenzyme of D-amino acid oxidase is in hydrophobic environment [9]. In such a circumstance, hydrogen bonding can be formed at definite hetero atoms. This is the case for flavo-proteins. In other words, the protein moiety of flavo-protein makes its coenzyme reactive, in addition to its role of fixing the flavin in proximity to the substrate.

REFERENCES

1. Kotaki, A., Naoi, M., and Yagi, K. (1970). Effect of

proton donors on the absorption spectrum of flavin compounds in apolar media. J. Biochem. 68, 287-292.

2. Yagi, K., Ohishi, N., Nishimoto, K., Choi, J. D., and Song, P.-S. (1980). Effect of hydrogen bonding on electronic spectra and reactivity of flavins. Biochemistry 19, 1553-1557.

3. Nishimoto, K., Watanabe, Y., and Yagi, K. (1978). Hydrogen bonding of flavoprotein. I. Effect of hydrogen bonding on electronic spectra of flavoprotein. Biochim. Biophys. Acta 526, 34-41.

4. Ludwig, M. L., Burnett, R. M., Darling, G. D., Jordan, S. E., Kendall, D. S., and Smith, W. W. (1976). The structure of Clostridium MP flavodoxin as a function of oxidation state: Some comparisons of the FMN-binding sites in oxidized, semiquinone and reduced forms. In: Flavins and Flavoproteins, T. P. Singer (ed). Elsevier, Amsterdam, pp. 393-404.

5. Watenpaugh, K. D., Sieker, L. C., and Jensen, L. H. (1976). A crystallographic structural study of the oxidation states of Desulfovibrio vulgaris flavodoxin. In: Flavins and Flavoproteins, T. P. Singer (ed). Elsevier, Amsterdam, pp. 405-410.

6. Watanabe, Y., Nishimoto, K., Kashiwagi, H., and Yagi, K. (1982). Ab initio MO study on hydrogen bonding in lumiflavin-water complex. In: Flavins and Flavoproteins, V. Massey and C. H. Williams (eds). Elsevier, Amsterdam, pp. 541-545.

7. Kawano, K., Ohishi, N., Takai Suzuki, A., Kyogoku, Y., and Yagi, K. (1978). Nitrogen-15 and carbon-13 nuclear magnetic resonance of reduced flavins. Comparative studies with oxidized flavins. Biochemistry 17, 3854-3859.

8. Nishimoto, K., Kai, E., and Yagi, K. (1984). Hydrogen bonding of flavoprotein. II. Effect of hydrogen bonding at hetero atoms of reduced flavin on its reactivity. Biochim. Biophys. Acta, in press.

9. Yagi, K. (1973) Hydrophobic interaction involved in D-amino acid oxidase and its complex. In: Oxidases and related redox systems, T. E. King, H. S. Mason, and M. Morrison (eds). University Park Press, Baltimore, pp. 217-225.

ON THE PROOFREADING MECHANISM OF LEUCYL-tRNA SYNTHE-TASES (LRS) FROM ESCHERICHIA COLI AND BAKER'S YEAST

S.ENGLISCH, U.ENGLISCH, F.VON DER HAAR[*] and F.CRAMER

Max-Planck-Institut für experimentelle Medizin, Abteilung Chemie, 3400 Göttingen, F.R.G.

INTRODUCTION

The high accuracy of aminoacylation of tRNAs can only be maintained by proofreading mechanisms. These mechanisms act either on the level of the aminoacyladenylate/enzyme complex (pretransfer proofreading) or on the level of the enzyme bound aminoacylated tRNA (posttransfer proofreading). The "chemical proofreading" model[1] for the post-transfer correction process postulates that the nonaccepting hydroxyl group of the 3'-terminal ribose serves as a general base for the activation of the hydrolysing water molecule.

[*] present address: B.Braun Melsungen AG, P.O.Box 110
3508 Melsungen, F.R.G.

Proceedings of the 16th FEBS Congress
Part A, pp. 101–107
© 1985 VNU Science Press

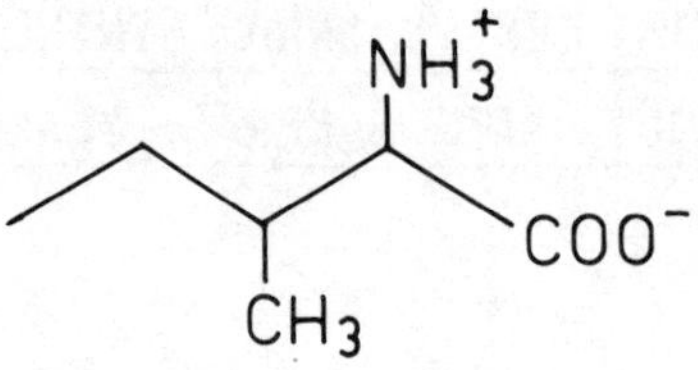

Isoleucine

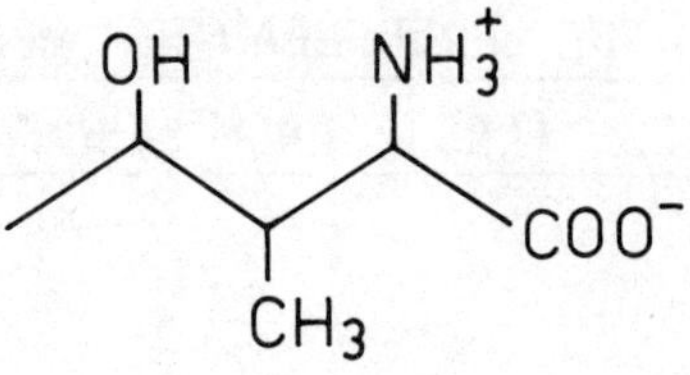

γ-Hydroxyisoleucine

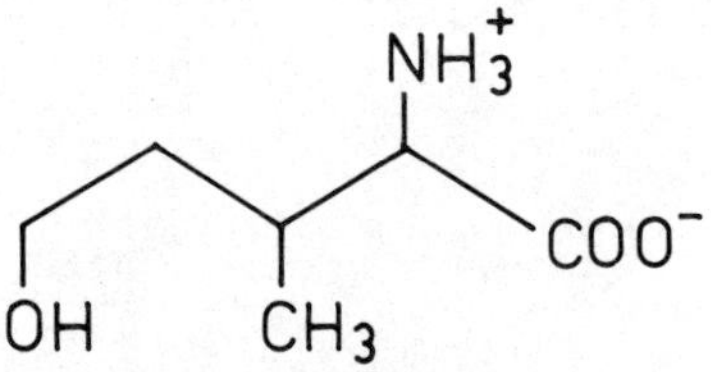

δ-Hydroxyisoleucine

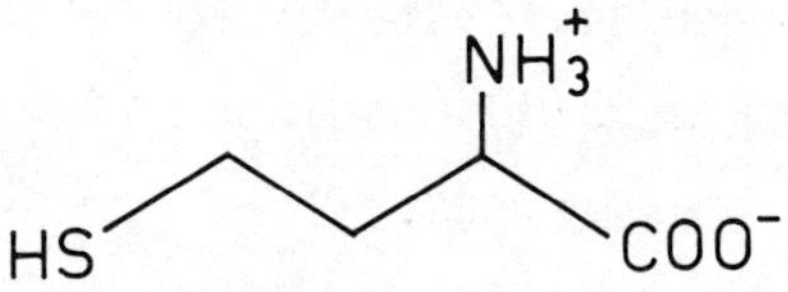

Homocysteine

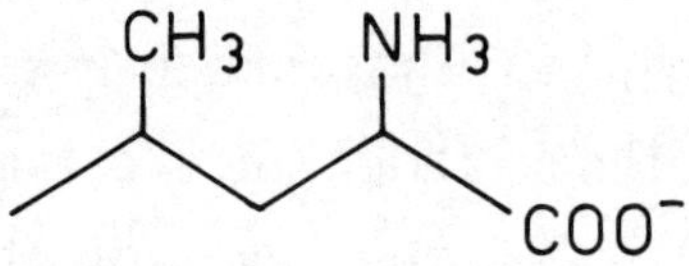

Leucine

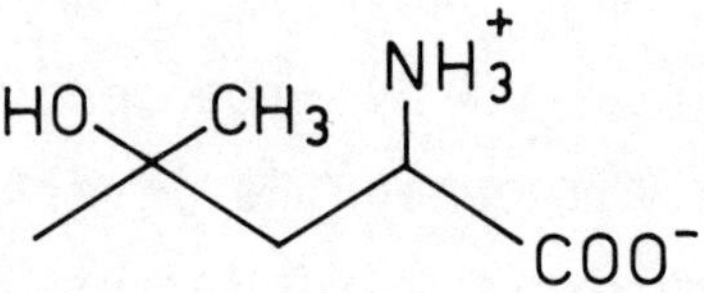

γ-Hydroxyleucine

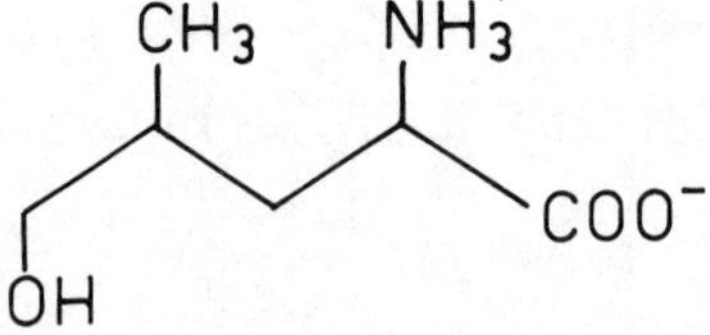

δ-Hydroxyleucine

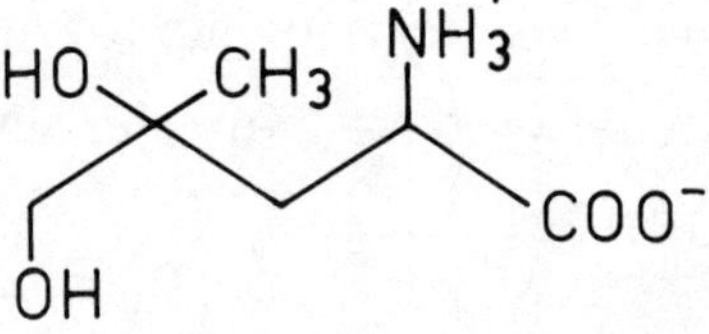

γ,δ-Dihydroxyleucine

Figure 1: Chemical structures of the analogues

In the present study we examine the activation and proof-reading of six different leucine and isoleucine hydroxyl-analogues (fig.1) and homocysteine by the leucyl-tRNA synthetases (LRS) from E.coli and baker's yeast. The approach using these analogues is based on the idea of simulating the "activated" water molecule by the hydroxyl- and thiol-groups and by their ability to form lactones which can be esaily detected by thin layer chromatography.

ACTIVATION OF THE AMINO ACID ANALOGUES BY THE LEUCYL-tRNA SYNTHETASES (LRS) FROM BAKER'S YEAST AND E.COLI.

Among the tested derivatives only γ,δ-dihydroxyleucine is not activated by either one of the LRS, as indicated by the ATP/PP$_i$ exchange. The other analogues however, although they are bulkier than leucine are activated most of them only by the yeast LRS. The E.coli LRS has a higher specificity towards the analogues, only γ-hydroxyleucine and homocysteine are accepted.

AMP FORMATION IN ABSENCE AND PRESENCE OF tRNA

Nonstoichiometric hydrolysis of ATP to AMP during enzyme catalysed formation of the aminoacyladenylate from ATP and aminoacid is characteristic for proofreading events[2,3]. In many cases the AMP formation is strongly dependent on tRNA, suggesting that the amino acid is transfered to tRNA prior to hydrolysis. However as noted for the valyl-tRNA

103

synthetases from lupin seeds and E.coli, the enzymes catalyse an appreciable AMP formation in the absence of tRNA[4,5]. The two LRSs investigated show a high AMP formation in presence of tRNA but in absence of tRNA only the yeast LRS splits ATP. This strongly indicates that the proofreading of the yeast LRS occurs on the aminoacyl adenylate level, while the E.coli LRS uses posttransfer hydrolysis to destroy these misactivated analogues.

AMINOACYLATION OF tRNA^{Leu} WITH LEUCINE ANALOGUES

The aminoacylation of tRNA^{Leu} with nonradioactive amino acids is followed by backtitration[6] of nonaminoacylated tRNA with ^{14}C-leucine. According to the AMP formation no aminoacylation of yeast tRNA^{Leu} was detectable, while the E.coli LRS aminoacylates the cognate tRNA with γ-hydroxyleucine and homocysteine. The hydrolysis of the other analogues might be too fast or they are despite the exclusive AMP formation in presence of tRNA proofred prior to transfer leading to a concerted pre- and posttransfer mechanism.

LACTONISATION OF HOMOCYSTEINYL-, γ-HYDROXYLEUCYL-tRNA^{Leu}

The cyclisation of homocysteine and γ-hydroxyleucine to the corresponding lactones is used as a marker for the posttransfer "chemical proofreading". The enzyme should rapidly hydrolyse the misaminoacylated tRNAs forming stable five membered lactones. In a typical experiment E.coli LRS is incubated with homocysteine or γ-hydroxyleucine, ATP and tRNA^{Leu} and samples of the reaction mixture are spotted on silica plates in time intervals of 10 minutes. The thin layer chromatography of homocysteinyl-tRNA^{Leu} (fig.2) clearly shows the increase of thiolactone with time until the spot reaches the intensity as the aminoacid (D-isomer as reference). The nonradioactive hydroxylactone could not unambigously be detected with this analytical technique, but incubation with ^{14}C-labeled γ-hydroxyleucine demonstrated the formation of the lactone.

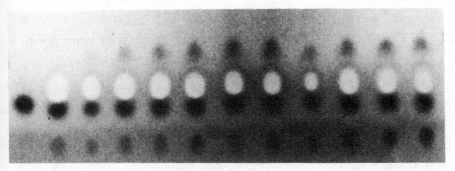

Figure 2: Thin layer chromatography of enzyme/tRNA dependent homocysteine lactonisation. Increasing spots of thiolacton appear after 10 minutes reactiontime.

DISCUSSION

Our examinations regarding the location of the hydrolytic mechanisms on the reaction pathway show that the LRS from yeast and E.coli use different ways to maintain the high

accuracy of aminoacylation. The yeast enzyme has a relatively poor initial substrate recognition and the AMP
formation in the absence of tRNA strongly suggests that
pretransfer hydrolysis is the main proofreading event.
The E.coli LRS exhibits a much better initial substrate
recognition regarding the analogues. Only two analogues
are activated; AMP formation occurs only in the presence
of tRNA favouring transfer of the aminoacyladenylate to
tRNA prior to hydrolysis. The E.coli LRS shows a typical
"chemical proofreading" in the posttransfer hydrolysis
of homocysteine and γ-hydroxyleucine. In both cases the
corresponding lactones are formed. The lactonisation is
enzyme dependent and occurs on the level of the mis-
charged tRNA. The thiol- and hydroxyl-groups are directly
activated by the nonaccepting hydroxyl-group of the tRNA
without a water molecule involved (fig.3). The two amino

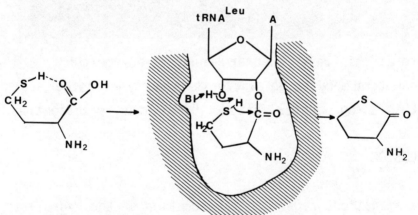

Figure 3: Proposed reaction mechanism for the thio-
lactonisation of homocysteine.

acids can mimick the "activated" water molecule which strongly supports the "chemical proofreading" model.

1. Von der Haar,F. and Cramer,F (1976). Biochemistry 15, 4131-4138.
2. Fersht,A.R. and Kaethner,M.M. (1976). Biochemistry 15, 3342-3346.
3. Hopfield,J.J. (1974). Proc.Natl.Acad.Sci. USA 71, 4135-4139.
4. Jakubowski,H. (1980). Biochemistry 19, 5071-5078.
5. Jakubowski,H. and Fersht,A.R. (1981). Nucleic.Acid Res. 9, 3105-3117.
6. Igloi,G.L., von der Haar,F. and Cramer,F. (1978). Biochemistry 17, 3459-3468.

CRYSTALLOGRAPHIC EVIDENCE FOR A MECHANISM OF ACTION OF ASPARTATE AMINOTRANSFERASE

J.N. JANSONIUS, M.G. VINCENT and D. PICOT
Biozentrum, University of Basel. Klingelbergstr. 70,
CH-4056 Basel, Switzerland.

Aspartate: 2-oxoglutarate aminotransferase (AAT; EC 2.6.
1.1), an α_2 dimeric enzyme, catalyses, in a ping-pong
mechanism, amino group transfer from aspartate or glutamate to oxaloacetate or 2-oxoglutarate. Its coenzyme
pyridoxal phosphate temporarily accepts the amino group
to become pyridoxamine phosphate. Different isoenzymes
are found in the cytoplasm and the mitochondria of higher animals with 412 and 401 amino acid residues per
chain respectively. The enzyme is the most extensively
studied representative of the class of vitamine B6 dependent enzymes, functioning in amino acid metabolism[1].
  The chemical pathway of the transamination reaction is
known (see Fig. 1). In the pyridoxal phosphate (or
PLP) enzyme, the coenzyme in its reactive bipolar ionic
form is bound to Lys 258 via an aldimine double bond.
The unprotonated species, absorbing at 360 nm, first accepts a proton from the substrate amino group, which
causes the absorption maximum to shift to 430 nm. Subsequently the transaldimination step can take place,
leading to the external aldimine intermediate, also absorbing at 430 nm. Lys 258 is released in uncharged
form. It is the prime candidate as proton acceptor in
the following α-deprotonation step, resulting in the
quinonoid intermediate, which absorbs at 490 nm. The
proton can subsequently be attached to the C4' carbon
atom (a 1,3 prototropic shift). The resulting ketimine
intermediate, absorbing at 340 nm can be hydrolysed to
pyridoxamine phosphate (PMP), absorbing at 330 nm, and
the oxoacid product.

Proceedings of the 16th FEBS Congress
Part A, pp. 109–120
© 1985 VNU Science Press

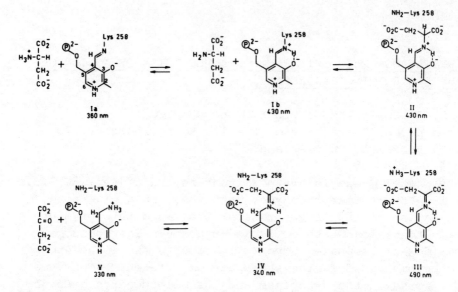

Fig. 1 Reaction scheme of the enzymatic conversion of aspartate to oxaloacetate.

Spatial structure of the chicken mitochondrial enzyme.
Crystallographic studies are being carried out on three different enzymes (2-6). The work described here was carried out with the mitochondrial isoenzyme from chicken. The structure of the native PLP holoenzyme was solved at 2.8 Å resolution in a triclinic crystal form, space group P1 (5,6). More recently, the structures of the PLP enzyme, liganded with maleate and 2-methylaspartate were solved in an orthorhombic crystal form, space group C222$_1$. Refinement to 2.3 Å resolution of this crystal form, the only one of all AAT's studied with only one subunit per asymmetric unit, nears completion.
The triclinic crystals of chicken mitochondrial AAT are enzymatically competent. The 360 nm absorption band of the PLP form can be transformed quantitatively into the 330 nm band of the PMP form by soaking a crystal in a solution of cysteine sulphinate. With oxaloacetate the process can be reversed. Both reactions occur without loss of crystalline order (7).

110

The overall structure of the dimeric enzyme (6,8) is
referred to in terms of a Cartesian coordinate system
with Z as the molecular 2-fold axis and the X-axis parallel to the longest dimension (~ 105 Å) of the dimer.
The subunits each consist of 16 α-helices, of which one
(residues 313-344) is 50 Å long. Another conspicious
feature is a 7-stranded, mainly parallel pleated sheet.
Each subunit can be subdivided into an amino terminal
arm, residues 3-14, which is hydrophobically attached
to the neighbouring subunit mainly through the indole
rings of Trp 5 and Trp 6, and two domains. The large
coenzyme binding domain consists of residues 48-325 and
interacts with its counterpart across the molecular 2-
fold axis. The second, "small" domain, contains residues 15-47 and 326-410.

The active sites are on opposite sides of the dimer
near the subunit interface. The coenzymes lie at the
back of the active site crevices, which can be approached from the Y (Fig.2) and -Y directions, respectively.
The aldimine double bond between coenzyme and Lys 258
is cisoid, i.e. cis with respect to the 3'-hydroxyl
group (Fig. 2). The protonated N1 makes an ion pair
with Asp 222. The ionized 3'-hydroxyl is hydrogen
bonded to Tyr 225. The bridging oxygen of the 5'-phos-
phate group lies behind the plane of the pyridine ring,
but the torsion angle around the C5-C5' bond is not
more than 25°, causing steric hindrance between C4' and
the bridging oxygen and favouring transaldimination.
The phosphate group is surrounded by 8 hydrogen bonding
ligands: Ser 107 Oγ, Gly 108 N, Thr 109 N and Oγ, Arg
266 Nη1 and Nη2, Ser 255 Oγ and Tyr 70* (from the neighbouring subunit) Oη. The double negative charge of the
phosphate group is compensated by Arg 266 and the positive side of an α-helix dipole (residues 108-122).
Thus the phosphate group is strongly fixed to the protein. In front of (and not above) the coenzyme there
is a pocket, surrounded by residues 37-39, Phe 360, Asn
194, Trp 140, Ser 296*, Asn 297* and Tyr 70*. At its
entrance one finds to the left Arg 292* and to the

111

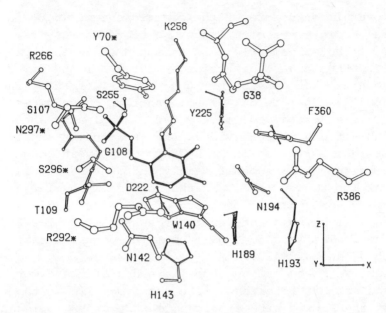

Fig. 2 Active site of mitochondrial AAT in its unliganded PLP form. The coenzyme is drawn with dark lines.
The substrate pocket is in front of the coenzyme.

right Arg 386. Clearly, this pocket forms the substrate binding site and the arginines compensate the
two carboxylate negative charges on the substrate.
This means, however, that during transaldimination the
coenzyme ring must rotate forward around one or more of
the three bonds between C5 and the phosphorus.

Other forms of the enzyme; conformational changes.
The first evidence of coenzyme rotation was provided by
an electron density difference map of the isomorphous
PMP enzyme. This map indicated a reorientation of the
(released) Lys 258 side chain, which forms hydrogen
bonds to both Tyr 70* and the PMP amino group, and an
increased tilt of ~20° of the pyridine ring with respect to the XZ plane, releasing strain around the
C5-C5' bonds. The main rotation is around C5-C5', but
additional small rotations around C5'-O5' and O5'-P

112

allow the hydrogen bond between N1 and Asp 222 to be retained (8,9). A coenzyme rotation around C5-C5' had already been postulated long ago in the dynamic model of
Karpeisky and Ivanov (10), a remarkable demonstration
of insight and intuition.

Conformational changes of the protein were first observed upon soaking apoenzyme crystals, also isomorphous with the holoenzyme (5), in a solution of N-(5'-
phosphopyridoxyl)-L-aspartate (PPL-Asp). This produced
an analogue of transamination intermediates (1). The
difference map at 3 Å resolution indicated an increase
in coenzyme tilt of ~30° and density corresponding to
the aspartate moiety in both active sites. In addition
a movement of the small domain towards the active site
was observed in one subunit. In the other, such a rearrangement is prevented by lattice contacts (5,8).
Although detailed interpretation of the difference map
was difficult, the PPL-Asp molecule could be built into
the density and the new position of Arg 386, which
moves with the small domain, located. The α-carboxyl-
ate group makes hydrogen bonds and an ion pair with Arg
386 while the distal carboxylate does the same with Arg
292*. Since N and Cα lie in the plane of the pyridine
ring, C and Cβ being equally close to it, this is a good
model for the external aldimine, and represents the
ideal conformation for α-deprotonation of a real external aldimine. This probably would cause a small (~10°)
additional tilt of the coenzyme, leaving the substrate
moiety in place. These constraints leave Lys 258 as
prime candidate for proton acceptor (as well as subsequent proton donor), with Tyr 70* as the only - and
less likely - alternative.

These results, complemented by model building with
computer graphics, suggested a mechanism of action of
the enzyme (8), which is briefly outlined below.

A mechanism of action.
In the Michaelis complex, aspartate is oriented through
charge interactions of its carboxylates with Arg 386 and

Arg 292*, and of its charged amino group with the ionized 3'-hydroxyl group of the coenzyme. Hydrogen bonds
are made between the β-carboxylate of aspartate and the
guanidinium group of Arg 292* as well as the indole nitrogen of Trp 140. The amino group is positioned at
van der Waals distance in front of C4' of the coenzyme.
pK-changes of the α-amino group and the coenzyme aldimine nitrogen due to the charge compensation cause proton
transfer from the former to the latter (10). This cre-
ates a situation favourable for nucleophilic attack of
the α-amino nitrogen on the C4' carbon atom. A 15° increase in tilt angle of the coenzyme ring allows a covalent bond to be made between the substrate nitrogen and
C4', while the Schiff base double bond to Lys 258 is
transformed into a single bond, which is rotated out of
the ring plane (geminal diamine). The substrate moiety
is pushed slightly in the X-direction and can now also
make a hydrogen bond to Arg 386 in the closed conformation which the enzyme takes up in the Michaelis complex. A further forward tilt of 15° brings the amino
nitrogen into the coenzyme ring plane and the lysine
ζ-nitrogen into the right position for release of its
bond to C4'. This process results in the external aldimine intermediate. During the transaldimination process the protonated pyridine nitrogen remains hydrogen
bonded to Asp 222. The released uncharged α-amino group
of Lys 258 forms a hydrogen bond with the phenolic
hydroxyl group of Tyr 70*, and is situated above the α-
proton of the substrate. The Cα-H bond is oriented
perpendicular to the conjugated double bond system of
the coenzyme-substrate aldimine, which favours α-deprotonation (11) leading to the quinonoid intermediate.
This transition probably is accompanied by a further
10° tilt of the pyridine ring plane, allowing the substrate carboxylate groups to remain essentially stationary. The pyridine ring is now oriented parallel to the
indole ring of Trp 140 at van der Waals distance. The
now charged Lys 258 ε-amino group may make an additional hydrogen bond to an oxygen of the double nega-

tively charged phosphate, thereby moving closer to the C4' carbon in a position where it can protonate the latter to produce the ketimine intermediate. The stereochemistry of the 1,3 prototropic shift, as proposed, corresponds to that observed experimentally. The tetrahedral coordination around C4' allows the coenzyme pyridine ring to rotate back into an intermediate orientation as observed in the PMP enzyme, which is also taken up in the PLP enzyme upon reduction of the Schiff base double bond and which presumably corresponds to the relaxed conformation of the coenzyme. Hydrolysis of the ketimine intermediate by a water molecule from above, probably assisted by Lys 258, results in the product complex of the PMP enzyme with oxaloacetate, the carbonyl group of which has an orientation similar to 2-oxoglutarate in nonproductive complexes with PLP enzyme (3,8). The product complex must take up the open conformation prior to product release.

Experiments on the cytosolic isoenzyme seem to confirm the two types of conformational change described above. Coenzyme rotation was observed for instance in the transition between the internal aldimine of the PLP enzyme and the external aldimine with 2-methylaspartate in cytosolic AAT of both pig and chicken, while a transition between open and closed conformations of the small domain was observed in this case as well as upon binding of non-covalent inhibitors like maleate and succinate to the cytosolic isoenzyme from chicken (2,4). Because of the sequence homology of about 50% and the strong structural homology between the cytosolic and the mitochondrial isoenzyme such similar behaviour is not unexpected. Rather, one would believe the same mechanism to be operative in both isoenzymes.

An alternative mechanism for transaldimination.
Arnone et al. (12) proposed an alternative mechanism for the transaldimination process, which they call "the oscillatory rotor mechanism". The origin of this proposal is the fact that in their model of the internal aldimi-

115

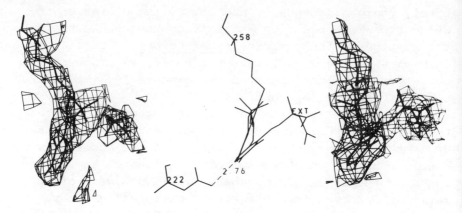

Fig. 3 The coenzyme, as internal aldimine, with the inhibitor maleate (left) and as external aldimine bound
to 2-methylaspartate (right) in their electron densities at 2.3 Å resolution. The left model (without maleate) and the right one (without Lys 258) are combined
in the centre. The hydrogen bond to Asp 222 is shown.

ne structure of the PLP enzyme, the bridging oxygen atom
to the phosphate group lies in front of the pyridine
ring. In a simple forward rotation of this ring as proposed above, it would have to pass through an eclipsed
conformation with strong steric hindrance between the
C4' carbon atom and the bridging oxygen (13). To overcome this problem, Arnone et al. propose a rotation of
the coenzyme around the P-O bond by 120° "over the top"
to give the geminal diamine and by another 120° to produce the external aldimine. The resulting model fits
their 3.5 Å resolution difference map of 2-methylaspar-
tate. This mechanism lacks the simplicity and elegance
of that of Ivanov and Karpeisky (10). A large movement
of the coenzyme ring, with release of the hydrogen bond
to Asp 222, would be necessary. Also, the coenzyme
would have to pass through two eclipsed conformations
of the C5'-O5' bond with P-O bonds in the process.
Recent quantum chemical calculations by J. Gerhards and
E.L. Mehler (Biozentrum, Basel) suggest that the energy
barriers involved might be higher than the one corres-

116

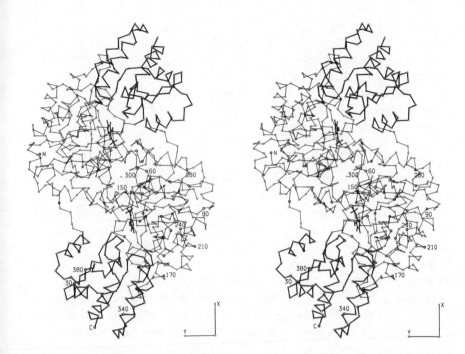

Fig. 4 Stereo view along the Z-axis of an α-carbon
model of the hybrid form of mitochondrial AAT with one
"open" (below) and one "closed" subunit. The coenzymes
and the small domains are emphasized by heavy dark
lines. For further information see text.

ponding to an eclipsed conformation of the bonds C5-C4
and C5'-O5' (bridging oxygen closest to C4').
    Recent electron density maps of the orthorhombic crys-
tal form at 2.3 Å resolution after partial crystallographic refinement confirm the mechanism of Kirsch et al.
(8). Figure 3 shows models of the internal aldimine
with maleate and of the external aldimine with 2-methyl-
aspartate in their densities. In the middle of the
Figure both models are combined. The 30° difference in
tilt and the hydrogen bond of pyridine N1 to Asp 222 in
both structures are evident.

117

Relevance of domain movement to catalysis.
Figure 4 is an α-carbon model of a hybrid structure
with one "open" subunit as in the unliganded PLP-enzyme
and one "closed" subunit, as in the liganded enzyme
forms observed in the orthorhombic crystals. As menti-
ioned above, the PPL-Asp derivative is forced into such
a hybrid structure, due to a different environment of
the two subunits in the Pl crystals. Comparison of the
two structures revealed that the conformational change
of the small domain can be described to a good approximation as a 13° rotation towards the active site around
an axis through Gly 325 $C\alpha$, parallel to Z. It encloses
the inhibitor in the active site and brings the small
domain into van der Waals contact with the adjacent subunit. Additional structural rearrangements occur in
the regions 12 to 17 and 37 to 47.

Although the function of this conformational change
is qualitatively understood, it is not clear how much
it contributes to catalysis. Experiments with micro-
crystals of the triclinic form (14) demonstrated an
overall activity of 10% of the soluble enzyme, with one
subunit transaminating five times faster than the
other. While an assignment of the "fast" and the
"slow" subunit to one of the two crystallographically
distinct subunits in the crystal has not been possible,
this result does not seem to be compatible with a gain
of much more than one order of magnitude in catalytic
efficiency due to the domain reorientation. Clearly,
the role of this conformational change has to be
studied further. Crystallographic studies and amino
acid sequence determinations of related aminotransferases, which likewise utilize the substrate pair glu-
tamate/2-oxoglutarate might shed more light on this
matter.

This work is part of a collaborative project on mitochondrial AAT structure and function with P. Christen
and colleagues, University of Zürich, Switzerland. Support by the Swiss National Science Foundation (Grant
3.224-0.82) is gratefully acknowledged.

118

References

1. Braunstein, A.E. (1973). Amino group transfer. In: The enzymes, 3rd edit., vol. 9, P.D. Boyer (ed.). Academic Press, New York, pp. 379-481.
2. Borisov, V.V., Borisova, S.N., Sosfenov, N.I. and Vainshtein, B.K. (1980). Electron density map of chicken heart cytosol aspartate transaminase at 3.5 Å resolution. Nature (London) 284, 189-190.
3. Harutyunyan, E.G., Malashkevich, V.N., Kochkina, V.M. and Torchinsky, Yu.M. (1984). Conformational changes in chicken heart cytosolic aspartate aminotransferase as revealed by X-ray crystallography. In: Chemical and Biological Aspects of Vitamin B6 Catalysis: Part B, A.E. Evangelopoulos (ed). Alan R. Liss, New York, pp. 205-212.
4. Arnone, A., Briley, P.D., Rogers, P.H., Hyde, C.C., Metzler, C.M. and Metzler, D.E. (1982). Changes in the tertiary structure of cytosolic aspartate aminotransferase induced by the binding of inhibitors and substrates. In: Molecular Structure and Biological Activity, J.F. Griffen and W.L. Duax (eds). Elsevier/North-Holland Inc., New York, pp. 57-74.
5. Eichele, G., Ford, G.C., Glor, M., Jansonius, J.N., Mavrides, C. and Christen, P. (1979). The three-dimensional structure of mitochondrial aspartate aminotransferase at 4.5 Å resolution. J.Mol. Biol. 133, 161-180.
6. Ford, G.C., Eichele, G. and Jansonius, J.N. (1980). Three-dimensional structure of a pyridoxal-phosphate-dependent enzyme, mitochondrial aspartate aminotransferase. Proc.Nat.Acad.Sci., USA 77, 2559-2563.
7. Eichele, G., Karabelnik, D., Halonbrenner, R., Jansonius, J.N. and Christen, P. (1978). Catalytic activity in crystals of mitochondrial aspartate aminotransferase as detected by microspectrophotometry. J.Biol.Chem. 253, 5239-5242.

8. Kirsch, J.F., Eichele, G., Ford, G.C., Vincent, M.G., Jansonius, J.N., Gehring, H. and Christen, P. (1984). Mechanism of action of aspartate aminotransferase proposed on the basis of its spatial structure. J.Mol.Biol. 174, 497-525.

9. Eichele, G. (1980) Three-dimensional structure of mitochondrial aspartate aminotransferase from chicken heart at 2.8 Å resolution. Doctoral thesis, University of Basel.

10. Ivanov, V.I. and Karpeisky, M.Ya. (1969). Dynamic three-dimensional model for enzymic transamination. Advan.Enzymol. 32, 21-53.

11. Dunathan, H.C. (1971). Stereochemical aspects of pyridoxal phosphate catalysis. Advan.Enzymol. 35, 79-134.

12. Arnone, A., Rogers, P.H., Hyde, C.C., Makinen, M.W., Feldhaus, R., Metzler, C.M. and Metzler, D.E. (1984) Crystallographic and chemical studies on cytosolic aspartate aminotransferase. In: Chemical and Biological Aspects of Vitamin B6 Catalysis: Part B, A.E. Evangelopoulos (ed). Alan R. Liss, New York, pp. 171-193.

13. Tumanyan, V.G., Mamaeva, O.K., Bocharov, A.L., Ivanov, V.I., Karpeisky, M.Y. and Yakovlev, G.I. (1974). On the conformation of pyridoxal phosphate imine in solution and in aspartate-aminotransferase active site. Eur.J.Biochem. 50, 119-127.

14. Kirsten, H., Gehring, H. and Christen, P. (1983). Crystalline aspartate aminotransferase: Lattice-induced functional asymmetry of the two subunits. Proc.Nat.Acad.Sci.,USA 80, 1807-1810.

STRUCTURAL FEATURES AND INHIBITORY PROPERTIES OF CYSTATHIONINE-β-SYNTHASE FROM BAKER'S YEAST

I. WILLHARDT, P. HERMANN, E.A. TOLOSA[+],
E.V. GORYACHENKOVA[+]
Institute of Physiological Chemistry, University of Halle, GDR, [+]Institute of Molecular Biology, Acad.Sci. USSR, Moscow, USSR

Baker's yeast contains an pyridoxal phosphate dependent enzyme activity which was originally designated as "serine sulfhydrase" for its ability to catalyze the synthesis of L-cysteine directly from L-serine and hydrogen sulfide (1).
More detailed studies on the specificity of the purified enzyme in our laboratory showed that with L-serine or L-cysteine as the substrates β-substitution reactions were cataly-

Table 1   Specificity of cystathionine-β-synthase from baker's yeast

$$\begin{array}{l} \text{L- H-Ser-OH} \\ \text{L- H-Cys-OH} \end{array} + RSH \longrightarrow \text{L- H-Cys-OH} + \begin{array}{l} H_2O \\ H_2S \end{array}$$

with R substituent on Cys:

RSH	Product	Name
H_2S	CH_2-SH ; $H_2N-CH-CO_2H$	L-cysteine
Alkyl-SH	$CH_2-S-Alkyl$; $H_2N-CH-CO_2H$	S-alkyl-L-cysteine
$HO-CH_2-CH_2-SH$	$CH_2-S-CH_2-CH_2-OH$; $H_2N-CH-CO_2H$	S-hydroxyethyl-L-cysteine
$H_2N-CH_2-CH_2-SH$	$CH_2-S-CH_2-CH_2-NH_2$; $H_2N-CH-CO_2H$	L-thialysine
$Acyl-HN-CH_2-CH_2-SH$	$CH_2-S-CH_2-CH_2-NH-Acyl$; $H_2N-CH-CO_2H$	$^\varepsilon$N-acyl-L-thialysine
$HO_2C-CH_2-CH_2-SH$	$CH_2-S-CH_2-CH_2-CO_2H$; $H_2N-CH-CO_2H$	S-carboxyethyl-L-cysteine
$HO_2C-CH-CH_2-CH_2-SH$; NH_2	$CH_2-S-CH_2-CH_2-CH-CO_2H$; $H_2N-CH-CO_2H$; NH_2	L-cystathionine

Proceedings of the 16th FEBS Congress
Part A, pp. 121–126
© 1985 VNU Science Press

zed with a group of alkyl thiols (or H_2S) which act as cosubstrates producing S-alkylated L-cysteine derivatives (2)(Table 1). The most effective enzyme-catalyzed reaction was the formation of cystathionine from L-serine and L-homocysteine as the cosubstrate. In accord with this specificity this enzyme activity should be named "cystathionine-β-synthase" (EC 4.2.1.22). Its rather broad cosubstrate specificity is likewise found in some other pyridoxal phosphate dependent lyases (3). The immobilized enzyme was used in the synthesis of labelled S-alkylated cysteine derivatives (e.g. thialysine, cystathionine)(4).

This paper describes some structural peculiarities of the yeast enzyme, studies on mechanism, participation of amino acid residues in the catalytic step and differention from other enzymes by the use of kinetic and inhibition experiments.

PURIFICATION AND STRUCTURAL FEATURES

The purification procedure (1) was modified by the use of protease inhibitors during the initial steps and continued by ion exchange chromatography, gel chromatography or hydrophobic chromatography. By PAGE it was revealed that in all cases 2 enzymatically active bands resulted with molecular masses of 71 000 and 66 000 respectively. By activity staining (5) after PAGE it was demonstrated that the enzyme activity in the initial purification steps (ammonium sulfate precipitation) was linked to a protein band with M_r=150 000. Up to now the mechanism of this change in the molecular masses is not clear. Both "subunits" behave similar due to kinetic constants, IP (4,6-4,7), specificity, pH-optimum (8-9) and the N-terminal His. Amino acid analysis is in agreement with M_r-determination by gelfiltration and PAGE and gave indication of different primary structure. This is also demonstrated by different immunological behavior of the "subunits".

EFFECT OF GROUP SPECIFIC REAGENTS, COENZYME SPECIFIC REAGENTS, COSUBSTRATE- AND SUBSTRATE ANALOGS

The following experiments were performed with the mixture of the "subunits". The SH blocker iodoacetamide, N-ethylmaleimide and p-chloromercuribenzoate were without influence on the enzyme activity, that means the about 12 cysteine residues per unit determined by the DTNB method do not participate in the catalytic reaction.

Modification of 4-5 tryptophan residues per unit by N-bromsuccinimide inactivats the enzyme completely. The influence of histidine and arginine is not clear from modification experiments. The results from inhibition studies are shown in table 2.

The cofactor blocking reagent hydroxylamine was used for the preparation of the enzymatic inactive apoenzyme which could be reconstituted by the addition of PLP. The dissoziation constant of the apoenzyme-PLP-complex was determined in this way and found to be 1,6 μmol/l.

The nucleophilic cosubstrate analogs CN$^-$ and SCN$^-$ behave competitive with respect to the thiol cosubstrate but do not participate in the reaction of cystathionine-β-synthase. Otherwise they are cosubstrates in the analogous β-replacement reaction catalyzed by cyanoalanine synthase (EC 4.4.1.9)(3).

In the group of the substrate analogs tested only β-chloroalanine is of importance. Its competitive mode of action is due to its substrate

Table 2   Inhibitors of cystathionine-β-synthase

Substance	K_i(mmol/l)	Type of inhibition
PLP-specific reagents:		
hydroxylamine	0,18	blocking of the cofactor
semicarbazide	5,7	
aminooxyacetic acid	0,006	
cosubstrate analogs:		
KCN	14,5	competitive
KSCN	20,6	competitive
substrate analogs:		
L-alanine	17,8	competitive
L-serine	3,5	competitive
L-threonine	4,8	competitive
L-allo-threonine	5,3	competitive
L-cysteic acid	4,3	competitive
L-methionine	13,5	competitive
L-chloroalanine	0,56	competitive

character in this reaction. The K_m-value in
the reaction of L-chloroalanine with NaHS is
in the order of serine as the substrate.

The ineffectiveness of cycloserine is in accord with the proposed mechanism which does
not imply a pyridoxamine-phosphate-ketimine
intermediate (3).

For the yeast enzyme was established earlier
(6) that the reaction proceeds via a ternary
enzyme-substrate-cosubstrate-complex according
to a Random Bi-Sequential Bi-mechanism. The
same kinetic mechanism was found for β-cyano-
alanine synthase by Tolosa et al. (7). Recently was observed for rat-liver cystathionine-β-
synthase (8) also a sequential mechanism.

This mechanism seems to be typical for the

exclusively β replacement reactions in contrast to the Ping-Pong mechanism for replacement reaction by α,β elimination-addition
steps as in the case with O-acetylserine sulfhydrase (9). Kinetic constants, pH-optimum and
mechanism differenciate cystathionine-β-synthase (EC 4.2.1.22) from O-acetylserine sulfhydrase (EC 4.1.99.8) in baker's yeast.

The proposed mechanism according Braunsteins
concept (3) is: The replacement of the β substituent proceeds via formation of an amino
acid-pyridoxal-phosphate aldimine to a ternary
complex whereby α-hydrogen exchange occurs
without formation of a ketimine and an α-amino-
acrylate intermediate (Fig. 1).

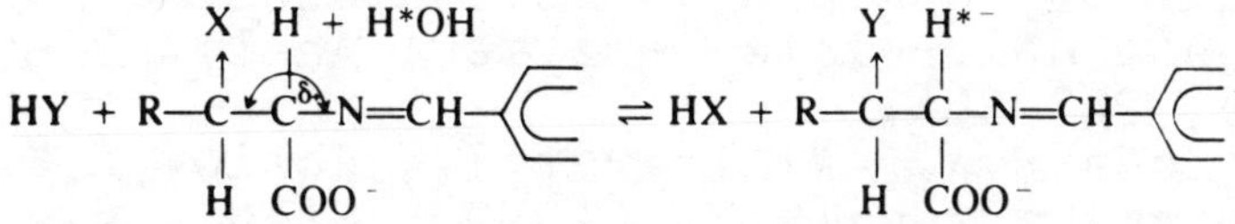

Fig. 1   Equation of the β-replacement
         reaction (3)

New results about the stereochemical course
of the replacement reaction, which demonstrate
a retention of configuration at the β-carbon
atom of the substrate were reported for cystathionine-β-synthase from rat liver (8).

Reference list

(1) Schlossmann,K., Lynen,F. (1957). Biosynthe-
    se des Cysteins aus Serin und Schwefelwas-
    serstoff. Biochem.Z. 328, 591-564.
(2) Willhardt,I., Hermann,P. (1974). Charakte-
    risierung der Cystathionin-β-synthase aus
    Hefe. 9.Ann.Meeting Biochem.Soc. GDR,
    (Dresden) Abstracts.
(3) Braunstein,A.E., Goryachenkova,E.V. (1984).
    The β-replacement-specific pyridoxal-P-de-
    pendent lyases. Adv.Enzymol.Relat.Areas
    Mol.Biol. 56, 1-98.
(4) Hermann,P., Willhardt,I. (1974). Verfahren
    zur Gewinnung von schwefelhaltigen radio-
    aktiv oder stabilisotop markierten Amino-
    säuren. DD WP 104293 Int.Cl.C 07 C 149/24.
(5) Willhardt,I., Wiederanders,B. (1975).
    Activity staining of cystathionine-β-syn-
    thase and related enzymes. Analyt.Biochem.
    63, 263-266.
(6) Tolosa,E.A., Willhardt,I., Kozlov,L.V.,
    Goryachenkova,E.V. (1979). Steady state
    kinetics of reactions catalyzed by serine
    sulfhydrase of Saccharomyces cerevisiae.
    Biokhimiya (USSR) 44, 453-459.
(7) Tolosa,E.A., Kozlov, L.V., Rabinkov,A.G.,
    Goryachenkova,E.V. (1978). Kinetics of
    β-cyanoalanine synthase reactions. Bioor-
    ganich.Khimiya (USSR) 4, 1334-1340.
(8) Borcsok,E., Abeles,R.H. (1982). Mechanism
    of action of cystathionine synthase. Arch.
    Biochem.Biophys. 213, 695-707.
(9) Cook,P.F., Wedding,R.T. (1976). A reaction
    mechanism from steady state kinetic stu-
    dies for O-acetylserine sulfhydrase from
    Salmonella typhimurium. J.Biol.Chem. 251,
    2023-2029.

REGULATION OF METABOLISM

POLYPHOSPHOINOSITIDE FORMATION: A POSSIBLE MECHANISM FOR THE MODULATION OF THE Ca^{2+} MESSENGER SYSTEM BY CYCLIC AMP

A.FARAGÓ, A.ENYEDI[+], B.SARKADI[+], G.FARKAS, and G.GÁRDOS[+]

1st Institute of Biochemistry, Semmelweis University Medical School, 1088 Budapest, and [+]National Institute of Haematology and Blood Transfusion, 1113 Budapest, Hungary

The cAMP and Ca^{2+} messenger systems are strongly interrelated. The ability of cAMP to influence the concentration of Ca^{2+} in the cytoplasm of cells is an important factor in this interrelation. However, the exact mechanism by which cAMP modulates the cytoplasmic Ca^{2+} concentration is not known. We have observed that the cAMP-dependent protein kinase participates in the regulation of phosphatidylinositol metabolism in the plasma membrane of the cells and we think that this effect of the protein kinase may play a significant role in the modulation of the Ca^{2+} messenger system.

Recently it is generally accepted that in those signal systems where Ca^{2+} serves as an intracellular mediator one of the first effects of the ligand-receptor complex is the stimulation of the breakdown of polyphosphoinositides. The hydrolysis of phosphatidylinositol-4,5-bisphosphate produces inositol triphosphate which has been suggested to act as a second messenger of Ca^{2+} mobilisation from internal stores. On the other hand the breakdown of both phosphatidylinositol bisphosphate and phosphatidylinositol monophosphate results in the formation of diacylglycerol which activates protein kinase C, an

Proceedings of the 16th FEBS Congress
Part A, pp. 129–137
© 1985 VNU Science Press

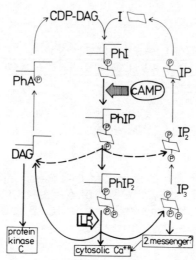

Fig.1. The site of the effect of the cAMP-de-
        pendent protein kinase on the polyphos-
        phoinositide metabolism

enzyme which is independent from the Ca^{2+} mediator system but may act in the same direction.
The hydrolysis of polyphosphoinositides is
followed by the resynthesis of these compounds.
However, the transient decrease in the amount
of polyphosphoinositides in the plasma membrane
may also have some role in the elevation of the
cytoplasmic calcium level.

While the breakdown of polyphosphoinositides
is involved in the signal transduction of the
Ca^{2+} messenger system, according to our observations (1,2) the cAMP-dependent protein kinase
stimulates the formation of polyphosphoinositides. In the present report we demonstrate
that the dissociated catalytic subunit of the
cAMP-dependent protein kinase stimulates the
phosphorylation of phosphatidylinositol to
phosphatidylinositol-4-phosphate in the isolated
plasma membranes of different cell types.

Our first observations derived from the investigation of the phosphorylation of the plasma
membranes isolated from human blood lymphocytes.

130

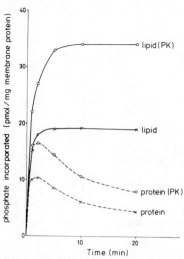

Fig.2. The phosphorylation of the plasma mem-
        brane of lymphocytes

The plasma membrane preparation was incubated
with $[\gamma-^{32}P]$ ATP in the presence or absence of
the dissociated catalytic subunit of the cAMP-
dependent protein kinase, and the amounts of
phosphate incorporated into the protein and
lipid fractions of the membrane were measured.
The catalytic subunit increased the amount of
phosphate incorporated into both the protein
and lipid fractions.

Similar results were obtained when the phosphorylation of the cell membranes of other cell
types was investigated. The catalytic subunit
increased the ^{32}P-incorporation into the protein
and lipid fractions of plasma membranes obtained
from human erythrocytes, thrombocytes and pig
granulocytes, as well. The heat stable inhibitor
protein of the cAMP-dependent protein kinase
abolished the stimulating effect of the protein
kinase in each case. The stimulating effect of
the cAMP-dependent protein kinase on the phosphorylation of certain membrane lipids seems to
be a general phenomenon in the different cell
types.

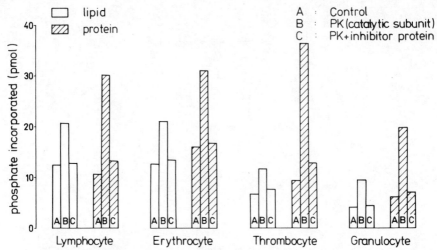

Fig.3. The effect of the protein kinase on the
plasma membranes of different cells

The ^{32}P-labelled membrane lipids were analysed
by thin layer chromatography. This chromatography was carried out in a system which separated the polyphosphoinositides from the other
phospholipids of the membrane /including phos-
phatidylinositol/, but in this system the phos-
phatidylinositol-4-phosphate and the phosphat-
idylinositol-4,5-bisphosphate were not separated from each other. In this thin layer chromatographic system we could demonstrate that the
cAMP-dependent protein kinase stimulated the ^{32}P
incorporation exclusively into the polyphosphoinositides of the membrane. In some membrane
preparations the traces of ^{32}P were found in
phosphatidic acid, but the cAMP-dependent protein
kinase had no effect on the ^{32}P-labbeling of
phosphatidic acid. Under the circumstances of
our experiments ^{32}P-phosphate was not incorporated into the other lipids of the membrane.
The ^{32}P-labelled lipids of the plasma membrane
of granulocytes were further investigated in a
high performance thin layer chromatographic
system. This system separated the two poly-

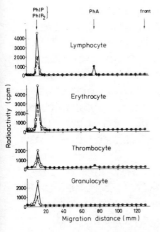

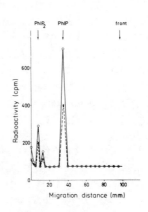

Fig.4. The analysis of the ^{32}P-labelled membrane-lipids in a TLC system

Fig.5. The analysis of the ^{32}P-labelled membrane-lipids of granulocytes in a HP-TLC system

phosphoinositides and we found that the protein kinase stimulated the incorporation of ^{32}P-phosphate into both polyphosphoinositides. This result shows that the cAMP-dependent protein kinase stimulates the phosphorylation of phosphatidylinositol to phosphatidylinositol-4-phosphate. The increased labelling of phosphatidylinositol bisphosphate may be the result of the increased formation of the ^{32}P-labelled substrate of that reaction which produces phosphatidylinositol bisphosphate. The small radioactivity in the position of an unidentified compound may correspond to a lyso-derivative of the ^{32}P-labelled phosphatidylinositol-4-phosphate.

This result was obtained with the membranes of a granulocyte population containing 90 per cent neutrophil granulocytes. It is known that the signals for the biological activation of neutrophils are mediated by the Ca^{2+} messenger system and the effects of these signals are antag-

133

onized by the elevation of the intracellular cAMP concentration, presumably because in neutrophils cAMP decreases the cytoplasmic Ca^{2+} concentration. The signal transduction of the Ca^{2+} messenger system in neutrophils is accompanied by the breakdown of polyphosphoinositides. It is conceivable that the stimulated formation of polyphosphoinositides is related to the ability of cAMP to decrease the cytoplasmic calcium level.

In our further work we tried to get some information about that target protein of the cAMP-dependent protein kinase which was responsible for the regulation of the phosphorylation of phosphatidylinositol. Since the stimulation of polyphosphoinositide formation by the protein kinase was a common property of membranes from different cell types, a protein which was phosphorylated by the protein kinase and which was responsible for the stimulated phosphorylation of phophatidylinositol was present in each membrane. The ^{32}P-labelled proteins of the membranes phosphorylated in the absence and presence of the catalytic subunit were analysed by SDS gelelectrophoresis. The phosphorylation of the erythrocyte membrane has been extensively studied by other investigators and it is known that spectrin and the protein fraction named band three are phosphorylated by the cAMP-dependent protein kinase. Beside these proteins we found only a 24 kD protein phosphorylated by the protein kinase. This was the single protein substrate of the protein kinase which was found in each membrane, hence we suppose that it may be that protein which is responsible for the stimulated formation of polyphosphoinositides.

In the plasma membrane of thrombocytes a 22 or 24 kD protein phosphorylated by the cAMP-dependent protein kinase has also been extensively studied by other investigators. It has been considered to be involved in the regulation

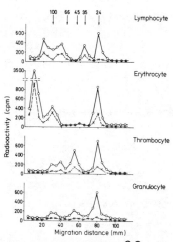

Fig.6. The analysis of the ^{32}P-labelled membrane
        proteins by SDS gel-electrophoresis

of the cytoplasmic calcium level and it has been
suggested to be similar to phospholamban. Phospholamban is the 22 or 24 kD protein substrate
of the cAMP-dependent protein kinase and a Ca^{2+}
+ calmodulin-dependent protein kinase in the
sarcoplasmic reticulum of heart and it is well
known that phospholamban plays an important role
in the regulation of the activity of the Ca^{2+}
pump of the heart sarcoplasmic reticulum. The
possible similarity between the functions of
phospholamban and the 24 kD phosphoprotein of
the thrombocyte plasma membrane led us to the
idea to investigate the regulation of polyphosphoinositide formation in the sarcoplasmic reticulum of heart. Here we present the results of
the high performance thin layer chromatography
of the ^{32}P-labelled lipids extracted from the
isolated sarcoplasmic reticulum membrane of rabbit heart which was phosphorylated by the cAMP-
dependent protein kinase or by a Ca^{2+} + calmodulin-dependent endogenous protein kinase.
    The chromatographic pattern shows that in the
presence of either the catalytic subunit of the

135

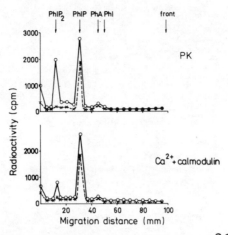

Fig.7. The HP-TLC analysis ot the ^{32}P-labelled lipids of the heart sarcoplasmic reticulum membrane

cAMP-dependent protein kinase or Ca^{2+} + calmodulin the phosphorylation of phosphatidylinositol to phosphatidylinositol-4-phosphate was stimulated and the formation of phosphatidylinositol-4,5-bisphosphate was also significantly increased. This effect coincided with the phosphorylation of phospholamban. Since cAMP and calcium + calmodulin are known to stimulate the activity of the sarcoplasmic reticulum to sequester Ca^{2+} our finding is consistant with the hypothesis that the stimulation of polyphosphoinositide formation may be related to the ability of cAMP to decrease the cytoplasmic Ca^{2+} level in different cell types.

REFERENCES

1. Sarkadi, B., Enyedi, A., Faragó, A., Mészáros, G., Kremmer, T. and Gárdos, G. /1983/ Cyclic AMP-dependent protein kinase stimulates the formation of polyphosphoinositides in the

plasma membranes of lymphocytes. FEBS Lett. 152, 195-198

2. Enyedi, Á., Faragó, A., Sarkadi, B., Szász, I. and Gárdos, G. /1983/ Cyclic AMP-dependent protein kinase stimulates the formation of polyphosphoinositides in the plasma membranes of different blood cells. FEBS Lett. 161, 158-162

TEMPORAL ORGANIZATION OF THE FRUCTOSE 6-PHOSPHATE/FRUCTOSE 1,6-BISPHOSPHATE CYCLE

EBERHARD HOFMANN, WOLFGANG SCHELLENBERGER AND KLAUS ESCHRICH
Institute of Physiological Chemistry, Karl-Marx-University, 7010 Leipzig, Liebigstrasse 16, GDR

The phosphofructokinase (PFK)/fructose 1,6-bisphosphatase (FBPase) cycle is of significance to the regulation of the carbohydrate metabolism. When the two enzymes are simultaneously active the capability of ATP homeostasis is reduced and the net flow through glycolysis and gluconeogenesis is decreased (1-3). For an efficient glycolytic regime it is necessary to suppress the activity of FBPase whereas for efficient gluconeogenesis a high ratio of the activities of FBPase to PFK must be attained (2). PFK and FBPase are controlled both by allosteric and epigenetic mechanisms (3).

Recently, the dynamic behaviour of a reconstituted open enzyme system containing PFK and FBPase has been investigated (4). In this system in addition to unique and stable stationary states multiple stationary states and sustained oscillations were found to occur. Oscillations and multiple stationary states were caused mainly by the reciprocal kinetic effects of AMP on PFK and FBPase.

This contribution will deal with the rate of futile substrate cycling in the stationary states and the effects of fructose 2,6-bisphosphate ($Fru(2,6)P_2$) on the stability and the metabolic efficiency of the stationary states. $Fru(2,6)P_2$ was found to be the most potent activator of PFK and to act as an inhibitor of FBPase (5).

MATERIALS AND METHODS

The experimental conditions, the purification and the properties of the individual enzymes, the experimental approach, and the mathematical modelling are described in (4,6).

Proceedings of the 16th FEBS Congress
Part A, pp. 139–146
© 1985 VNU Science Press

RESULTS AND DISCUSSION

The reaction network

The cooperation of the enzymes in the reaction chamber is shown in Fig. 1.

Fig. 1. Reaction scheme of the enzyme system.

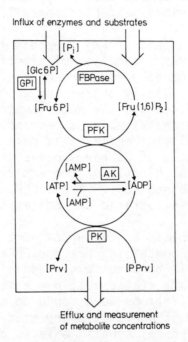

Influx of enzymes and substrates

Efflux and measurement
of metabolite concentrations

In addition to PFK and FBPase the system contains pyruvate kinase (PK), adenylate kinase (AK), and glucose 6-phosphate isomerase (GPI). The influx concentrations of the substrates ($[ATP]_{IN}$, $[PPrv]_{IN}$, $[Fru(1,6)P_2]_{IN}$, $[Fru(2,6)P_2]_{IN}$), the rate of flow through the reaction chamber (τ), and the concentrations of the enzymes (V_{PFK}, V_{FBPase}, V_{PK}) are adjusted experimentally, while the metabolite concentrations in the reactor result from the enzymatic conversions and the flow processes.

Functional states of the Fru6P/Fru(1,6)P$_2$ cycle in the absence of Fru(2,6)P$_2$

Fig. 2 shows a parameter plane formed by the maximum activities of PFK and FBPase as well as from the influx concentrations of Fru6P and Fru(1,6)P$_2$. For calculation the sum of the influx concentrations of the hexosephosphates and the sum of V_{PFP} and V_{FBPase} were held constant.

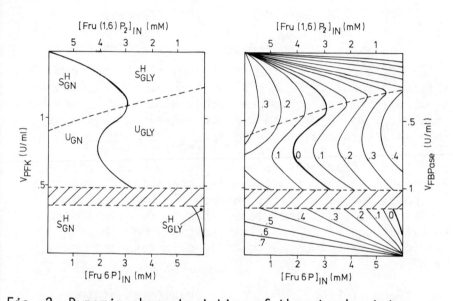

Fig. 2. Dynamic characteristics of the steady states (absence of Fru(2,6)P$_2$)
$[ATP]_{IN}$ = 3 mM, $[PPrv]_{IN}$ = 9 mM, τ = 40 min, V_{PK} = 7.5 U/ml, $[Fru6P]_{IN}$ + $(Fru(1,6)P_2]_{IN}$ = 6 mM; V_{PFK} + V_{FBPase} = 1.5 U/ml.
A. Character of the stationary states (for explanation see the text). S and U designate actually the stable and unstable states, GLY means glycolytic and GN gluconeogenic states. With H high energy and with L low energy steady states are denoted.
B. Contour plot indicating the efficiency of the stationary states.

In the small hatched band alternate steady states occur, while outside of this region unique states exist. By the solid curve glycolytic ($v_{PFK} > v_{FBPase}$) and gluconeogenic ($v_{PFK} < v_{FBPase}$) states are separated. The dashed curves limit a domain of unstable steady states which correlate to the appearance of sustained oscillations (4).

For characterizing the rate of substrate cycling the efficiency of the stationary states is defined according to eq. (1):

$$\eta = \begin{cases} (v_{PFK} - v_{FBPase})/v_{PFK} & \text{if } v_{PFK} > v_{FBPase} \\ (v_{FBPase} - v_{PFK})/v_{FBPase} & \text{if } v_{PFK} < v_{FBPase} \end{cases} \tag{1}$$

The efficiencies of the stationary states in the absence of $Fru(2,6)P_2$ are shown in Fig. 2B. Efficient glycolytic states arise preferably at high V_{PFK} and high $[Fru6P]_{IN}$, while efficient gluconeogenic states come into appearance only at high V_{FBPase} and high $[Fru(1,6)P_2]_{IN}$. A high ratio in the activities of PFK and FBPase has to be applied to obtain efficient glycolytic states of high energy character. This indicates incompatibility between ATP homeostasis and efficiciency of either state. This is related to the fact that the $Fru6P/Fru(1,6)P_2$ cycle under these particular experimental conditions is regulated mainly by AMP.

The effect of $Fru(2,6)P_2$ on the properties of the stationary states

As already pointed out the dynamic structures as described in the previous section are mainly caused by the reciprocal kinetic effects of AMP on the activities of the two cycle enzymes. It is now well established (5) that PFK and FBPase are oppositely influenced and very efficiently controlled by $Fru(2,6)P_2$.

Yeast PFK is strongly activated by this effector. It increases both the apparent affinity of the enzyme to Fru6P and its maximum activity (7). $Fru(2,6)P_2$ is capable of increasing the AMP sensitivity of the enzyme and its extent of activation by AMP. Similarly, the half

142

activation constant of yeast PFK for Fru(2,6)P$_2$ is significantly decreased by AMP (8). FBPase at low substrate level is strongly inhibited by Fru(2,6)P$_2$ (9,10). Because of the interactions of AMP and Fru(2,6)P$_2$ with PFK and FBPase a rather complex dynamic pattern in the Fru6P/Fru(1,6)P$_2'$ cycle may arise when both effectors are present.

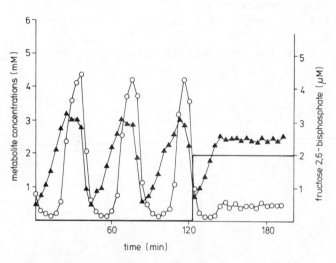

Fig. 3. The effect of Fru(2,6)P$_2$ on a state exerting sustained oscillations.
[Fru6P]$_{IN}$ = [Fru(1,6)P$_2$]$_{IN}$ = 3 mM, V$_{PFK}$ = V$_{FBPase}$ = 0.75 U/ml. The other parameters are as in Fig. 2.
▲ : [ATP], ○ :([Fru6P]+[Glc6P]).

In Fig. 3 an experiment is shown in which the parameters fit to the centre of the parameter plane demonstrated in Fig. 2. At first Fru(2,6)P$_2$ is absent. According to the instability of the respective steady state sustained oscillations emerge. After 120 min Fru(2,6)P$_2$ was added and a constant concentration (2 µM) of this metabolite in the second phase of the experiment maintained. After addition of Fru(2,6)P$_2$ the

oscillations are rapidly extinguished and a stable
steady state with low ATP (S_{GLY}^L) is approached.
    In the experiment shown in Fig. 4 initial conditions
were used which correspond to the region of stable
gluconeogenic states according to Fig. 2. As
demonstrated, in the first phase of the experiment
($[Fru(2,6)P_2] = 0$) a stable gluconeogenic state
(S_{GN}) was approached. Then the concentration of the
Fru(2,6)P_2 was stepwise increased. When the
concentration of this effector is 0.3 µM the states
become unstable and sustained oscillations emerge. At
increasing concentration of this effector the
oscillation frequency is enhanced and the amplitude
decreased. At a critical level of Fru(2,6)P_2 the
metabolites evolve to a stable glycolytic state (S_{GLY}^L).

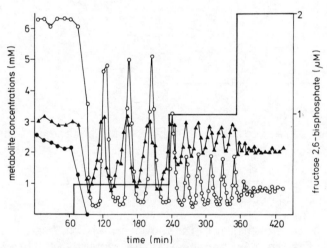

Fig. 4. The effect of Fru(2,6)P_2 on a stationary state.
$[Fru6P]_{IN}$ = 5 mM, $[Fru(1,6)P_2]_{IN}$ = 1 mM, V_{PFK} = 0.3
U/ml, V_{FBPase} = 1.2 U/ml. The other parameters are as in
Fig.2.
▲: [ATP], O ([Fru6P]+[Glc6P]),●: [PPrv].

144

These experiments show that depending on the initial conditions Fru(2,6)P$_2$ is capable of either generating or of extinguishing oscillations. In general, due to the stimulation of PFK by Fru(2,6)P$_2$ glycolytic states are favoured.

Influence of Fru(2,6)P$_2$ on the functional states of the Fru6P/Fru(1,6)P$_2$ cycle

In this paragraph the consequences of the addition of Fru(2,6)P$_2$ are discussed under the condition of a linear relation between the influx rate of Fru6P and the level of Fru(2,6)P$_2$ in the reaction chamber. This is a first attempt to analyse the rather complex kinetic effects of Fru(2,6)P$_2$. The conditions resemble the physiological situation insofar as the intracellular level of Fru(2,6)P$_2$ is correlated to the supply of glucose.

It is shown in Fig. 5 that Fru(2,6)P$_2$ reduces the

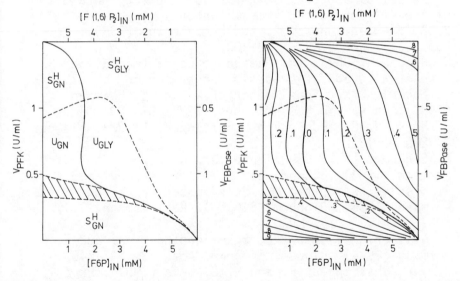

Fig. 5. The dynamic characteristics of the steady states in the presence of Fru(2,6)P$_2$.
The control parameters and the construction of the plane are as in Fig. 2. Fru(2,6)P$_2$ was added in a predetermined proportion to F6P: $[Fru(2,6)P_2]_{IN} = 0.33 \cdot 10^{-4} [Fru6P]_{IN}$.

parameter region in which oscillations arise, whereas the domain is expanded in which glycolytic states are occurring. A comparison of Figures 2 and 5 shows, that $Fru(2,6)P_2$ augments the efficiency of the glycolytic states. However, as in the system without $Fru(2,6)P_2$, efficient states come into being only when the supply of the substrates as well as the maximum activities of the enzymes correspond with either the glycolytic or the gluconeogenic mode. Hence, transitions between efficient glycolytic and gluconeogenic states can only be attained by simultaneous changes of both the enzyme concentration as well as the substrate supply.

To get a deeper insight into the regulation of the $Fru6P/Fru(1,6)P_2$ cycle the enzyme which forms and degrades $Fru(2,6)P_2$ (PFK-2/FBPase-2)(11) should be integrated into the reaction network.

REFERENCES

1. Reich, J. and E.E. Selkov (1981). Energy Metabolism of the Cell. Academic Press, London.
2. Boiteux, A., Hess, B. and E.E. Selkov (1980). Curr. Top. Cell. Regul. 17, 171-203.
3. Hue, L. (1982). In: Metabolic Compartmentation, H. Sies et al. (eds.). Academic Press, London, pp. 71-97.
4. Eschrich, K., Schellenberger,W. and E. Hofmann (1983). Arch. Biochem. Biophys. 222, 657-660.
5. Hers, H.-G. and E. Van Schaftingen, (1982). Biochem. J. 206, 1-12.
6. Schubert, Ch., Schellenberger, W., Eschrich K. and E. Hofmann (1983). Biomed. Biochim. Acta 42, 597-608.
7. Nissler, K., Otto, A., Schellenberger, W. and E. Hofmann (1983). Biochem. Biophys. Res. Commun. 111, 294-300.
8. Nissler, K., Otto, A., Schellenberger, W. and E. Hofmann (1984). Biomed. Biochim. Acta 43, 535-540.
9. Van Schaftingen, E. and H.-G. Hers (1981). Proc. Natl. Acad. Sci. 78, 2861-2863.
10. Mc Grane, M.M., El-Maghrabi, M.R. and S.J. Pilkis (1983). J. Biol. Chem. 258, 10445-10454.
11. Pilkis, S.J., Walderhaug, M., Murray, K., Beth, A., Venkataramu, S.D., Pilkis, J. and M.R. El-Maghrabi (1983). J. Biol. Chem. 258, 6135-6141.

THE ROLE OF PROTEIN-PROTEIN INTERACTIONS IN THE CONTROL OF ENZYME ACTIVITY (GLYCERALDE-HYDE-PHOSPHATE DEHYDROGENASE)

N.K. NAGRADOVA[1]
A.N. Belozersky Laboratory of Molecular Biology and Bioorganic Chemistry, Moscow State University, Moscow 119899, USSR

This paper is devoted to the problem of site-site cooperativity in catalysis and its possible role in the regulation of enzyme activity. We have investigated this problem using as an object glyceraldehyde-phosphate dehydrogenase (GPDH) - a tetrameric enzyme composed of identical subunits which exhibit a marked cooperativity. It will be shown that the behavior of this model enzyme is consistent with the idea that the activity of an individual subunit can be regulated by its interaction with other subunits within the oligomeric enzyme molecule, as well as by specific protein-protein interactions with another, functionally related enzyme.

Using the technique of matrix immobilization we have prepared Sepharose-bound tetra, trimeric, dimeric and monomeric forms of the enzyme (1-4). All enzyme species proved to be catalytically active. These results clearly indicate that subunit interactions in the GPDH molecule are not necessary for catalysis. An isolated subunit of the dehydrogenase is fully catalytically competent.

THE DEMONSTRATION OF SUBUNIT COOPERATIVITY IN CATALYSIS

The catalytic properties of immobilized monomeric and tetrameric enzyme species were

---

[1]This study was carried out in collaboration with Drs L.I. Ashmarina and V.I. Muronetz

Proceedings of the 16th FEBS Congress
Part A, pp. 147-153
© 1985 VNU Science Press

compared in the reverse reaction (1,3,-diphos-
phoglycerate reductive dephosphorylation).
Fig. 1 shows the plot of the reciprocal initial
velocities versus reciprocal substrate concentrations. It is seen that the monomeric species
is nearly twice as active as the tetrameric
one. It seemed important to elucidate if
catalytic cooperativity persists in an isolated

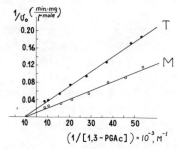

Fig. 1. Reductive dephosphorylation of 1,3-
diphosphoglycerate catalyzed by a monomeric (M)
or tetrameric (T) immobilized enzyme species.
For details see (5).

dimeric species. The results of a comparative
study carried out with different enzyme forms
and summarized in Table 1, show that this
really is the case. Immobilized tetrameric
and dimeric forms have similar specific activities, corresponding to nearly one-half of the
activity of the monomer.

This indicates that interdimeric interactions
are not a prerequisite for the appearance of
cooperativity between the subunits composing
each of the functional dimers. A question
arises: what is the mechanism of the decrease
in the catalytic activity of monomers upon
their association into a dimer or a tetramer?
The experimental data are consistent with the
suggestion that only one-half of the active
centers of the oligomer are functioning simultaneously as a consequence of their alternating
participation in catalysis. This interpretation

Table 1. Specific activity of various enzyme forms in the reverse reaction. The reaction was carried out at 25°C in 100 mM triethanol amine buffer pH 7.5 containing 0.6 mM NADH, 6 mM ATP, 16 mM MgSO$_4$, 16 mM 3-phosphoglycerate. Each sample contained, in addition to the indicated species immobilized phosphoglycerate kinase. Open circles, native GPDH subunits; dotted circles, peroxide-inactivated GPDH subunits.

Enzyme species	Specific activity, μmole / min·mg of the native enzyme
	7.85
	8.0
	17.95
	7.42
	19.7

is supported by the results obtained with a hybrid dimer composed of a peroxide-inactivated and a native monomer. As shown in Table 1, the unmodified subunit within this dimer is twice as active as a native dimer. It appears that the decrease in catalytic activity is a result of interactions between the functioning active centers in the oligomeric enzyme molecule.

We also studied the behavior of a hybrid tetramer containing one peroxide-inactivated subunit. As seen in Table 1, the specific activity of the unmodified subunits in this tetramer was similar to that of a native tetramer. This indicates that subunit interactions in catalysis extend over the two dimeric pairs per tetramer. Otherwise, specific activity of the hybrid tetramer (calculated with respect to the native enzyme) should be markedly higher than those of the native tetrameric or dimeric forms, since it is composed of a native functional dimer and of a dimer possessing one active and one inactive subunit. The latter dimer, if acting independently, exhibits specific activity (calculated with respect to the native enzyme) equal to the activity of a monomeric form of the enzyme.

It seemed reasonable to suggest that some factors capable of specifically changing the enzyme conformation can also influence the character of subunit cooperativity in catalysis. Our interest was focused in this connection on the investigation of a possible effect of specific protein-protein interactions between two functionally linked enzymes. It was decided to study the catalytic properties of GPDH·phosphoglycerate kinase complex in order to find out whether catalytic subunit cooperativity persists in the complex.

THE EFFECT OF PHOSPHOGLYCERATE KINASE ON THE CATALYTIC COOPERATIVITY OF GPDH SUBUNITS

Preparation of GPDH·phosphoglycerate kinase complexes

Immobilized tetrameric or dimeric GPDH species (40-160 µg/ml gel) was incubated in 50 mM sodium phosphate pH 8.0, 1 mM EDTA, 0.5 mM glyceraldehyde-3-phosphate, 1.2 mM NAD^+ in the presence of soluble PGK taken in a 32-fold excess with respect to GPDH protein content. After 20 min incubation under gentle stirring the gel was washed with 50 mM sodium phosphate pH 8.0. The protein content of the complex was determined. Three kinase molecules were bound per tetramer of GPDH and one per a dimer. The monomeric species of the dehydrogenase formed no complex. We suppose that the matrix-bound subunit is incapable of binding PGK, and hence - the structure of the complexes

can be schematically represented as shown
on Fig. 2.

The catalytic properties of GPDH in complex with PGK

The activity of GPDH bound in a complex with
PGK was measured in a reaction mixture containing the substrates of PGK (3-phosphoglycerate,
ATP), as well as NADH, and followed by the
disappearance of NADH (see Table 1 for details).
Fig. 2 shows that the binding of PGK markedly
affects the catalytic properties of GPDH. In
fact, the specific activities of the hybrid
tetrameric and dimeric enzyme forms become

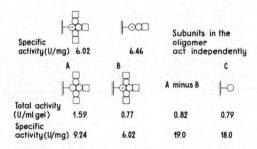

Fig.2. The catalytic activity of GPDH subunits
in the complex with PGK. Specific activities
are calculated with respect to the unmodified
protein. See text for details. Open circles,
native GPDH subunits, dotted circles, peroxide-
inactivated GPDH subunits, squares, PGK molecules.

nearly equal in complexes with PGK in sharp
contrast with the results obtained with similar
species free of PGK. As was discussed above
(see Table 1), in the latter case the unmodified
subunits within the tetramer had about one-half
of the activity of the unmodified monomer
within the dimer probably due to subunit cooperativity. Our data suggest therefore that
the binding of PGK affects subunit interactions

151

in the oligomeric enzyme. It appears that the subunits become independent in catalysis and capable of functioning simultaneously.

Let us now consider the results obtained with a tetramer comprising a subunit free of PGK (form A on Fig. 2). It is seen that the total activity of this tetramer is markedly higher than the total activity of a partially modified tetramer (form B). The difference (A minus B) is to be attributed to the activity of a matrix-bound unmodified monomer. Since it is free from PGK, these results indicate that the 1,3-diphos-phoglycerate produced by PGK bound in a complex with other subunits can come out into solution and be utilized by this subunit. If we calculate the specific activity of this subunit, we obtain a value (19 U/mg) which is close to the specific activity of an isolated immobilized monomer. This indicates once again that subunit coopera-tivity in catalysis is abolished in the tetramer when it is bound to PGK and functions in the bienzyme complex.

REFERENCES
1. Muronetz, V.I., Zueva, V.S., Nagradova, N.K. (1979) Half-of-the-sites reactivity in immobi-lized hybrids of glyceraldehyde-3-phosphate dehydrogenase. FEBS Lett. 107, 277-280.

2. Ashmarina, L.I., Muronetz, V.I., Nagradova, N.K. (1980) A monomer of glyceraldehyde-3--phosphate dehydrogenase is catalytically active. Biochem. Int. 1, 47-54.

3. Ashmarina, L.I., Muronetz, V.I., Nagradova, N.K. (1981) Immobilized D-glyceraldehyde-3--phosphate dehydrogenase can exist as a tri-mer. FEBS Lett. 128, 22-26.

4. Muronetz, V.I., Golovina, T.O., Nagradova, N.K. (1982) Use of immobilization to study glyceraldehyde-3-phosphate dehydrogenase. Immobilized dimers. Biokhimiya (in Russian) 47, 3-12.

5. Ashmarina, L.I., Muronetz, V.I., Nagradova,
   N.K. (1982) Evidence for a change in catalytic properties of glyceraldehyde-3-phosphate
   dehydrogenase monomers upon their association in a tetramer. FEBS Lett. 144, 43-46.

TYPE-2 CASEIN KINASES: STRUCTURE, METABOLIC INVOLVEMENTS AND REGULATION.

LORENZO A. PINNA, FLAVIO MEGGIO, ARIANNA DONELLA-DEANA
AND ANNAMARIA BRUNATI.
Istituto di Chimica Biologica, Università di Padova,
Via Marzolo 3 - 35131 Padova, Italy.

INTRODUCTION.

The operational term casein kinase is widely used to indicate a class of ubiquitous protein kinases which are independent of cAMP, Ca^{2+} and any other known second messenger, and display their activity in vitro toward casein and phosvitin, while they are inactive on histones and protamines. It is generally accepted that casein kinases can be grouped into two distinct subsets: on one side monomeric enzymes using only ATP as phosphate donor and affecting Ser residues of β-casein, on the other oligomeric kinases, using also GTP besides ATP as phosphate donor and chiefly affecting Thr residues in casein fractions. After these properties casein kinases of the former type were designated A or S and those the latter type G (1) or TS (2). Regrettably however a merely conventional nomenclature of casein kinases, based on their order of elution from DEAE-cellulose, is more widely adopted, referring to casein kinases A (S) as type-1 (or NI if isolated from nuclei) and to casein kinases G (TS) as type-2 (or NII). Although it is commonly held that both families of casein kinases are multi-substrate enzymes playing relevant roles in many biological processes, their physiological significance and regulation mechanism remain unclear. The most relevant properties of casein kinases

Proceedings of the 16th FEBS Congress
Part A, pp. 155-163
© 1985 VNU Science Press

have been reviewed in (3). This paper will focuse on some new features of type 2 (G, TS) casein kinases, emerged in the last two years.

SUBUNIT STRUCTURE.

In most cases the quaternary structure of casein kinases-2 has been reported to be either $\alpha\alpha'\beta_2$ or $\alpha_2\beta_2$, the α-subunits being the larger ones (Mr 35,000-44,000) and the β-subunits the smaller ones (24-26,000), to give holoenzymes with Mr around 130,000 (3). The feeling that the α' subunits and, more in general, the α subunits with relatively low Mr, could be generated by limited proteolysis of larger α-subunits has been now suffragated by experiments showing that by limited digestion with trypsin the α subunit or rat liver cytosol casein kinase TS can be converted into slightly smaller α' and α'' derivatives with a parallel partial loss of activity (Fig. 1). Since the β-subunits are unaffected it should be concluded that the catalytic activity resides in the α-subunits. Such a conclusion is also supported the demonstration that isolated α-subunits, but not β-subunits, still exhibit detectable casein kinase activity (4) and by the recent report of casein kinases-2 from yeast (5) and Dictyostelium (6) which are lacking the β subunits.

On the other hand it should be recalled that a casein kinase-2 purified from pig liver nuclei has a Mr of about 200,000 and is composed by two identical subunits of 95,000 KDa, very different from the α-subunits of typical casein kinase-2 (7). The recent observation that the cytosolic counterpart of this enzyme is a typical casein kinase-2, with 37 KDa α-subunits (8) discloses the possibility that there might exhist two

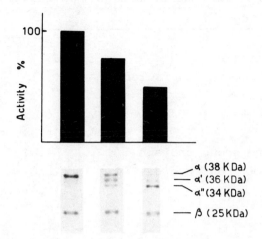

Fig. 1 - Effect of limited digestion on the structure and activity of casein kinase-2. Rat liver casein kinase TS was incubated for 2 min with 0, 0.5 and 1 µg trypsin (from left to right). Reaction was stopped with PMSF and aliquots were either tested for casein kinase activity or analyzed for their subunit composition by PAGE-SDS (Coomassie staining).

distinct forms of type 2 casein kinases in the cytoplasmic and nuclear compartments of the same cells.

POTENTIAL TARGETS AND SITE SPECIFICITY.

The number of potential physiological targets of casein kinase-2 is continuously increasing. A list of proteins which can be phosphorylated by casein kinase-2 is reported in Table I: it includes key enzymes of different metabolic pathways, factors involved in gene expression and proteins implicated in specialized functions. This confirms the view that casein kinases-2 represent a class of multifunctional protein kinases.

Table I: Proteins which are phosphorylated by casein kinase-2.

Proteins	References
Glycogen synthase	(9, 10)
Translation initiation factors	(11)
RNA polymerase	(12)
Spectrin	(13)
Glycophorin	(13)
High mobility group protein 17	(14)
High mobility group protein 14	(15)
Troponin-T	(16, 17)
R_{II}	(18, 19)
Calsequestrin	(20)
Acetyl CoA carboxylase	(21)
Acidic ribosomal proteins	(22)
Myosin light chain	(23)
T-substrate (wheat germ)	(24)
C-proteins (hn RNP-particles)	(25)
Ornithine decarboxylase	(26)

Two points however should be outlined: 1) in several cases the phosphorylation of potential substrates has been tested only in vitro and no evidence has been provided as yet corroborating the occurrence of such a process in vivo. 2) Many of the proteins listed undergo "silent" phosphorylation, i.e. their biological activity is not apparently modified. On this matter however it should be mentioned the recent finding that the per se silent phosphorylation of glycogen synthase at site 5 by casein kinase-2 makes easier the subsequent phosphorylation of site-3 by glycogen synthase kinase-3 which promotes a remarkable inactivation (27). It is possible therefore that also in other instances casein kinase-2 may induce indirect modifications of the biological properties of the target proteins.

The amino acid sequences around three residues affected by casein kinase-2 both _in vitro_ and _in vivo_ is already known (table II): the most remarkable recurring

Table II: Phosphorylation sites of proteins and related peptides affected by casein kinase-2.

Substrate	Amino acid sequence	Km(uM)	Ref.
R_{II}	-Asp-<u>Ser</u>-Glu-<u>Ser</u>-Glu- -Asp-Glu-Glu-Glu-(18)	13	(18)
Troponin-T	Ac-<u>Ser</u>-Asp-Glu-Glu-Val- -Glu-(16)	39	(16)
Glycogen synthase	-Glu-<u>Ser</u>-Glu-Asp-Glu- -Glu-Glu-(10)	11	unp.
Synthetic peptide	<u>Ser</u>-Glu-Glu-Glu-Val-Glu	1,600	(29)
Synthetic peptide	<u>Ser</u>-Glu-Glu-Glu-Glu-Glu	2,600	unp.
β-casein A	-Gln-Gln-Gln-<u>Thr</u>-Glu- -Asp-Glu-	60	(28)
Synthetic peptide	Arg-Arg-Arg-Glu-Glu- -Glu-<u>Thr</u>-Glu-Glu-Glu	500	(30)

feature is a cluster of several acidic residues on the C terminal side of the phosphorylated one. The actual importance of the acidic residues has been recently confirmed by using synthetic peptides reproducing the structure of such phosphorylation sites. It has been shown that these peptides can be phosphorylated with aproximately the same Vmax of the corresponding protein substrates (29, 30) though the Km values are 1 to 2 orders of magnitude higher (see table II).

REGULATION.

Although the physiological effectors of casein kina-

ses-2 remain unknown, several compounds have been reported to either inhibit or stimulate this class of enzymes. (see table III). Inhibition by heparin is especial-

Table III: Effectors of casein kinase-2 activity.

Inhibitors	References
Heparin	reviewed in (3)
Inositol hexosulphate	(31)
2,3 diphosphoglycerate(DPG)	(32)
Pyridoxal phosphate(PLP)	(31)
Quercetin	(33)
Polyglutamyl (aspartyl) peptides	(34)
Stimulators	
Polyamines	(1,35,36)
Polybasic peptides	(26,37)

ly effective and often used as a criterion for distin-
guishing casein kinase-2 from casein kinase-1 and other
protein kinases. Recently however a glycogen synthase/-
casein kinase-1 very sensitive to heparin has been
described (38). A newly discovered class of powerful
competitive inhibitors of casein kinase-2 is represented by polyglutamyl peptides (34): this discloses the
possibility that naturally occurring very acidic polypeptides may act as regulators of casein kinase-2.
Finally the inhibition by PLP (31) warrants attention
as PLP is required as a cofactor of ODC, whose phosphorylation by a rat liver cytosol casein kinase-2 has
been recently reported (26). Furthermore ODC is a key
enzyme in the biosynthesis of polyamines which are
stimulators of casein kinases-2 (Table III). Apparently
they exert their effect by decreasing the concentration
of Mg^{2+} required for optimal activity (36). Since however polyamines interact with the protein substrates

160

altering their conformation (35), the use of simple peptide substrates, lacking tertiary structure, could be useful for insighting the mechanism by which polycations stimulate casein kinase-2. Actually, the phosphorylation of the hexapeptide Ser-(Glu)$_5$ by casein kinase--2 from rat liver cytosol is enhanced by spermine through an increase of Vmax; on the contrary basic peptides (e.g. protamine, polylysine and polyarginine) increase the phosphorylation by lowering the Km for the peptide substrate (F. Meggio and L.A. Pinna, unpublished data). Thus both polyamines and polybasic peptides may play independent physiological roles in the regulation of casein kinase-2 by making the intracellular concentrations of Mg^{2+} and protein substrates, respectively, compatible with the operation of this enzyme.

Acknowledgement: The excellent secretarial aid of Miss Monica Vettore is gratefully acknowledged.

REFERENCES.

1. Cochet C., Job D., Pirollet F. and Chambaz E.M. (1980) Endocrinology 196, 750-757.
2. Meggio F., Donella-Deana A., Pinna L.A. and Moret V. (1977) FEBS Lett. 75, 192-196.
3. Hathaway G.M. and Traugh J.A. (1982) Curr. Top. Cell. Regul. 21, 101-127.
4. Cochet C. and Chambaz E.M. (1983) J. Biol. Chem. 258, 1403-1406.
5. Kudlicki W., Szyszka R. and Gasior E. (1984) Biochim. Biophys. Acta 784, 102-107.
6. Ranart M.F., Sastre L. and Sebastian J. (1984) Eur. J. Biochem. 140, 47-54.
7. Baydoun H., Hoppe J., Jacob G. and Wagner K.G. (1980) FEBS Lett. 122, 231-233.

8. Baydoun H., Feth F., Hoppe J. and Wagner K.G. (1984) Eur. J. Biochem., submitted.

9. De Paoli Roach A.A., Ahmad Z. and Roach P.J. (1981) J. Biol. Chem. 256, 8955-8962.

10. Cohen P., Yellowlees D., Aitken A., Donella-Deana A., Hemmings B.A. and Parker P.J. (1982) Eur. J. Biochem. 124, 21-35.

11. Hathaway G.M. and Traugh J.A. (1979) J. Biol. Chem. 252, 2691-2697.

12. Dahmus M.E. (1981) J. Biol. Chem. 256, 3332-3339.

13. Hosey M.M. and Tao M. (1977) Biochemistry 16, 4578-4583.

14. Inoue A., Tei Y., Hasuma T., Yukioka M. and Morisawa S. (1980) FEBS Lett. 117, 68-72.

15. Walton G.M. and Gill G.N. (1983) J. Biol. Chem. 258, 4440-4446.

16. Pinna L.A., Meggio F. and Dediukina M. (1981) Biochim. Biophys. Res. Commun. 100, 449-454.

17. Villar-Palasi C. and Kumon A. (1981) J. Biol. Chem. 256, 7409-7415.

18. Carmichael D.F., Geahlen R.L., Allen S.M. and Krebs E.G. (1982) J. Biol. Chem. 257, 10440-10445.

19. Hemmings B.A., Aitken A., Cohen P., Rymond M. and Hofmann F. (1982) Eur. J. Biochem. 127, 473-481.

20. Meggio F., Donella-Deana A. and Pinna L.A. (1981) J. Biol. Chem. 256, 11958-11961.

21. Tipper J.P., Bacon G.W. and Witters L.A. (1983) Arch. Biochem. Biophys. 227, 386-396.

22. Meggio F., Brunati A.M., Donella-Deana A. and Pinna L.A. (1984) Eur. J. Biochem. 138, 379-385.

23. Matsamura S., Murakami N., Tashiro Y., Yasuda S. and Kumon A. (1983) Arch. Biochem. Biophys. 227, 125-135.

24. Yan T-F. J. and Tao M. (1982) J. Biol. Chem. 257, 7044-7049.

25. Holcomb E.R. and Friedman D.L. (1984) J. Biol. Chem. 259, 31-40.
26. Meggio F., Flamigni F., Caldarera C.M., Guarnieri C. and Pinna L.A. (1984) Biochim. Biophys. Res. Commun., in press.
27. Picton C., Woodgett J., Hemmings B. and Cohen P. (1982) FEBS Lett. 150, 191-196.
28. Meggio F., Donella-Deana A. and Pinna L.A. (1981) Biochim. Biphys. Acta 662, 1-7.
29. Pinna L.A., Meggio F., Marchiori F. and Borin G. (1984) FEBS Lett. 171, 211-214.
30. Kuenzel E.A. and Krebs E.G. (1984) Fed. Proc. Fed. Am. Soc. Exp. Biol. 43, 1469 (Abstr.).
31. Hathaway G.M. and Traugh J.A. (1983) Methods in Enzymology 99, 317-331.
32. Hathaway G.M. and Traugh J.A. (1984) J. Biol. Chem. 259, 2850-2855.
33. Cochet C., Feige J.J., Pirollet F., Keramidas M. and Chambaz E.M. (1982) Biochem. Pharmacol. 31, 1357-1361.
34. Meggio F., Pinna L.A., Marchiori F. and Borin G. (1983) FEBS Lett. 162, 235-238.
35. Hara T. and Endo H. (1982) Biochemistry 21, 2632-2637.
36. Hathaway G.M. and Traugh J.A. (1984) J. Biol. Chem. 259, 7011-7015.
37. Meggio F., Brunati A.M. and Pinna L.A. (1983) FEBS Lett. 160, 203-208.
38. Ahmad Z., Camici M., De Paoli-Roach A.A. and Roach P.J. (1984) J. Biol. Chem. 259, 3420-3428.

BALANCE OF ATP-PRODUCING AND CONSUMING REACTIONS IN THE RED CELL

S. RAPOPORT, W. DUBIEL, D. MARETZKI, W. SIEMS

Institute of Physiological and Biological Chemistry, Humboldt University, DDR - 104 Berlin, GDR

Regulation is a basic property of all biological systems. Their regulatory properties are expressed in the precise determination of kind, amount, distribution in space and kinetics of most of their components. Regulation constitutes the teleonomic response of biological systems to external and internal signals and ensures their adaptability to changes of inner and outer conditions. It is characterized by the circumstance that the needs of a biological system determine its performance within the limits of its capacities.

A. THE ERYTHROCYTE

I shall omit the discussion of ATP production in the erythrocyte since these studies have been published (1 - 4), and will turn to the main subject of my discourse, the ATP consuming processes.

The ATP consuming processes of the erythrocyte

Production and consumption of ATP are closely geared to each other. From a functional point of view consumption governs ATP production. Therefore it is an essential task to identify and quantify the various ATP-consuming

Proceedings of the 16th FEBS Congress
Part A, pp. 165–176
© 1985 VNU Science Press

processes of the cell and to elucidate their interrelations. The first question we asked concerned the kinetics of ATP consumption by the erythrocyte. We followed the changes of ATP and ADP in glucose free cells taking into account residual sources of ATP production. From the data (fig. 1) it is evident that the rate of overall ATP consumption declines

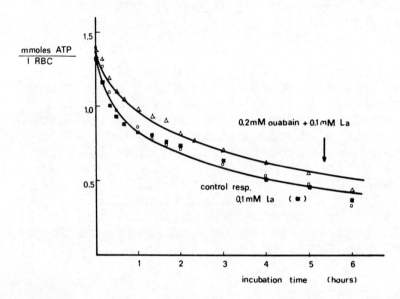

<u>Fig. 1</u> ATP in glucose-free human red cells at 37°, pH 7.4

approximately exponentially, dropping to one half at a concentration of ATP of 0,8 mM. This behaviour indicates that the bulk of the ATP consuming processes have a low affinity for ATP. Most ATP-consuming reactions so far described such as transport ATPases and various phosphokinases have high affinities for ATP with K_m values of less than 0,1 mM.
    Therefore our strategy to find the main ATP consuming processes consisted in a search for

reactions with high K_m-values for ATP. Experiments on membrane-free hemolysates under conditions closely approximating those in the cell indicated clearly that no more than 10 % of the ATP consumption in the steady state could occur in the cytosol. Therefore the bulk of ATP consumption resides in the cell membrane.

The best known consumer of ATP is the Na^+K^+ ATPase. The course of decline of ATP in the presence of Ouabain, which inhibits the Na^+K ATPase, is shown in the upper curve of fig. 1. This enzyme contributes about 25 % to the ATP consumption, in consonance with older work in which other methods were employed. Also shown is the effect of lanthanum which inhibits the Ca^+ATPase. This system contributes under normal conditions despite its high capacity only about 1 % because of the slow permeation of Ca-ions through the cell membrane.

Thinking that it was essential to keep as close as possible to cellular conditions we prepared erythrocyte membranes maintaining isotonicity throughout the entire isolation procedure. It was found that the Ca^{++}ATPase of isotonic membranes has a several fold higher capacity than that of hypertonically prepared membranes and that its K_m-value with 0,8 mM is more than one order of magnitude higher. The reason for this difference is the presence of a protein which we have called the ATP affinity modulator (5). It is removed under hypotonic conditions or by EGTA, whereby the membranes are converted to a high affinity state for ATP. The modulator protein has a molecular weight of 120 KD. and consists apparently of 3 types of subunits one of which appears to be calmodulin.

Let us turn to the phosphorylation of lipids and proteins, in experiments on intact erythrocytes with labelled phosphate the bulk of radioactivity was found in the phospholipids

with more than 80 %, whereas the proteins contribute a minor share. Among the proteins spectrin is most prominent but all of them contribute only about 5 % to the total ATP consumption.

The phosphate turnover in the phospholipids
is practically limited to the di- and tri-
phosphatidylinositols. The ATP dependence of
the phosphorylation of phosphoinositol appears
to belong to the class of processes with low
ATP affinity with a K_m-value of 0,4 mM ATP
without differentiation between di- and tri-
phosphoinositide. Thus the turnover of the
phosphotidylinositols fits the characteristics
we have been searching for. Careful assessment
of the specific radioactivity of the phosphoinositides indicates that the phosphatidylinosi-
tol-cycle accounts for about 20 % of the ATP
consumption (6).

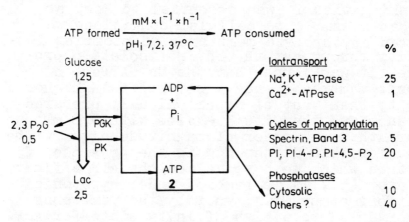

Fig. 2 Balance of ATP formation and consumption
        in erythrocyte of man

In Fig. 2 is shown the status of our present
knowledge. It depicts the balance of ATP formation and consumption for the normal in vivo
condition of human erythrocytes with an intracellular pH of 7,2. On the left side are

summarized the data for ATP production which
amounts to 2 mmoles per 1 cells and hour. On
the right side are listed the processes of ATP
consumption so far determined. 40 % remain unaccounted for. What could they be?

There are some indications of interactions
between cytosol and membranes, which so far
have escaped precise manipulation; there is the
thought of another type of ATPase connected
with the maintenance of the shape of the erythrocyte; there is also the possibility of
ultralabile phosphates which are destroyed in
the process of analysis. These are the directions of current work.

B. THE RETICULOCYTE

Let me turn now to the reticulocyte, a more
complex system but still much simpler than most
other types of cells.

The reticulocyte is a well-defined intermediate stage of the differentiation of ery-
throid cells. It is characterized by the inactivation or elimination of the cell nucleus
of the erythroblast on the one hand, and on
the other by the presence of functional mitochondria and ribosomes.

A comparison of the metabolic pathways
between reticulocytes and erythrocytes shows
that the reticulocyte lacks DNA replication,
RNA synthesis, the pathways of glycogen formation and breakdown as well as lipid synthesis.
On the other hand it performs actively the synthesis of proteins - mostly globin and cor-
respondingly of heme.

During the maturation of the reticulocyte
there occurs extensive re-building. The mitochondria and ribosomes and parts of the cell
membrane are destroyed, while about one third
of the final complement of hemoglobin is

169

synthesized, partly from the amino acids
furnished by the breakdown of the organelles.

ATP production in the reticulocyte
The first aim of our study was the determination of the metabolic sources and the amount of
ATP production. The main conclusions of this
phase of our work are as follows (7). Glucose
is the main substrate of reticulocyte energy
metabolism (fig. 3). The citrate acid cycle

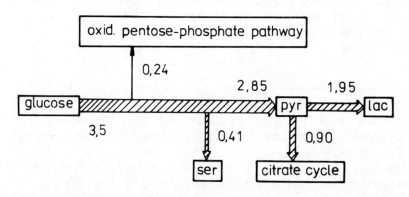

Fig. 3 Utilization of glucose in reticulocytes
μmoles x ml cells^{-1} x hour^{-1}; 37°C, pH 7,4

and lactate formation account for most of the
glucose consumption while the pentose phosphate
pathway and serine formation account for minor
shares. The ATP production, which may amount to
120 to 200 mM/l cells·h ist about 100-fold
larger than in erythrocytes. About 80 % are
derived from respiration; oxydation of fatty
acids contributes about 15 % to the ATP production.

The ATP consuming processes in reticulocytes
What about the balance of ATP consuming processes in reticulocytes?

- For this purpose the coupled respiration, the extent of globin synthesis, of ATP-dependent proteolysis, of ATP-dependent transport of Na^+, K^+ and Ca^{++} ions and of heme synthesis were determined (8).

Based on the reasoning that production of ATP is determined by its consumption and that most of the energy is derived from respiration we looked for the effect of selective inhibitors on the coupled respiration of reticulocytes. The use of selective inhibitors for specific processes involves several preconditions. Firstly it has to be shown that the inhibitor affects only one pathway, secondly it should not interfere with the viability of the cell for the period studied; thirdly the process inhibited should not be indirectly coupled to another pathway, e.g. by supply or removal of a substrate or product. Therefore it is imperative to check the result obtained in an indirect manner by direct determination of the activity of the pathway, if possible. The effects of ouabain on respiration indicate that the Na^+K^+ATPase accounts for about 25 % of the ATP consumption, which in absolute terms is two orders of magnitude higher than in erythrocytes. The effect of lanthanum is distinctly higher than in erythrocytes.

Next we studied the share of protein synthesis. From the inhibition of the coupled respiration by cycloheximide a share of about 30 % for protein synthesis was estimated. To make sure of our conclusions we determined the protein synthesis directly from the amount of radioactive lysine incorporated and also from the changes of intracellular lysine concentration.

There is another ATP consuming process in reticulocytes, the ATP dependent proteolysis. This system is primarily directed to the degradation of the mitochondria during the

maturation of the reticulocytes and is triggered by a preceding attack of their cell-
specific lipoxygenase (9). According to Hershko
and Ciechanover (10, 11) the proteolytic
system is quite complex; it involves as an
initial step the activation and attachment of
ubiquitin - a large peptide - to the exposed
lysine residues of its substrate.

We have evidence that ubiquitin is obligat-
ory for the proteolytic attack on mitochondria,
whereas ubiquitin-unrelated proteolysis, which
has been postulated by Goldberg (12), may be
an artefact which is demonstrable only in
reticulocytes produced by phenylhydrazine administration (12).

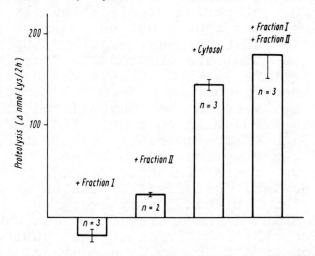

Fig. 4 Protein breakdown of reticulocyte
stroma (mitochondria) in the presence
of ATP (5 mM) and Mg^{2+}(5 mM). Cytosol
was fractionated in Fraction I
(ubiquitin) and Fraction II (10). All
components used corresponded to 0.8 ml
cells

In fig. 4 is shown the proteolysis of mito-

chondria - containing stroma of reticulocytes.
It is evident that stroma with ubiquitin alone
(fraction I) or with the rest of the proteolytic system (fraction II) undergoes little if
any proteolysis, whereas the combination of
both fractions produces proteolysis which may
be even larger than that effected by the lysate
of reticulocytes.

According to our data there is a surprisingly large ATP consumption for the ubiquitin-
dependent proteolysis amounting to about
1 mole of ATP, per peptide bond.

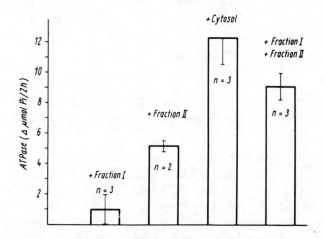

Fig. 5 ATPase activity stimulated by stroma in
Fraction I, Fraction II, Cytosol and
Fraction I + Fraction II. Conditions
as in Fig. 4

In fig. 5 the corresponding data on the P-
liberation from ATP are presented. While there
is some unspecific ATP degradation by fraction
II, it is quite clear that there is a sizeable
ATP breakdown connected with proteolysis. This
is far in excess of the amount needed for the
activation and transfer of ubiquitin and would
indicate that the steps beyond its attachment,

i.e. the breakdown of the ubiquitin-protein-
conjugates, require also ATP.
A synopsis of the results is presented in
fig. 6. It shows that three processes are
major consumers of ATP in the reticulocyte:for

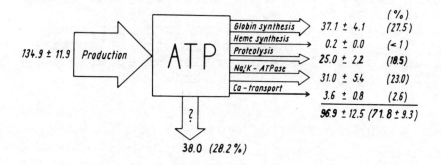

Fig. 6 Balance of ATP production and con-
        sumption in the rabbit reticulocyte

one protein synthesis with about 30 %, secondly Na^+K^+ ATPase with about 25 % and
thirdly ATP dependent proteolysis with 15 %.
About 30 % of ATP consumption are unaccounted
for. These processes behaved in an independent
manner. It appears as if they do not compete
with each other for ATP and would thus be regulated independently.
    However in an amino acid medium designed for
maximal hemoglobin synthesis ATP production is
greatly increased, on account of a nearly four-
fold protein synthesis, whereas under reduced
ATP supply there is a disproportionate reduction of both protein synthesis and proteolysis,
possibly caused by inhibitors arising from the
breakdown of adenine nucleotides.

REFERENCES

1. Rapoport, T. A., Heinrich, R., Jacobasch, G., and Rapoport, S. (1974). A linear steady-state treatment of enzymatic chains. A mathematical model of glycolysis of human erythrocytes. Eur. J. Biochem. 42, 107-120
2. Rapoport, T. A., Heinrich, R. and Rapoport, S. M. (1976). The regulatory principles of glycolysis in erythrocytes in vivo and in vitro. Biochem. J. 154, 449-469
3. Heinrich, R., Rapoport, S. M. and Rapoport, T. A. (1977). Metabolic regulation and mathematic models. Prog. Biophys. Molec. Biol. 32, 1-82
4. Schauer, M., Heinrich, R. und Rapoport, S. M. (1981). Mathematische Modellierung der Glykolyse und des Adeninnukleotidstoffwechsels menschlicher Erythrozyten. II. Simulation des Adeninnukleotidabbaus bei Glukoseverarmung. Acta biol. med. germ. 40, 1683-1697
5. Maretzki, D., Klatt, D., Reimann, B. and Rapoport, S. (1982). Isolation of A 120 KD Modulator protein of $(Ca^{2+}+Mg^{2+})$-ATPase which contains calmodulin from membranes of human erythrocytes. Biochem Inf. 4, 323-329
6. Maretzki, D., Reimann, B., Klatt, D. and Schwarzer, E. (1983). Involvement of polyphosphoinositides in the ATP turnover of intact human erythrocytes and in the ATPase activity of purified membranes. Biomed. Biochim. Acta 42, 72-76
7. Siems, W., Müller, M., Dumdey, R., Holzhütter, H.-G., Rathmann, J. and Rapoport, S.M. (1982). Quantification of pathways of glucose utilization and balance of energy metabolism of rabbit reticulocytes. Eur. J. Biochem. 124, 567-576

8. Siems, W., Dubiel, W., Dumdey, R., Müller, M. and Rapoport, S. M. (1984). Accounting for the ATP-consuming processes in rabbit reticulocytes. Eur. J. Biochem. 139, 101-107

9. Müller, M., Dubiel, W., Rathmann, J. & Rapoport, S. (1980). Determination and characteristics of energy-dependent proteolysis in rabbit reticulocytes. Eur. J. Biochem. 109, 405-410

10. Ciehanover, A., Hod, Y. and Hershko, A. (1978). A heat-stable polypeptide component of an ATP-dependent proteolytic system from reticulocytes. Biochem. Biophys. Res. Com. 81, 1100-1105

11. Hershko, A., and Ciechanover, A. (1982). Mechanisms of intracellular protein breakdown. Annu. Rev. Biochem. 51, 335-364

12. Tanaka, K., Waxman, L., and Goldberg, A. L. (1984). Vanadate inhibits the ATP-dependent degradation of proteins in reticulocytes without affecting ubiquitin conjugation. J. Biol. Chem. 259, 2803-2809

13. Rapoport, S. and Dubiel, W. (1984). The effect of phenylhydrazine on the protein breakdown in rabbit reticulocytes. Biomed. Biochim. Acta 43, 23-27

ROLE OF SECONDARY MESSENGERS IN THE REGULATION OF CELL FUNCTIONS

E.S.SEVERIN, T.V.BULARGINA, S.M.DUDKIN, A.V.ITKES,
S.N.KOCHETKOV, M.V.NESTEROVA, V.L.TUNITSKAYA

Institute of Molecular Biology, USSR Academy of
Sciences, Moscow 117984 USSR

This paper reviews the recent studies on the enzymes involved in metabolism and regulation by secondary messen-
gers. It also develops some ideas about the mechanism of
regulation of various metabolic processes in some cell
cultures. We were mostly concerned with the studies on
the mechanism of action and substrate specificity of
cAMP-dependent protein kinase and biological effects of
cAMP. In each part of the present article we tried to
give a brief outline of the investigations which were
carried out in several directions.

THE MOLECULAR MECHANISM OF ACTION OF cAMP-DEPENDENT
PROTEIN KINASE

In our previous communications we reported on the mechanism of action of cAMP-dependent protein kinase. One
of the main results of our studies was the discovery of
the phosphointermediate of the phosphotransferase reaction which was found to be the phosphoform of the catalytic subunit of protein kinase. We also assumed that
the histidine residue of the enzyme active site acts as
the phosphoryl acceptor [1].
It was established that the phosphoryl residue transfer from histidine to the substrate is catalized by a
specific functional group of the active site. By a num-

Proceedings of the 16th FEBS Congress
Part A, pp. 177–182
© 1985 VNU Science Press

ber of methods, the latter was found to be a carboxyl group. The main function of this group is to form a hydrogen bond with the proton of the substrate attacking group. The formation of such bond permits to avoid the production of the thermodynamically unfavourable H_3^+O ion and to stabilize the transition state of the reaction, which sufficiently increases the reaction rate.

If the specific protein substrate interacts with the phosphoenzyme, the formation of the enzyme - substrate complex first takes place, which lowers the energy of activation by approximately 5 kcal/mol. To study this complex and the character of protein-protein interaction during its formation, we used a number of histone H1 fragments and synthetic peptide substrates as substrates and inhibitors of the reaction. These experiments suggested that there are two orders of specificity of the enzyme-histone H1 interaction. The first one is evidently conditioned by the spatial structure of the substrate, and the second - by the amino acid sequence of histone H1 phosphorylation site. The specificity of the second order is mostly determined by the positively charged amino acid residues, which are located at the N-terminus of the phosphorylation site. The structures of the C-terminal sequence and, moreover, the phosphorylating residue itself are not determining for the effective binding of the substrate.

REGULATION OF ADENYLATE CYCLASE ACTIVITY BY cAMP-DEPENDENT PROTEIN KINASE

cAMP-dependent protein kinases do not only control numerous processes, occuring in the cytoplasm, but regulate a great number of the membrane enzymes as well. In particular, they regulate the activity of the membrane adenylate cyclase from pigeon erythrocytes, thus being directly involved in the process of desensitisation.

Preincubation of pigeon erythrocytes with $10^{-5}M$ adrenaline causes the progressive decrease in adenylate cyclase sensitivity to the repeated action of a hormone. The similar effects were observed when erythrocytes

were preincubated with dibutyryl-cAMP and isobutylme-
thylxanthine. This indicates that cAMP-dependent protein kinases are involved in this process. Thus, preincubation of plasmatic membranes from pigeon erythrocytes with the catalytic subunit of cAMP-dependent protein kinase leads to the desensitisation of adenylate
cyclase.

The experiments on the reconstruction of the adenylate cyclase complex from individual components demonstrated that β-adrenoreceptor is the substrate of protein kinase. cAMP-dependent protein kinase phosphory-
lates the membrane protein with $M_r \sim 49000$, which corresponds to the molecular weight of β-adrenoreceptor,
identified by Lefkowitz by the method of affinity modification [2]. The phosphorylation of the receptor im-
paires the interaction between the receptor and N_S-
protein and decreases the constant of binding of adrenaline with the receptor.

cAMP-DEPENDENT REGULATION OF THE ENZYMES OF THE
2',5'-OLIGOADENYLATE SYSTEM

At present we know a number of the regulatory systems,
involved in the control of cell growth and differentiation. Two of them - the systems of cAMP and 2',5'-
oligoadenylate were the objects of our study.

We have earlier demonstrated that the rise in the
intracellular level of cAMP causes an increase in 2-5A
synthetase activity and a decrease in 2'-phosphodieste-
rase activity [3].

To prove the concept that cAMP effect on 2'-phospho-
diesterase is mediated by the activation of cAMP-dependent protein kinase, the cell homogenate was treated with the catalytic subunit of cAMP-dependent protein kinase. The control homogenate retained 70% of
its 2'-phosphodiesterase activity during 8 hours incubation. During incubation in the presence of protein
kinase, the enzyme activity decreased 5 fold. Thus,
phosphorylation of cell homogenate proteins in vitro
produced the same effect on 2'-phosphodiesterase acti-

vity as the increase in the intracellular level of cAMP, which is consistent with the above concept.

The activity of cAMP-dependent protein kinase increased significantly in resting cells. During 9 days of incubation it increased 5-7 fold. At the same time, the activity of the heat-stable protein inhibitor of cAMP-dependent protein kinase in resting cells was noticeably lower than in proliferating cells. This suggests that the observed increase in protein kinase activity can be accounted for by the decrease in the level of its specific protein inhibitor.

The activity of 2-5A synthetase increased continuously when cells were incubated in the medium with 0.5% serum, increasing 8 fold during 9 days of observation. The activity of 2'-phosphodiesterase first fell during 5 days and then rose again. These two enzymes are known to regulate the level of 2-5A. The latter was found to increase significantly in resting cells (from $0.3 \cdot 10^{-14}$ to $1-4 \cdot 10^{-14}$ mol per mg cell protein).

Thus, the variations in the activities of the enzymes of 2-5A metabolism in cells, deepening into the resting state, were similar to those, occuring in cells after the increase in the intracellular level of cAMP.

A sufficient activation of cAMP-dependent phosphorylation is observed in cells, sinking into the resting state. Hence, it is reasonable to suggest that cAMP-dependent protein kinase is involved in the regulation of 2-5A synthetase and 2'-phosphodiesterase activities in resting cells.

The results obtained are summarized in the scheme, depicted in Figure 1. The scheme presents the data, described in the present paper, as well as the earlier discovered fact of phosphodiesterase of cAMP activation by 2-5A [4].

In view of this, it is reasonable to consider cAMP and 2-5A as the agents, involved in cell regualtion.

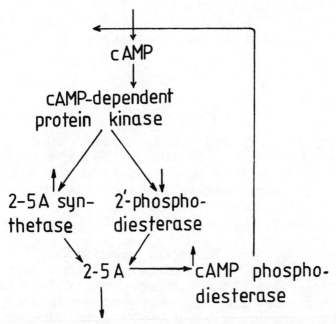

Fig.1   Scheme of interconnections between cAMP and
         2-5A systems.

cAMP-REGULATION OF NGF SECRETION BY L 929 CELLS

It was earlier established that the conditioned medium
of L 929 cells contains NGF - the protein growth factor of nervous cells. cAMP regulation of the production of this factor was the purpose of our study.
    To test the secreted NGF we used pheochromacytoma
cells, line PC 12. It was discovered   that after
the treatment with NGF these cells developed an ability to grow neurites. The conditioned medium of L 929
cells contained low quantities of NGF. However, after
the treatment of these cells with dibutyryl-cAMP, the
secretion of NGF increased about 10 fold. The electrophoresis of the proteins of the conditioned medium
showed the appearance of the protein with $M_r \sim 13000$,
which was identified as β-subunit of NGF.

The above findings suggested that cAMP-dependent processes control NGF production , thus demonstrating that there is a novel way of cAMP-dependent regulation of cell activity.

REFERENCES

1. Kochetkov,S.N., Bulargina,T.V., Saschenko,L.P., Severin,E.S. (1977). Studies on the mechanism of action of histone kinase dependent on adenosine 3',5'-monophosphate. Evidence for involvement of histidine and lysine residues in the phosphotransferase reaction. Eur.J.Biochem. 81, 111-118.
2. David R.Sibley, Jack R.Peters, Ponnal Nambi, Mark J.Caron, Robert J.Lefkowitz. (1984). Photoaffinity labelling of turkey erythrocyte β-adrenergic receptors: degradation of the M_r 49000 protein explains apparent hydrogenity. Biochem. Biophys.Res.Commun. 119, 458-464.
3. Itkes,A.V., Turpaev,K.T., Kartasheva,O.N., Kafiani,C.A., Severin,E.S. (1983). Cyclic AMP-dependent regulation of activities of synthetase and phosphodiesterase of 2',5'-oligoadenylate in NIH 3T3 cells. Mol.Cell.Biochem. 58, 165-171.
4. Itkes,A.V., Kochetkova,M.N. (1981), Activation of phosphodiesterase of adenosine monophosphate by 2',5'-oligoadenylate. Biochem.Int. 3, 341-347.

MEDICAL BIOCHEMISTRY

MAPPING OF EPITOPES ON IgG Fc INTERACTING WITH Fc RECEPTORS ON K CELLS

J. GERGELY,* GABRIELLA SÁRMAY,* D.R. STANWORTH°
and R. JEFFERIS°

*Department of Immunology, L. Eötvös University,
 Göd, Hungary
°Department of Immunology, The University of
Birmingham, U.K.

Fc Receptors (FcR) are immunoglobulin binding
structures which interact with the C-terminal
domains of the antibody molecules. The receptors
are expressed on the membranes of a wide range of
cells, most of them belonging to the immune system. FcR-s are structurally and functionally
very heterogenous, i.e. they interact with different classes and subclasses of immunoglobulins,
mediate various signals, trigger several functions.
   The fascinating heterogeneity of these receptors may mean either that
   - the different binding specificity is the function of molecules differing in their primary
structure, or that
   - the binding specificity of different conformational forms of the same molecule is different.
   The class and subclass specificity of FcR-s may
be the consequence of the former type of heterogeneity. On the other hand, another form of IgG
FcR heterogeneity was described by us which may
reflect the latter type (1-8).
   In the present paper we summarize our results
showing some functional consequence of this type
of IgG FcR heterogeneity and present data which
enabled us to localise the submolecular sites on
IgG Fc reacting with the binding sites of the FcR-s.

Proceedings of the 16th FEBS Congress
Part A, pp. 185–195
© 1985 VNU Science Press

Monomeric and polymeric forms of IgG FcR-s on human lymphocytes

The observation that a population of the human peripheral lymphocytes shed their IgG FcR-s after 4-37°C temperature shift in contrast to another population which does not shed the FcR under identical experimental conditions allowed us to distinguish between two forms of IgG binding structures.

Evidence was provided showing that (1-10)
- the shed FcRI molecules are mobile, soluble and monomeric, while the FcRII molecules are crosslinked,
- the binding specificity of the two types of receptors are not identical which is the consequence of differing binding sites,
- the monomeric FcRI molecules possess only one active binding site interacting with the CH3 domain of IgG,
- the crosslinking of the monomeric FcRI molecules in model experiments results in the expression of a second active binding site, specific for the CH2 domain of IgG,
- as a consequence of various stimuli "receptor conversion" can take place on the cell surface, and both FcRI to FcRII and FcRII to FcRI conversion can be induced.

The functional importance of IgG FcR conversion

IgG FcR-s expressed on K (killer) cells have been shown to be directly involved in the antibody dependent cell mediated cytotoxicity (ADCC). The IgG FcR-s on K cells serve as recognizing units for the target-cell bound antibody molecules and the target cell lysis is triggered by the interaction of Fc-structures of the antibody and IgG FcR-s of the K cells (9).

Regarding our results showing that two categories of IgG FcR-s can be distinguished it seem-

186

ed reasonable to study, which type can be found on K cells.

The temperature shift from 4-37°C is a very simple way to induce shedding of the mobile FcRI molecules and to get a cell population having temporarily only the crosslinked FcRII molecules on the cell surface. We found that neither the shedding nor the reappearance of the FcRI molecules affected the structures on K cells responsible for ADCC. On the other hand, the depletion of either: both types of IgG FcR-bearing cells or only that of the FcRII$^+$ subset resulted in significant decrease of ADCC activity. These observations indicated that *only cells belonging to the FcRII$^+$ subset are active in ADCC*, i.e. cells bearing the polymerised form of the IgG binding receptors interacting both with the CH2 and CH3 domains of the sensitizing antibody (4).

The two binding-site model of IgG FcR-mediated killing in ADCC

It is generally accepted that K cells in ADCC need functionally intact IgG FcR-s. On the other hand, the data dealing with the localisation of submolecular sites on IgG reacting with the FcR-s on K cells are conflicting, and the preferential role either of the CH2 or CH3 domains is still an unsettled question. Our approach to this problem was based on our observations summarized above. We supposed that if the prerequisite of the transfer of the killing signal in ADCC would be the simultaneous binding of both domains to both receptor binding sites, the killing could be abolished when the binding of the domains to the corresponding binding sites is inhibited separately.

Since the first complement component (Clq) binds to the CH2 domain of IgG and the isolated FcRI molecules interact with the CH3 domain, the application of these substances allowed us to demonstrate a selective inhibition of the interaction of CH2 and CH3 domains with the corresponding sites of FcRII on the K cells and test its effect on ADCC. Since Clq and the soluble FcRI dose-dependently inhibited the ADCC, we could conclude that the simultaneous binding through both binding sites is really the precondition for the FcR-mediated killing in ADCC (4).

Inhibition of receptor-domain interaction by synthetic polypeptides

These results came up to our expectations concerning our "two binding sites" FcR model, however, these experiments were not suitable for the finer mapping of the interacting sites on the IgG Fc domains. In order to localize sites within the Fc region of IgG responsible for the interaction with the binding sites of the FcRII on K cells, the effect of synthetic peptides comprising sequences of the human γ 1 chain (Listed in Table I) on ADCC was studied by us.

Three peptides (Y48, Y51 and Y91), representatives of CH2 domain sequences, and one peptide (Y98), a slightly modified CH3 sequence showed dose dependent inhibitory activity in ADCC (Fig. 1). To control whether this inhibitory effect was to the consequence of a stable binding of the peptides to the FcR binding sites, the effector cells were spun down after the peptide treatment, and both the killing capacity of the washed cells and the effect of the supernatants on ADCC activity of fresh lymphocytes were tested. We found that the washing of the pretreated K cells did not abolish the inhibitory effect of the peptides and the preincubation of the peptide solution with the FcR bearing lymphocytes resulted in the loss of their ADCC-inhibitory capacity. These point to a stable interaction of the peptides and the K cells, and may mean that a portion of the synthetic peptides adopted the biologically active conformation which allowed the high affinity binding to the receptor binding sites.

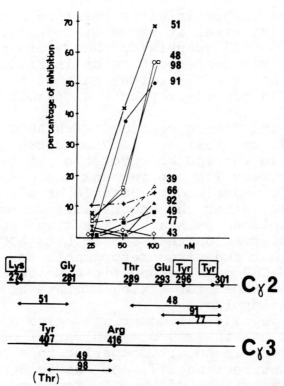

Fig. 1. Effect of synthetic peptides on ADCC

Table I AMINO ACID SEQUENCES OF THE SYNTHETIC PEPTIDES STUDIED

PEPTIDE No.	N terminus /sequence/ C terminus	Location on chain
Y 51	Lys-Phe-Asp-Trp-Tyr-Val-Asn-Gly	IgG CH2 domain 274-281
Y 48	Thr-Lys-Pro-Arg-Glu-Gln-Gln-Tyr-Asp-Ser-Thr-Tyr-Arg	IgG CH2 domain 289-3o1
Y 91	Glu-Gln-Gln-Tyr-Asp-Ser-Thr-Tyr-Arg	IgG CH2 domain 293-3o1
Y 77	Gln-Tyr-Asp-Ser-Thr-Tyr-Arg	IgG CH2 domain 295-3o1
Y 49	Tyr-Ser-Lys-Leu-Thr-Val-Asp-Lys-Ser-Arg	IgG CH3 domain 4o7-416
Y 98	(Thr)-Ser-Lys-Leu-Thr-Val-Asp-Lys-Ser-Arg	IgG CH3 domain (4o7)-416
Y 66	Val-Phe-Ser-Arg-Leu-Gln-Thr-Arg-Ala-Glu	IgE CH4 domain 5o5-515
Y 92	Tyr-Tyr-Ser-Glu-Thr-Asp-Arg	nonsense peptide
Y 39	Gly-Trp-Met-Asp-Phe-Gly	C terminal end of gastrin

As to the subdomain sites reacting with the FcRII binding sites it seems of significance that peptide Y77 comprising the C-terminal part of peptide Y48 turned out to be ineffective. This suggests that the N-terminal part of the ADCC-blocking Y48 peptide may be responsible for the inhibitory activity.

The two CH2 domain peptides with ADCC blocking effect (Y48 and Y51) are located close to each other within the IgG Fc. Moreover, the only difference between Y51 peptide and the C1-binding octapeptide described by Boackle et al. (11) is that in the latter the Phe residue in position 275 was replaced by Ala. Taken together these and our observation that C1q ihibits ADCC, we may conclude that the sites responsible for the binding to the CH2 domain-specific site of FcRII on K cells and those for fixing C1q are at least partly overlapping.

The nonapeptide Y91 comprising also a sequence of the CH2 domain (293/Glu/-301/Arg/) proved to be inhibitory in ADCC. Comparing this peptide with the ineffective Y77, one has to consider the possible importance of the Glu residue in position 293 in forming the conformation which allows the high affinity binding to the corresponding site of FcRII. Moreover, one may speculate on the role of residues characteristic for the γ1 subclass in this respect. We point to the Lys residue in position 274 (present in peptide Y51) and on the Tyr residues in positions 296 and 300 (present in peptides Y48 and Y91).

Based on these one may suggest that the *groups which react with one of the binding sites of FcRII are situated within the CH2 domain in the region of residues 274/Lys/ - 301/Arg/. The interacting groups on CH3 domain may comprise the region of 408/Ser/ - 416/Arg/ residues (Fig. 1).*

Inhibition of receptors-domain interaction by monoclonal antibodies

Monoclonal antibodies with defined specificity

proved to be excellent tools for definition of
epitopes localised within individual domains of
IgG Fc. A panel of monoclonal antibodies detecting epitopes expressed within the Cγ3 or Cγ2 domains, or others dependent on the native conformation of the intact Fc region of IgG (listed in
Table II) were used in the present study to localise the interacting groups with the binding
site(s) of FcRII-s on K cells. Labelled anti-D
IgG sensitized human red blood cells were pretreated with dilutions of ascitic fluid containing monoclonal antibodies and the ADCC activity
of lymphocytes to pretreated target cells was
measured. Fig. 2 shows that some antibodies having specificity for Cγ2 or Cγ3 domain epitopes
inhibited dose dependently and significantly the
ADCC, whilst others gave no inhibition. Similar
inhibition was obtained with antibodies specific
for IgG1 subclass, while anohter monoclonal antibody having specificity for a Cγ1 domain epitope
exerted no inhibitory effect.

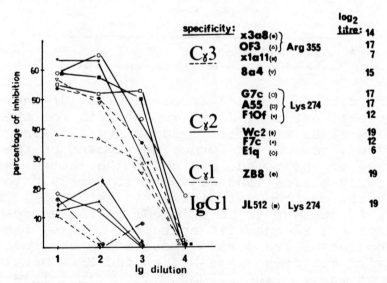

Fig. 2   Effect of Cγ2 and Cγ3 specific mono-
        clonal antibodies on ADCC

Table II

INHIBITION OF ADCC BY ASCITES FLUIDS CONTAINING MONOCLONAL
ANTIBODIES AGAINST HUMAN IgG

Monoclonals	% ADCC INHIBITION				$\log_2$ titres
Dilutions:	1	10^2	10^3	10^4	(hemagglutination)
anti-Cγ3					
8a4	57	49	25	o	15
x1a11	11	o	-	-	7
x3a8	54	5o	35	o	14
OF3	38	37	28	o	16
anti-Cγ2					
G7c	59	65	43	17	17
F1oF	64	63	28	11	12
A55	55	52	53	o	17
QF1	56	38	3o	o	15
JD 312	35	37	34	28	16
F7c	13	16	nd	nd	9
JD 79	32	17	nd	nd	13
E1g	18	13	nd	nd	6
WC2	14	23	nd	nd	19
anti-Cγ1					
Z86	17	o	8	nd	16
anti-IgG1					
JL512	59	58	5o	o	8
NL 16	41	19	o	o	12

Target:effector ratio in ADCC: 1:1o

The numbers represent the average % inhibition of ADCC of 6 donors

According to Nik Jaafar et al. (12-13) the monoclonal antibody JL512 is specific for the IgG1 subclass specific residues Lys/274/ and Tyr/296/. Since the former is exposed on the surface of the molecules, while the latter is partially buried (and adjacent to Asp/297/ to which the carbohydrate moiety is attached), the Lys/274/ appears to be critical to the expression of the γ1 specific epitopes. Hence, the antibodies of Cγ2 domain specificity are reactive with epitopes expressed on the N-terminal region of the Fy face of the Cγ2 domain. This is in good agreement with the inhibitory effect of peptide Y51 containing the Lys/274/ and allows

the site for the FcR recognition to be localised
to the N-terminal region of the CH2 domain.
   Both CH3 and CH2 domain specific monoclonal
antibodies inhibited separately the killing activity of K cells supporting our "two binding site
FcR model" in agreement with the results obtained
with Clq and soluble FcRI. Moreover, these observations are consistent with the synthetic polypeptide findings, that the simultaneous interaction of the two Fc-domains with two binding sites
is the prerequisite of killing.

SUMMARY

Crosslinked (anchored) IgG Fc receptors possessing two binding sites, one of which interacting
with the Cγ2, the other with the Cγ3 domain of
the IgG molecule characterise the effector cells
(K cells) of the antibody-dependent cell-mediated
cytotoxicity (ADCC). The simultaneous interaction of the Fc-domains of the sensitizing antibody with both binding sites of FcR-s on K cells
is the prerequeisite of triggering of killing
activity. Clq or Cγ2 specific monoclonal antibodies, as well as synthetic polypeptides comprising sequences of the Cγ2 domain dose-dependently inhibited the ADCC. Similar inhibition was
found when soluble FcRI and monoclonal antibodies
which bind to the Cγ3 domain, or a synthetic
polypeptide representative of a slightly modified
Cγ3 sequence was used. Evidence was provided
suggesting that the groups reacting with one of
the FcRII binding sites are situated within the
Cγ2 domain in the region of residues 274/Lys/ -
301/Arg/. The interacting groups on Cγ3 domain
may involve the residues of 408/Ser/ - 416/Arg/.

REFERENCES

Sármay G., István L. and Gergely J. (1978) Shedding and reappearance of Fc, C3 and SRBC receptors on peripheral lymphocytes from normal

donors and chronic lymphatic leukaemia (CLL) patients. Immunology 34, 315-321.

Sármay G., Iványi J. and Gergely J. (1980) The involvement of preformed cytoplasmic Fc receptor pool in the expression of Fc receptors following their interactions with various antibodies Cell Immunol. 56, 452-464.

Sármay G. and Gergely J. (1983) Activation of lymphocytes alters Fc receptor and β-2-microglobulin interrelationship on the lymphocyte surface. Cell. Immunol. 78, 73-81.

Sármay G., Benczur M., Petrányi Gy., Klein E., Kahn M., Stanworth D.R. and Gergely J. (1984) Ligand inhibition studies on the role of Fc receptors in antibody-dependent cell-mediated cytotoxicity. Molec. Immunol. 21, 43-51.

Sándor M., Füst G., Medgyesi G.A., Erdei A. and Gergely J. (1978) Isolation and characterisation of Fc receptors shed from human peripheral mononuclear blood cells. Immunology 35, 559-566.

Sándor M., Füst G., Medgyesi G.A., Erdei A. and Gergely J. (1979) The heterogeneity of Fc receptors on human peripheral mononuclear blood cells. Immunology 38, 553-560.

Gergely J., Erdei A., Sándor M., Sármay G. and Uher F. (1982) The Fc receptor model of membrane cytoplasmic signalling. Molec. Immunol. 19, 1223-1228.

Gergely J., Sándor M., Sármay G. and Uher F. (in press) Fc receptors on lymphocytes and K cells. Transactions of the Biochemical Society.

Fésüs L., Sándor M., Erdei A. and Gergely J. (1982) The influence of tissue transglutaminase on the function of Fc receptors. Molec. Immunol. 19, 39-43.

Uher F., Jancsó Á., Sándor M., Pintér K., Biro E.N.A. and Gergely J. (1981) Interaction between actomyosin complexes and Fc receptors of human peripheral mononuclear cells. Immunol. Lett. 2, 213-217.

Boackle R.J., Johnson B.J. and Caughman G.B. (1980) An IgG primary sequence theory for complement activation using synthetic peptides. Nature, London 282, 742-743.

Nik Jafaar M.I., Lowe J.A., Ling N.R. and Jefferis R. (1983) Immunogenic and antigenic epitopes of Immunoglobulins - V. Reactivity of a panel of monoclonal antibodies with sub-fragments of human Fc and abnormal paraproteins having deletions. Molec. Immunol. 20, 679-686.

Nik Jafaar M.I., Lowe J.A., Ling N.R. and Jefferis R. (1984) Immunogenic and antigenic epitopes of immunoglobulins - VII. Distribution of Fc epitopes and the relationship of and iso-allotypic specificity to the presence of histidine 435. Molec. Immunol. 21, 137-145.

APPLICATIONS OF RADIOIMMUNOASSAY IN ANTENATAL CARE

R.J.S. HOWELL & T. CHARD,
Departments of Obstetrics, Gynaecology and Reproductive
Physiology, St. Bartholomew's Hospital Medical College
and the London Hospital Medical College, London, UK.

Present day antenatal care consists largely of diagnosis.
Three means are available for detecting an increased
risk to the life or health of the fetus. The first lies
in the clinical facts of the situation, interpreted from
epidemiological data. The second is in biophysical
examination of the fetus by ultrasound or cardiotoco-
graphy, and the third is biochemical measurement of feto-
placental products in maternal body fluids. The technique of radioimmunoassay (RIA) has played a major role
in the biochemical assessment of fetal well-being and
here we will discuss the more important pregnancy protein
molecules to which this technique has been applied.

HUMAN CHORIONIC GONADOTROPHIN (hCG)

Chorionic gonadotrophin consists of two amino acid chains
(alpha and beta subunits) linked by non-covalent bonds,
both chains having carbohydrate residues. The alpha
subunit is the common subunit of all the glycoprotein
hormones; the beta subunit is similar to that of
luteinising hormone (LH) but has an additional 30 amino
acids at the carboxy-terminus. Chorionic gonadotrophin
may play an important role in maintenance of the corpus
luteum in early pregnancy. Radioimmunoassays for hCG
use antibodies either to the whole molecule or to the
beta subunit. The latter are considerably more specific
with respect to LH and are now the assays of choice.

Qualitative hCG measurement by particle agglutination
is the most commonly used pregnancy test. Quantitative
measurement by RIA is used in a variety of clinical
situations: (1) monitoring of trophoblastic tumours;
(b) prognosis of threatened abortion. For example, in
one study on 198 patients, normal levels of hCG were
associated with a satisfactory outcome in 92% of

Proceedings of the 16th FEBS Congress
Part A, pp. 197–205
© 1985 VNU Science Press

cases (1). The doubling time of hCG in the first few weeks of pregnancy is 2-3 days, and small dating errors make a critical difference to interpretation of values. For this reason, serial measurements are more predictive than single measurements; (c) estimation of gestational age in the first 60 days of pregnancy. This estimate has a confidence interval of 12-15 days (Fig. 1);

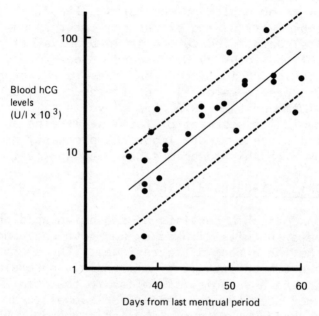

FIGURE I: ESTIMATION OF GESTATIONAL AGE

(d) differential diagnosis of ectopic pregnancy (2). Measurement of hCG has been advocated as an investigation in cases of lower abdominal pain in young women.

HUMAN PLACENTAL LACTOGEN (hPL)

This is a placental hormone consisting of a single 191 amino acid chain, two disulphide bonds and no carbo- hydrate residues. It is chemically and functionally similar to pituitary growth hormone and prolactin, but with less biological activity.

198

Clinical measurement of maternal blood levels of hPL
are usually performed by RIA or non-isotopic variants of
this technique. The levels in maternal blood show a progressive rise with a plateau after 35 weeks. It may play
a role in the control of carbohydrate and lipid metabolism, though this function cannot be crucial since in
rare cases hPL is absent with no apparent detrimental
effects (3).

Measurement of hPL has been used in a variety of clinical situations: (a) threatened abortion: low maternal
hPL levels after the 10th week of pregnancy indicate a
poor prognosis (4); (b) growth retardation: levels of
hPL detect this condition with a sensitivity of around
40% (5). Levels of hPL are lower in small babies with
evidence of dysmaturity than in small but normal babies
(Fig. 2). Placental lactogen levels are also reduced in

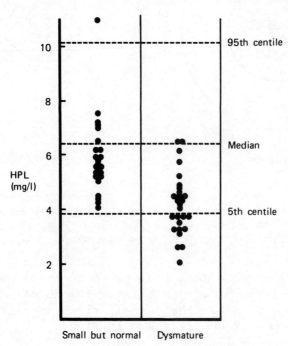

FIGURE 11: hPL LEVELS IN DYSMATURITY

cases of placental insufficiency with apparently normal
delivery weight (6). The low levels of hPL associated
with growth retardation are independent of the cause of
the condition or of other complications; (c) diabetic
pregnancies are associated with elevated hPL levels but
these are reduced below the 'normal range' for diabetics
when placental dysfunction supervenes (7); (d) fetal
distress: low levels of hPL may be predictive of acute
problems in labour (fetal distress) (5) when due to
long-term placental insufficiency (Fig. 3).

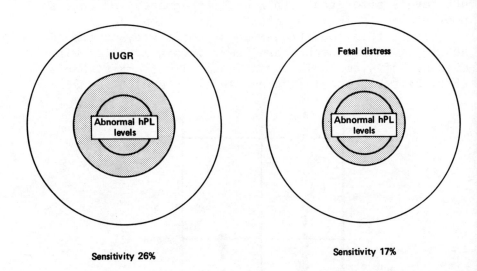

FIGURE III: hPL AS A PREDICTOR OF FETAL DISTRESS

 As with all other biochemical tests of fetal well-
being, there is much overlap between the normal and
abnormal range of hPL. The overall risk associated with
different ranges of hPL is shown in figure 4.

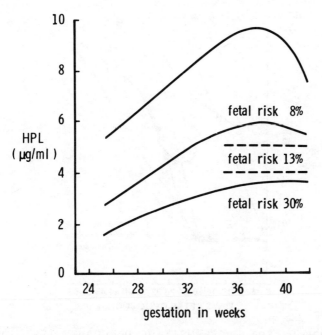

FIGURE IV: FETAL RISK AT DIFFERING hPL LEVELS

SCHWANGERSCHAFTS PROTEIN 1 (SP1)

This placental protein, first characterised by Bohn in
1971 (8) is a beta-1 globulin; 30% of the molecule
consists of carbohydrate including sialic acid. The biological activity, if any, is unknown. High levels of
SP1 are present in maternal plasma in late pregnancy (9)
and can readily be detected by immunoprecipitation
methods. The low levels in early pregnancy require an
RIA (10), but it appears at a very early stage and may
have value as a sensitive pregnancy test (Fig. 5).
Measurement of SP1 has been evaluated in a number of
clinical situations: (a) threatened abortion: low levels
have a predictive value of 96% (11); growth retardation:
Levels of SP1 are reduced in this condition (Fig. 6).
This reduction is seen in the presence or absence of
hypertension, i.e. like hPL it is unrelated to the cause

201

of growth retardation.

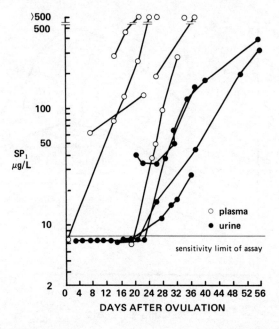

FIGURE V: SP1 - A SENSITIVE PREGNANCY TEST

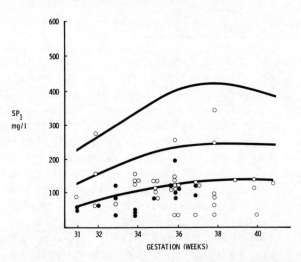

FIGURE VI: SP1 LEVELS IN GROWTH RETARDATION
WITH (●) AND WITHOUT (○) HYPERTENSION

202

PLACENTAL PROTEIN 5 (PP5)

Placental protein 5 is a beta-1 globulin with a carbohydrate content of 12%. It may exist in a number of
different molecular forms (12). The concentration in
maternal blood is relatively low and can only be measured
by RIA. Placental protein 5 has activities analogous to
antithrombin III and it may act as a natural anticoagu-
lant at the placental site (13).

Although levels in late pregnancy are unrelated to
fetal weight, it is not a good test for fetal growth
retardation as the sensitivity is only 17% (14). However, it may have some predictive value in cases of placental abruption; elevated levels are sometimes found
prior to the incident (13). Elevated levels are also
found at 16 weeks gestation in patients subsequently
developing preterm labour (15); if this can be confirmed
it would provide a uniquely useful test in antenatal
care.

ALPHAFETOPROTEIN (AFP)

Alphafetoprotein is physicochemically similar to albumin
and is present in large amounts in fetal tissues and
certain tumours. It was first identified in 1956 and
its relationship to fetal neural tube defects emerged in
the early 1970's (16). In the presence of such a defect,
AFP leaks across exposed fetal capillaries and reaches
high levels in amniotic fluid and, secondarily, in
maternal blood (Fig. 7). Measurement in the latter site
forms the basis of a population screening programme
which leads to the identification and termination of
80-98% of these defects.

A recent finding of great potential interest is the
observation of low maternal AFP levels in association
with Downs' syndrome of the fetus. This may prove to
be as good a predictor of this condition as advanced
maternal age.

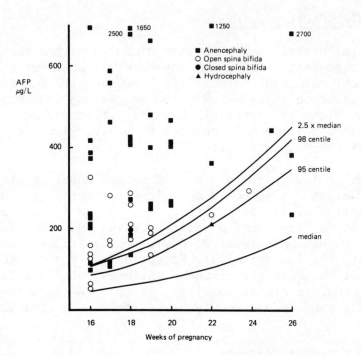

FIGURE VII: MATERNAL AFP LEVELS IN NEURAL TUBE DEFECTS

REFERENCES

1. Jouppila P, Tapanainen J, Huhtanieni I (1979). Plasma
   hCG levels in patients with bleeding in the first and
   second trimester of pregnancy. Br J Obstet Gynaecol.
   86: 343.
2. Seppala M, Tontti K, Ranta T, Stenman UH, Chard T
   (1980). Use of a rapid hCG-beta-subunit radioimmunoassay in acute gynaecological emergencies. Lancet. i,
   165.
3. Nielsen PV, Pedersen H, Kampmann E-M (1979). Absence
   of human placental lactogen in an otherwise unevent-
   ful pregnancy. Am J Obstet Gynecol. 135: 322.
4. Niven PAR, Landon J, Chard T (1972). Placental
   lactogen levels as a guide to outcome of threatened
   abortion. Br Med J. ii, 799.
5. Morrison I, Green P, Oomen B (1980). The role of
   human placental lactogen assays in antepartum fetal

assessment. Am J Obstet Gynecol. 136, 1055.
6. Daikoku NH, Tyson JE, Graf C, Scott R, Smith B, Johnston JWC, King TM (1979). The relative significance of human placental lactogen in the diagnosis of retarded fetal growth. J Obstet Gynecol. 135, 516.
7. Ursell W, Brudenell M, Chard T (1973). Placental lactogen levels in diabetic pregnancy. Br Med J. i, 80-82.
8. Bohn H (1971). Nachweis und charakteriserung von schwangerschaftsproteinen in der menschilichen plazenta sowie ihre quantitative immunologische bestimmung in serum schwangerer frauen. Arch Gynaekol 210, 440-457.
9. Klopper A, Masson G, Wilson G (1977). Plasma oestriol and placental proteins: a cross-sectional study at 38 weeks gestation. Br J Obstet Gynaecol 86, 648-655.
10. Grudzinskas JG, Gordon YB, Jeffrey D, Chard T. (19 Specific and sensitive determination of pregnancy specific β1 glycoprotein (SP1) by radioimmunoassay: a new pregnancy test. Lancet, i, 333-335.
11. Jouppila P, Seppala M, Chard T (1980). Pregnancy specific β1 glycoprotein in complications of early pregnancy. Lancet, i, 667.
12. Salem HT, Obiekwe BC, Al-Ani ATM, Seppala M, Chard T (1980). Molecular heterogeneity of placental protein 5 (PP5) in late pregnancy serum and plasma: evidence for a heparin-PP5 polymer. Clin Chim Acta 107, 211.
13. Salem HT, Westergaard JG, Hinderson P, Seppala M, Chard T (1981). Placental protein 5 (PP5) in placental abruption. Br J Obstet Gynaecol 80, 500.
14. Obiekwe BC, Grudzinskas JG, Chard T (1980). Circulating levels of placental protein 5 in the mother: relation to birthweight. Br J Obstet Gynaecol. 87, 302-304.
15. Salem HT, Lee, JN, Seppala M, Vaara L, Aula P, Al-Ani ATM, Chard T (1981). Measurement of placental protein 5 (PP5), placental lactogen and pregnancy specific β1 glycoprotein in mid trimester as a predictor of outcome of pregnancy. Br J Obstet Gynaecol 88, 371.
16. Brock DJH, Sutcliffe RG (1972). AFP in the antenatal diagnosis of anencephaly and spina bifida. Lancet ii, 197-199.

COMPETITION BETWEEN THYROXINE 5' MONODEIODINASE ENZYME AND THE OXIDATIVE PROCESSES OF NEUTROPHILS IN AN AUTOIMMUNE DISEASE

J.T. NAGY, I. SZOTJKA, M. HAUCK, G. FÓRIS,
A. LEÖVEY.
1. Dept. of Medicine, Medical University of
Debrecen, Pf. 19. Debrecen, Hungary

INTRODUCTION

The evidence that triiodothyronine $/T_3/$ and reverse triiodothyronine $/rT_3/$ are produced in substantial quantities from peripheral metabolism of thyroxine $/T_4/$ was among the most interesting developments of thyroidology in the last ten years. 60-90 % of the physiologically more active hormone T_3 is the result of peripheral enzymic monodeiodination of T_4 which process is strongly NADPH dependent and the importance of reduced form of glutathione was also reported. Inner or outer ring deiodination resulting rT_3 or T_3 are not random processes. The decreased level of T_3 with simultaneous increase or normal values of serum rT_3 in systemic illnesses such as chronic renal failure, hepatic cirrhosis indicated that close correlation between tissue catabolism and deiodination can be expected. The in vitro experiments demonstrated that human tissues including liver, heart, kidney, fibroblasts and peripheral blood neutrophils have significant monodeiodinase activity. Recently the immunmodulatory role of thyroid hormones was demonstrated /1,2/.

The possible correlation between the T_4 to T_3 conversion and the immune system turned our attention to the deiodinating function of peripheral blood neutrophils.

Human neutrophils have an intensive reactive oxygen species generating system for defense

Proceedings of the 16th FEBS Congress
Part A, pp. 207–215
© 1985 VNU Science Press

against invading micro-organisms and host tissues. The production of highly reactive oxygen metabolits for example superoxide, hydrogen peroxide, hydroxyl radical, hypochlorous acide the so called oxidative burst has been the focus of interest for the last years because of its central role in the mechanisms by which granulocytes kill micro-organisms /3/.

The key role of NADPH, NADPH oxidase, reduced and oxidized forms of glutathione in the reactive oxygen species generating system is evident but the same enzymes and molecules are also involved in the in vitro monodeiodination of T_4 to T_3. Therefore it seemed for us probable that there is a competition between the oxidative burst of human neutrophils and the monodeiodinating function of these cells.

EXPERIMENTAL RESULTS

In a preliminary study we have found that living suspensions of human granulocytes are able to convert T_4 to T_3 in our in vitro system. The monodeiodinase activity was measured as the amount of T_3 produced by the cells /8/ while significant enzymic activity was found.

In order to demonstrate the effect of monodeiodination on the effector function of granulocytes two generally accepted indicators: antibody dependent cellular cytotoxicity /ADCC/ that is extracellular killing and intracellular killing was detected on the effect of thyroxine /Fig. 1-2/. Both markers were significantly decreased representing the alteration of the effector functions of granulocytes during the possible activation of the granulocyte monodeiodinase enzyme by its substrate thyroxine.

Therefore in the next series of the experiments we examined whether this decrease of the effector functions is in correlation with the NADPH linked oxidative burst or not. A speci-

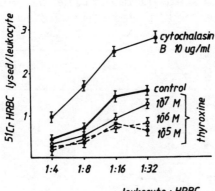

Fig. 1. The effect of thyroxine on the ADCC activity of human neutrophils. The number of lysed ^{51}Cr labelled human red blood cells /^{51}CrHRBC/ is the indicator of the ADCC. The measurement was carried out at different target: effector cell ratios /4/.

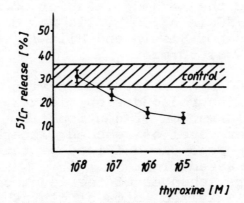

Fig.2. The effect of thyroxine on the intracellular killing activity of human neutrophils measured by ^{51}Cr labelled Candida albicans. The indicator of the killing activity is the amount of released activity which was expressed as the percentage of total phagocytosed activity according to Yamamura et al. /5/.

fic indicator of the granulocyte oxidative burst the superoxide production as well as reduced and oxidized glutathione /G-SH, GS-SG/ content of the cells were measured. It was

T_4	O_2^-	G-SH	GS-SG
none	$44,8 \pm 2,0$	295 ± 7	$22 \pm 1,8$
$10^{-5}M$	$23,7 \pm 1,5^x$	172 ± 5^x	$49 \pm 2,1^x$
$10^{-6}M$	$28,4 \pm 1,7^x$	-	-
$10^{-7}M$	$37,1 \pm 1,9$	-	-

mean $\pm$ SEM of 5 experiments
x p 0,01

Table I. Glutathione levels and superoxide /O_2^-/ production of granulocytes on the effect of thyroxine. O_2^- production in nmol ferricytochrome C/30 min/5x10^6 cells was measured according to the method of Babior et al. /6/, G-SH and GS-SG in ng/10^6 cells was detected by the method of Hissin and Hilf /7/. Incubation time was 60 min.

found that 60 min preincubation with 10^{-5}- 10^{-6}M thyroxine reduced significantly the superoxide formation of neutrophils. Intracellular level of reduced glutathione decreased whereas the oxidized glutathione content increased /Table I./.
Furthermore, changes of the level of reduced and oxidized forms of glutathione were measured in human neutrophils as well as monodeiodinase activity of these cells were detected during yeast cell phagocytosis. A similar effect on the glutathione level was found as on the effect of thyroxine.

Simultaneous decrease of monodeiodinase enzyme activity was observed /Table II./.

Time /min/	G-SH	GS-SG	Deiodinase activity
0	298 ± 6	$19\pm2,1$	$46,1\pm1,8$
30	112 ± 9^x	$27\pm2,0$	$29,9\pm3,0^x$
60	125 ± 8^x	$49\pm1,7^x$	$20,5\pm2,8^x$
120	206 ± 8	$41\pm1,8^x$	$31,4\pm2,7$

mean$\pm$SEM of 5 experiments
x p 0,01

Table II. Glutathione levels and monodeiodinase activity during yeast cell phagocytosis. Enzymatic activity was measured according to the method of Ozawa et al. /8/ as the amount of produced T_3 /pmol/30 min/ 10^7 cells/. For glutathione determination see the legend of Table 1.

Such effect of phagocytic stimuli on the level of oxidized and reduced forms of glutathione is wellknown but our data suggest that not only excitation of granulocytes by such stimuli but monodeiodinase activation by its substrate thyroxine /Table I./ is able to increase the intracellular conversion of reduced glutathione to the oxidized form.

In the last series of our experiments some clinical aspects of our in vitro results were studied. Two groups of patients: one with autoimmune thyroiditis and the other with chronic renal failure were compared to healthy subjects whether any correlation between the oxidative burst of their granulocytes and the monodeiodinase activity of them exists or not.

Parameter	Contr. /20/	Immune thyr. /19/	Chr. renal failure /15/
Deiodinase act./prod. T_3 in pmol/ 30 min/10^7 cells/	$36\pm2,0$	$17\pm1,5$	$21\pm1,9$
O_2 consumption /nmol/ min/10^6c/	$5,9\pm0,2$	$9,3\pm0,2$	$2,2\pm0,1$
Chemiluminescence /count/ 40 min/	$5,6 \times 10^6$	$18,7 \times 10^6$	$1,2 \times 10^6$
O_2^- prod. during phagocytosis nmol cytochromeC/30 min/5×10^6 cells/	$68,7\pm1,2$	$22,4\pm0,9$	$10,8\pm0,5$
Glutathione peroxidase /nmol NADPH/ min/10^6cells[x] /	147 ± 6	168 ± 5	52 ± 5
Glutathione reductase /nmol NADPH /min/10^6cells[x] /	105 ± 3	67 ± 2	56 ± 3
GS-SG/ G-SH	$0,13\pm 0,02$	$0,30\pm 0,02$	$0,28\pm 0,01$

Table III. Comparison of parameters of human neutrophils separeted from healthy donors and patients. [x]Methods see as ref.7

Data obtained from the chronic renal failure group are relatively easy to explain. The granulocytes of these patients are characterized by decreased activity of the reactive oxygen species generating system. The signs of this are demonstrated on Table III. On the other hand a significant fall in the monodeiodinase enzyme activity was found which is characterized by the decrease in the amount of T_3 produced by the granulocytes.

It is more difficult to explain the results of the immune thyroiditis group. Data shows the increased oxygen consumption, spontaneous chemiluminescencewhich are signs of the excited state of the reactive oxygen species generating system. In contrast superoxide production stimulated by phagocytosis decreased significantly. It means that despite of this excited state, the NADPH-linked oxidative burst is functionally insufficient. Furthermore, a significant decrease of the activity of glutathione reductase enzyme was accompanied with the elevated ratio of the oxidized/reduced glutathione as well as in the chronic renal failure group. A measurable fall in the monodeiodinase activity was detected in this group of patients too.

DISCUSSION

In vitro monodeiodination of thyroxine in granulocytes has an inhibitory effect on their superoxide formation, diminishes the reduced glutathione content of them and decreases the effector function of the cells characterized by ADCC and intracellular killing. Granulocytes with an excited oxidative burst caused by phagocytosis partially loose their capability for enzymatic monodeiodination of T_4. Therefore we conclude that a unique form of correlation exists betweem the immune and endocrine regulation of human granulocytes. The competition between the catabolism of T_4 and the respiratory burst is an example of this correlation and it could be explained by the NADPH dependency of both processes.

Impaired granulocyte oxidative burst in patients with chronic renal failure and decrease of glutathione reductase enzyme activity in the autoimmune thyroiditis patients group is accompanied with measurable fall of monodeiodinase activity. We can conclude that the hypothesis of the competition and correlation between the granulocyte oxidative burst and monodeiodinase activity was strenghthened by the investigations which were carried out in these two groups of patients.

REFERENCES

1. Chopra, I.J., Solomon, D.H., Chopra, O., Wu, S-y., Fisher, D.A., Nakamura, Y./1978/. Pathways of metabolism of thyroid hormones. Rec.Progr.Horm.Res. 34, 521-567.
2. Gupta, M.K., Chiang, T., Deodhar, S. /1983/. Effect of thyroxine on immune response in C57Bl/6J mice. Acta Endocrinol. /Copenh/. 103, 76-80.
3. Babior, B.M. /1984/. The respiratory burst of phagocytes. J.Clin.Invest. 73, 599-601.
4. Cordier, G., Samarut, C., Revillard, J.P. /1981/. Distinct functions of surface receptors in the induction of neutrophil-mediated cytotoxicity. Ann. Immunol. 132, 3-14.
5. Yamamura, M., Boler, J., Valdimarsson, H. /1976/. A [51]chromium release assay for phagocytic killing of Candida albicans. J.Immunol.Meths. 13, 227-233.
6. Babior, B.M., Kipnes, R.S., Curnutte, J.T. /1973/. The production by leucocytes of superoxide, a potential bactericidal agent. J.Clin.Invest. 52, 741-744.

7. Hissin, P.J., Hilf, R. /1976/. A fluorometric method for determination of oxidized and reduced glutathione in tissues. Anal. Biochem. 74, 214-226.
8. Ozawa, Y., Shimizu, T., Shishiba, Y. /1981/. effect of sulfhydryl reagents of the conversion of thyroxine to 3,5,3'-triiodothyronine:direct action on thyroxine molecules. Endocrinology 110, 241-245.
9. Beutler, E. /1975/. Red cell metabolism. In: A Manual of Biochemical Methods. Grune and Stratton, New York, pp. 69-73.

THE ROLE OF THE VARIOUS LIVER CELL TYPES IN LDL AND MODIFIED LDL CATABOLISM

THEO J.C. VAN BERKEL[1], LEEN HARKES[1], J. FRED NAGELKERKE[1] AND HERMAN JAN M. KEMPEN[2]

[1] Department of Biochemistry I, Erasmus University Rotterdam, P.O. Box 1738, 3000 DR Rotterdam, The Netherlands.
[2] Gaubius Institute, Health Research Division TNO, Herenstraat 5d, Leiden, The Netherlands.

High levels of low density lipoproteins (LDL) are correlated with an increased occurrence of atherosclerosis. Because the liver is the only organ where cholesterol, carried in LDL, can be removed irreversibly from the blood, we were interested in the quantitative role of the liver in LDL turnover. Furthermore it is important to know the specific cellular sites inside the liver which are involved in the LDL uptake. In order to attach this problem we labeled LDL with ^{14}C-sucrose. After cell-binding and uptake of LDL the ^{14}C-labeled degradation products of LDL remain for several hours entrapped intracellularly and form during this time a cumulative measure for uptake (1). Fig. 1. indicates that upto 4.5 hours after intravenous injection into rats accumulation of LDL in the liver occurs and that upto 35% of the injected LDL is then recovered in liver. With iodinated LDL never more than 2% is found at any time in liver (2). Because at 4.5 hours after LDL injection about 50% of the LDL is removed from serum the 35% accumulation indicates that the liver is responsible for at least 70% of the removal of LDL from the blood.
Fig. 2 illustrates the relative importance of the different liver cell types. At the indicated times after injection of LDL parenchymal and non-parenchymal liver cells were isolated and the uptake was determined. Notice the different scales for parenchymal cells (left side) and non-parenchymal cells (right side). It can be seen that non-parenchymal cells accumulate at least 60 times higher amounts of ^{14}C-sucrose LDL then parenchymal cells. However because non-parenchymal cells contain only 7.5% of the

total liver protein and parenchymal cells 92.5% (4) the
low specific uptake in the parenchymal cells has to be
multiplied by a high contribution of these cells to total
liver protein in order to assess the contribution of these
cells to the total liver uptake. Such a calculation indicates that 29% of the liver uptake of LDL is exerted by
parenchymal cells while the non-parenchymal liver cells
are responsible for 71% of the total liver uptake of ^{14}C-
sucrose LDL.

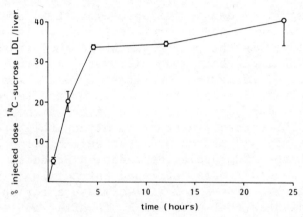

Fig. 1
Association of ^{14}C-sucrose LDL with liver at different
times after injection.
Values are means of 3 experiments ± SEM

Although the regulation of the level of LDL is important
for lowering the risk for atherosclerosis, current theo-
ries do not directly relate the native LDL uptake with
the formation of foam cells. A hypothetical mechanism involved in the conversion of mononuclear phagocytes to foam
cells was proposed by Goldstein and Brown (5) and in this
theory native LDL is converted to a modified form either
chemically with malondialdehyde or acetic anhydride or
biologically upon incubation with umibilical vein endothelial cells (6). These modified forms of LDL are then
supposed to induce formation of foam cells in the atherosclerotic plaque. In order to determine to what extent

the liver could form a protection system against these
modified and so-called atherogenic forms of LDL we determined the uptake of acetylated and biologically modified
LDL in the various liver cell types. The endothelial-
cell modified LDL, when injected in vivo into rats, is
more rapidly cleared from the blood than native LDL and
it is quantitatively recovered in the liver (6).

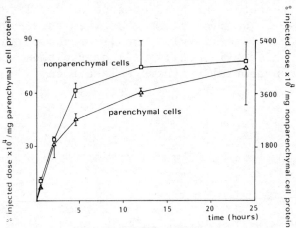

Fig. 2
Cell association of ^{14}C-sucrose LDL with parenchymal and
non-parenchymal cells at different times after intravenous injection.
[14]C-sucrose LDL association with cells was determined
after a low temperature (8°C) isolation and purification
procedure (3). Values are from 2-3 experiments ± SEM.

The cell types which are responsible for the increased
disappearance of EC-modified LDL from the blood are indicated in Fig. 3. It can be seen that upon incubation of
LDL with umbilical vein endothelial cells specifically the
uptake in parenchymal and endothelial liver cells increases. These uptake values are expressed as % of the injected dose/mg cell protein but notice the 20 fold difference
in scale needed to quantify the endothelial cell uptake.
For comparison also the uptake of chemically modified LDL
(upon acetylation) is indicated and this figure suggests
that the relative uptake of acetyl-LDL in the various
liver cell types is similar to EC-modified LDL and is

possibly mediated by a single receptor. To investigate
this point more clearly, rat liver endothelial cells were
incubated in vitro with radiolabeled EC—modified LDL and
different quantities of unlabeled acetyl-LDL and it is
found that acetyl-LDL very effectively competes with EC-
modified LDL (7). These data indicate that both acetylated
and endothelial-cell modified LDL interact with the active
scavenger receptor which is present on rat liver endothelial cells. It will be clear that when these modified LDL
forms are generated in vivo the liver and in particular
the liver endothelial cells will entrap them and so prevent their potentially atherogenic action.

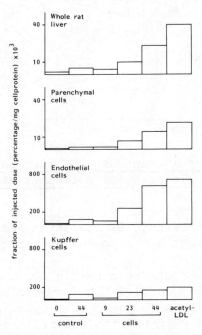

Fig. 3
Cell association of ^{125}I-labeled LDL with liver, parenchymal, endothelial and Kupffer cells at 10 minutes after
injection.
LDL was incubated with human umbilical vein endothelial
cells for 9, 23 or 44 hours. Thereafter the LDL or acetylated LDL was injected into rats, the cells were purified as
in ref. 6 and the cell-associated radioactivity was determined.

Whatever the direct toxic form of LDL will be, it is clear that lowering the level of native LDL will either directly or indirectly lead to a lowered occurrence of atherosclerosis. This is especially important for patients with LDL receptor deficiency as in these persons myocardial infarction usually occurs before age 20. In order to lower the LDL level therapeutically, a cholesterol derivative was synthesized (8) which contains a triantennary galactose recognition mark (diagram I). The cholesterol is coupled to 3 galactose groups by an intermediate succinyl, and glycyl connection. This compound is highly soluble in water and upon mixing with LDL it is immediately incorporated.

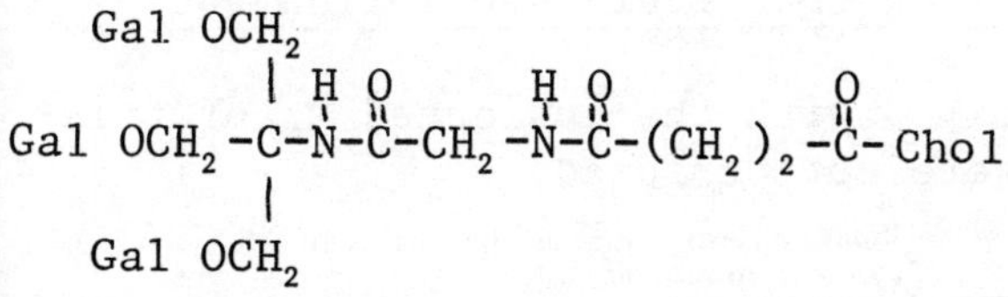

$$\text{Gal OCH}_2$$

Gal OCH$_2$-C-N-C-CH$_2$-N-C-(CH$_2$)$_2$-C-Chol

$$\text{Gal OCH}_2$$

Diagram I
The structure of N-(tris (β-D-galactopyranosyloxymethyl) methyl)-N$^\alpha$-(4-(5-cholesten-3β-yloxy-succinyl)-glycinamide (abbreviated tris-gal-chol).

Fig. 4 shows that with incorporation of 5, 13 or 200 µg of tris-gal-chol into LDL (20 µg) a marked increased uptake of LDL by the liver is achieved. Inside the liver the Kupffer cells appear to be mainly responsible for the increased uptake of tris-gal-chol loaded LDL (Fig. 5.).

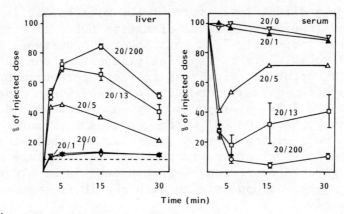

Fig. 4

Effect of tris-gal-chol on the liver-association and serum-decay of LDL

^{125}I-LDL (20 µg) was mixed with the indicated µg of tris-gal-chol. The livers were not perfused.

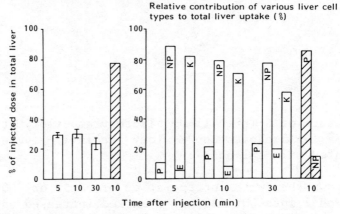

Fig. 5

Relative contribution of various liver cell types to total liver uptake (%).

At various times after injection of tris-gal-chol LDL (20/13) or asialofetuin (hatched blocks) the cell association to purified parenchymal (P), non-parenchymal (NP), endothelial (E) and Kupffer (K) cells was determined. The relative contribution of the various cell types to total liver uptake was calculated as in ref. 9.

The increased uptake of tris-gal-chol loaded LDL (20/13) by parenchymal cells is inhibited (Fig. 6) by preinjection of 5 or 25 mg asialofetuin. N-acetyl galactoseamine but not N-acetylglucosamine blocks the increased uptake of LDL both by parenchymal and non-parenchymal cells completely.

This indicates that the increased interaction of LDL with the cells is caused by the exposure of a galactose-recognition marker on these particles. The increased interaction is coupled to a transport of LDL to the lysosomes as determined by a subcellular distribution performed 60 min after injection of tris-gal-chol LDL, labeled with ^{14}C-sucrose.

These data lead to the conclusion that incorporation of tris-gal-chol into LDL leads to a markedly increased catabolism of LDL by the liver which might provide a strategy for treating hypercholesterolemia.

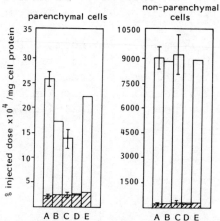

Fig. 6

The effect of preinjection of asialofetuin, GalNAc or GlcNAc on the cell-association of LDL and tris-gal-chol LDL.

The injection of ^{131}I-LDL (hatched blocks) and tris-gal-chol ^{125}I-LDL (open blocks) was preceded at -1 min by injection of 5 or 25 mg of asialofetuin (B resp. C), 0.5 m mole GalNAc (D) or 0.5 mmole GlcNAc (E). Ten minutes after injection the cell association was determined.

REFERENCES

1. Pittman, R.C., Green , S.R., Attie, A.D. and Steinberg, D. (1979). J. Biol. Chem. 254, 6876-6879.
2. Harkes, L. and Van Berkel, Th.J.C. (1983). FEBS Letters, 154, 75-80
3. Harkes, L. and Van Berkel, Th.J.C. (1984). Biochem. J. in press.
4. Van Berkel, Th.J.C. (1982) in "Metabolic Compartmentation" (H. Sies ed.). Academic Press Inc. London pp 437-482.
5. Goldstein, J.L. and Brown, M.S. (1977). Ann. Rev. Biochem. 46, 897-930.
6. Henriksen, T., Mahoney, E.M. and Steinberg, D. (1982). Ann. N.Y. Acad. Sci. 401, 102-116.
7. Nagelkerke, J.F., Havekes, L., Van Hinsbergh, V.W.M. and Van Berkel, Th.J.C. (1984). Arteriosclerosis 4, 256-264.
8. Kempen, H.J.M., Hoes, C., Van Boom, J.H., Spanjer, H.H., De Lange, J., Langendoen, A. and Van Berkel, Th.J.C. (1984). J. Medicin. Chem. in press.
9. Nagelkerke, J.F., Barto, K.P. and Van Berkel, Th.J.C. (1983). J. Biol. Chem. 258, 12221-12227.

PLASMA LIPOPROTEINS, APOLIPOPROTEINS, AND ATHEROSCLEROSIS

ANTONIO M. GOTTO, Jr., M.D., D. Phil.
HENRY J. POWNALL, Ph.D.
GABRIEL PONSIN, Ph.D.
JOSEF R. PATSCH, Ph.D.
JAMES T. SPARROW, Ph.D.
Baylor College of Medicine and The Methodist Hospital
Department of Medicine
6565 Fannin, A601
Houston, Texas 77030 USA

Five major classes define the plasma lipoproteins: the chylomicrons, very-low-density lipoproteins (VLDL), intermediate-density lipoproteins (IDL), low-density lipoproteins (LDL), and high-density lipoproteins (HDL). Furthermore, the HDL are subdivided into HDL_2 and HDL_3. High levels of LDL are known to correlate with accelerated atherogenesis, while the HDL are anti-atherogenic. Some evidence suggests that HDL_2 is the subclass of HDL associated with protection against atherosclerosis, but this point is not yet firmly established. Whether the stastical inverse relationship of HDL with coronary heart disease represents an inhibition of atherogenesis by HDL or is a secondary relationship is not known. The major pathways of lipoprotein catabolism are shown in Figure 1.

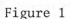

Figure 1

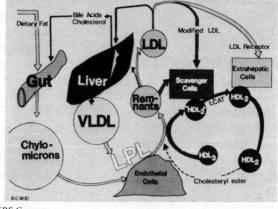

Proceedings of the 16th FEBS Congress
Part A, pp. 225–232
© 1985 VNU Science Press

Chylomicrons are made in the gut and VLDL in the liver. They are attacked by an enzyme called lipoprotein lipase which catalyzes the hydrolysis of triglycerides. This enzyme specifically requires apoC-II as an activator. The enzyme is attached to the surface of endothelial cells, is released by intravenous heparin, is increased by exercise and estrogen and depends on insulin for its synthesis. It is a key enzyme involved in regulating lipoprotein catabolism. The smaller particles produced by lipoprotein lipase are called remnants and may be atherogenic. Chylomicron renmants are rapidly removed by the liver by a receptor that recognizes apoE and/or apoB.

VLDL remnants are further catabolized to LDL, which may be removed through receptor mediated endocytosis by cells which contain a specific LDL receptor. These include the liver, endothelial cells, smooth muscle cells, the adrenal cortex, the gonads, fibroblasts, and various other cellular tissues. The classical LDL receptor recognizes apoB or apoE. Receptors for apoB and/or apoE also exist in the liver. Hypertriglyceridemic VLDL and modified LDL may be taken up directly by scavenger cells; such a mechanism could contribute to the pathogenesis of atherosclerosis.

LDL may also be catabolized via a non-specific scavenger pathway involving tissue macrophages. The macrophage contains a receptor which binds and internalizes LDL that has been altered, as by acetylation, or by acting with malondialdehyde. This receptor has very poor binding activity toward "normal" LDL.

The hepatic cell contains receptors which regulate cellular LDL removal and intracellular levels of cholesterol and HMG CoA reductase. The classical LDL receptor activity is deficient in familial hypercholesterolemia. The removal of bile acid by a sequesterant results in an increase in the number of LDL receptors. This treatment was used in the Coronary Primary Prevention Trial in the 12 North American Lipid Research Clinics. As compared to the placebo group, the treatment group receiving cholestyramine had a 12.5% reduction in LDL cholesterol. The hard end points for measuring coronary heart disease risk were myocardial infarction and coronary heart disease death.

In the model structure of HDL (Figure 2) and for any lipoprotein, the central interior contains neutral lipid, consisting of triglyceride and cholesteryl ester. A surface monolayer of apolipoproteins or

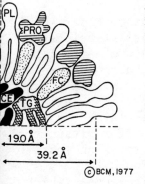

proteins, and the polar head groups of phospholipids interact with the aqueous environment and protect the neutral lipid interior. The apolipoproteins contain specific binding regions called amphipathic or amphiphilic helices which enable them to interact with the fatty acyl chains to phospholipids. The principal apolipoproteins are given in Table 1. The apolipoproteins are intimately involved in regulating the metabolism of the lipoproteins. This is accomplished in at least three major ways: the apolipoproteins bind the lipid and form stable complexes; they are activators of the enzymes which regulate lipoprotein catabolism; and they serve as recognition sites for the removal of lipoproteins by receptors located on the surface of cells.

TABLE 1. CHARACTERISTICS OF PLASMA APOLIPOPROTEINS IN NORMAL FASTING HUMANS

	Plasma Concentration µM	mol %*	Distribution in Lipoproteins HDL	LDL	IDL	VLDL mol %**	Tissue Source	Mol. Weight (daltons)
apoA-I	46	38	100				liver	28,000
apoA-II	23	20	100				intestine	17,000
apoA-IV							intestine	46,000
apoB-48	} 5	} 4	} 82	} 8	} 2		intestine	264,000
apoB-100							liver	550,000
apoC-I	18	16	97		1	2	liver	5,800
apoC-II	3	3	60		10	30	liver	9,100
apoC-III	13	12	60	10	10	20	liver	8,750
apoD	5	4	100					22,000
apoE-II								
apoE-III	2	2	50	10	20	20	liver	35,000
apoE-IV								
β-glycoprotein-1 (apoH)							liver	54,000

*Based on total plasma concentration.

**For each apoprotein.

These combined parameters were reduced by 19% with a P value of less than 0.05. This is the most definitive evidence to date supporting the lipid hypothesis in man and indicating that reducing cholesterol lowers coronary heart disease risk.

HDL are snythesized as incomplete or nascent particles by liver and gut, and they contain no cholesteryl esters at this point. They are converted to mature particles through the action of the enzyme, lecithin:cholesterol acyl transferase, or LCAT. This enzyme specifically requires apoA-I or apoC-I as an activator. The anti-atherogenic mechanism of HDL has not been explained; a postulated one is that it acts as a scavenger for tissue cholesterol and, directly or indirectly, promotes cholesterol transfer to the liver. HDL_2 have been found to be a substrate for a liver enzyme, called hepatic lipase, which catalyzes the hydrolysis of phospholipid and triglyceride.

The plasma apolipoproteins bind and solubilize lipids. In addition, they exert a number of specific actions. ApoA-I and apoC-I activate LCAT; apoC-II activates lipoprotein lipase; and apoB and apoE are ligands for the cellular recognition of lipoproteins. ApoD may be involved in catalyzing the transfer of cholesteryl ester between HDL and other lipoproteins, and apoA-II may be the activator of hepatic lipase.

APOLIPOPROTEINS AND LIPID BINDING

The most atherogenic apolipoprotein appears to be apoB and the most anti-atherogenic apoA-I. The lipid binding regions of apolipoproteins reside in a part of the protein called the amphipathic or amphiphilic helix. (Figure 3) The polar amino acids are oriented to the outside of the lipoprotein, the hydrophobic to the inside. There are alternating charged acidic and basic groups on the polar surface. This property probably keeps the apolipoproteins at the surface of the lipoprotein so they can be transferred between lipoprotein families and can influence metabolic events. ApoA-I has 7 to 22 amino acid length amphipathic units, which Fitch has postulated have devised by gene duplication and which have preserved the

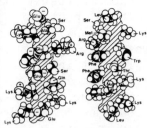

POLAR FACE   NON-POLAR FACE

Figure 3
(copyright BCM)

function of lipid binding.(1)   ApoA-I is also an activator of LCAT. We have found that lipid binding is a prerequisite for the function. We undertook on a theoretical basis to prepare a series of lipid binding peptides, using the theoretical concept of Eisenberg, in which hydrophobic and hydrophilic forces along a peptide are summed by vectors. (2)   This gives a directional value to the amphipathic helix, and is called the amphipathic moment.

SYNTHETIC, LIPID ASSOCIATING PEPTIDES

A lipid associating peptide (LAP)-20 is shown with its hydrophilic and hydrophobic face.(3) (Figure 4)   On a plot of hydrophobicity versus amphipathic moment, this synthetic peptide and all of the naturally occurring apolipoproteins are found in the cluster of surface-seeking peptides. The charged amino acid groups most likely function to keep the membrane seeking peptides on the surface of the lipoprotein.

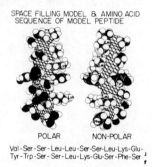

SPACE FILLING MODEL & AMINO ACID
SEQUENCE OF MODEL PEPTIDE

POLAR   NON-POLAR

Val-Ser-Ser-Leu-Leu-Ser-Ser-Leu-Lys-Glu-
Tyr-Trp-Ser-Ser-Leu-Lys-Glu-Ser-Phe-Ser

Figure 4
(copyright BCM)

We devised a series of experiments to determine the effect of disrupting the helix while keeping the hydrophobicity constant. We substituted a helix breaker, namely, a single proline in the peptide backbone. Single substitutions were made at residues 1, 5, 8, 11, and 15 of LAP-20. The 8 and 11 substituted peptides did not bind lipid, the 1 and 15 substituted did bind, while the 5 was intermediate in its binding activity. We conclude that location of helix breakers near the middle of a lipid-binding region of a peptide lowers its affinity for a lipid water interface. This is strong evidence for the importance of the alpha helix to apolipoprotein structure.

A second series of experiments was designed to test the importance of hydrophobicity to the affinity of peptides for lipid surfaces. We kept the helicity constant and increased hydrophobicity by adding saturated acyl groups to the amino terminal serine of LAP-15. The intrinsic helical potential of this series of peptides remained constant while the hydrophobicity increased with the number of carbons in the acyl chain. Tyrosine could be labelled with iodine 125 and tryptophan used for fluorescence analysis. The peptides associate almost exclusively with HDL both in-vitro and in-vivo. These peptides associate in solution, form amphipathic helices on binding to HDL, and activate LCAT. Thus, the peptides exhibit a number of the characteristics of apoA-I.

The rates of serum clearance of 125 I-labelled peptides were measured in the rat. The clearance curves were consistant with a 2-compartment model. The clearance rates decreased as the acyl chain length increased. The curve of the C_{16} derivative was very similar to that of apoA-I. The inset shows that the apparent half-life of the long-lived component increased with the length of the acyl chain and therefore, the hydrophobicity. This finding was consistent with the concept of an in-vivo binding of the peptide to HDL, increasing in proportion to acyl chain length. (Figure 5) We calculated the organ distribution volumes of the free peptide and HDL-bound peptide. The distribution volumes were expressed per gram of organ. The distribution volumes of the free peptide were the same in all organs except the kidney, which appeared to be the preferential site of catabolism. The HDL-associated peptide was associated to a significant extent with only three tissues: liver, adrenal, and ovaries.

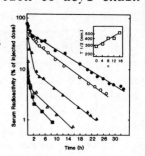

Figure 5
(copyright BCM)

Using an adequate mathematical model, we have been able to estimate the in-vivo partitioning of synthetic peptides between HDL and the aqueous phase. The in-vivo and in-vitro data are highly correlated and support the concept of in-vivo

230

equilibrium regulated by hydrophobicity. Thus, the hydrophobic properties of a lipophile can be expressed in-vivo and likely represent a major determinant of in-vivo behavior.

METABOLISM OF HDL

HDL contain a more lipid-rich HDL_2 and a lipid-poor HDL_3. HDL_2 levels in plasma correlate positively with HDL-cholesterol, show the greatest variability among lipoproteins, are high in females, runners and hyperalphalipoproteinemics, and are inversely related to postprandial lipemia. We undertook a study to determine if postprandial lipemia influences HDL_2 levels. The following changes occurred in HDL_2 after a fatty meal: an increase in flotation rate, an increase in phospholipid content, a decrease in protein content, and a variable increase in triglyceride content. We identified three species of HDL_2: a post-absorptive one low in triglyceride (PA), a postprandial one low in triglyceride (PP), and a postprandial one high in triglyceride (PP). From a great deal of work in-vitro and in-vivo, we speculate that these three species are substrates for hepatic lipase. We suggest that PA HDL_2 and triglyceride-poor PP HDL_2 are converted by hepatic lipase to HDL_2-like particles and triglyceride-rich PP HDL_2 to HDL_3. This scheme is summarized in Figure 6.

In summary, the structure of the apolipoproteins contain determinants which are important in regulating lipoprotein metabolism. LAP's which have been snythesized are analogs of apoA-I. Studies with these analogs have permitted a fractionation of the effects of helicity and hydrophobicity. The hydrophobicity of a peptide

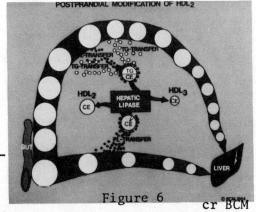

Figure 6

231

was shown to influence the metabolism. We have presented evidence which suggests that lipemia and hepatic lipase may influence the metabolic pathways of HDL. Our hope is that by gaining a greater knowledge of lipoprotein and apolipoprotein structure and metabolism, we may be able to devise innovative and more effective approaches for the treatment and prevention of atherosclerosis.

REFERENCES

(1) Pownall, H.J., Gotto, A.M., Jr., Sparrow, J.T. (1980) Activation of lecithin:cholesterol acyl transferase by a synthetic model-associating peptide. Proc. Natl. Acad. Sci. 77, 3154-3158.

(2) Fitch, W.M. (1977) Phylogenics constrained by the crossover process as illustrated by human hemoglobins and a thirteen-cycle, eleven-amino acid repeat in human apolipoprotein A-I. Genetics. 86, 623-644.

(3) Eisenberg, D., White, R.M., Terwilliger, T.C. (1982) The helical hydrophobic moment: a measure of the amphiphilicity of a helix. Nature. 299, 371-374.

AUTOIMMUNE THEORY OF PATOGENESIS OF ATHE-ROSCLEROSIS

A.N.KLIMOV
Institute for Experimental Medicine, Le - ningrad, USSR

INTRODUCTION

At present it is considered generally accepted that the development of athero -sclerosis is connected with the ingress and accumulation in the arterial wall of plasma lipoproteins containing apoprotein (apo) B as the major protein. Low density (LDL) and very low density (VLDL) lipoproteins pertain to the latter; they were called atherogenic lipoproteins in contrast to antiatherogenic high density lipoproteins (HDL).

One of the new trends in the investiga - tion of pathogenesis of atherosclerosis is studing it from the immunological point of view, according to which apo B containing lipoproteins possess autoantigenic proper- ties.

Autoimmune complexes lipoprotein-antibo- dy were detected in the blood of patients with hyperlipoproteinemia (1-5), ischemic heart disease patients (5,6), and also in rabbits with experimental atherosclerosis (7,8). It is significant that autoimmune complexes containing LDL or VLDL and IgG were detected also in the arterial wall impaired with atherosclerosis of man and animals (4,5,9).

The presence of autoantigenic properties in lipoproteins and the appearance of auto-

Proceedings of the 16th FEBS Congress
Part A, pp. 233–249
© 1985 VNU Science Press

immune complexes lipoprotein-antibody in
the blood of animals during the develop -
ment of atherosclerosis underlies the autoimmune theory of pathogenesis of athero -
sclerosis (10-12). According to this theory,
autoimmune complexes LDL-IgG or VLDL-IgG
possess a more pronounced atherogenicity
than native lipoproteins and, consequently,
their formation in an organism leads to the
initiation and/or aggravation of the athe -
rosclerotic process.

A ponderable argument in favour of the
autoimmune theory were the experiments in
which it was managed to produce a resistance to atherosclerosis by means of immunization of newborn rabbits with homologous apo
B containing lipoproteins isolated from the
plasma of adult rabbits having had experi -
mental atherosclerosis (12,13). The immunological effect of such a resistance mani -
fested itself in a low production in the
animals of antibodies to apo B containing
lipoproteins (the absence of an autoimmune
complex circulating in the blood), and the
biochemical effect - in an increased oxidation of the cholesterol administered into
the organism into bile acids (13).

It is presumed that the following chain
of successive events underlies the autoimmune theory of pathogenesis of atherosclerosis (10-12): a) the appearance of auto -
antigenic properties in plasma lipoproteins
(LDL and VLDL); b) the formation of immune
complexes lipoprotein-antibody circulating
in the blood in excess antigen; c) the fixation of complexes on the surface of the
arterial wall, and the injury of the endothelial lining, contributing to the penet-
ration of both the complexes themselves and

234

the atherogenic lipoproteins into the in -
tima.
    In the present review we shall dwell upon
two questions: 1. why do autoimmune complexes lipoprotein-antibody form? and 2. in
what way do these complexes interact with the
cell and accomplish the transport of cholesterol into the latter?

FORMATION OF AUTOIMMUNE COMPLEXES.

    Speaking about lipoprotein autoantigenic
properties one should stress that it is
difficult to name other high-molecular compounds circulating in the blood which are
subjected to such considerable changes de -
pending upon the character of nutrition and
other conditions of environmental and in -
ternal medium, as lipoproteins are. In this
case we have in mind not only changes of
the lipid composition, but also of the apoprotein composition, accompanied by changes
of the size, charge, fluidity, and other
parameters of the lipoprotein particle.
    The most pronounced changes in the lipo-
proteins are observed in cases of hypercholesterolemia. Even in experimental conditions, hypercholesterolemia in rabbits is accompanied by an abrupt increase of apo E
content in VLDL, by the appearance of a new
lipoprotein subclass in the blood designated
as β-VLDL (14), and, besides, by a notice-
able increase of IgG content (15). Moreover,
a lipoprotein subclass of high density -
HDL_c appears in the blood of man and animals
in cases of hypercholesterolemia (16). Pa-
thologic lipoproteins, designated as LP-X
(17), have been detected in patients with
obstructive liver disease (17). Glucosylated

LDL were found in some diabetic individuals
(18).Evidently, partially degraded lipoproteins that have been subjected to the action
of proteolytic enzymes in the extracellular
medium of the organism may find way into the
blood-flow. The ability of apo B containing
lipoproteins to form soluble complexes with
glycosaminoglycanes of the connective tissue
of arteres is known. A considerable change
of lipoprotein structure and apoprotein conformation brings about peroxidation of lipids
constituting the lipoproteins. And finally,
lipoproteins can bind some substances of
exogenous origin, particularly fat-soluble
ones, which in one way or another got into
the blood. In this case exogenous substances,
as well as lipid peroxides, may, on the one
hand, bring about apoprotein conformation
changes and, on the other hand, serve as
haptens.

This enumeration, evidently, does not ex-
haust the whole diversity of altered or modified lipoproteins. We cannot exclude also
the appearance of apoprotein phenotypes in
the composition of lipoproteins.

Antibodies to lipoproteins, apparently,
are formed in two cases: a) in response to
the appearance of altered or modified in vivo lipoproteins that have acquired autoantigenic properties; b) in response to the ac -
tion of pathogenic or some other factors,
when the immunocompetent system of the organism synthesizes antibodies, which form complexes with ordinary plasma lipoproteins.
Both in the first and in the second case the
formed immune complex lipoprotein-antibody
may be regarded as a peculiar modified lipoprotein, which must differently interact
with the cell in comparison with the native

lipoprotein.

INTERACTION OF LIPOPROTEIN-ANTIBODY IMMUNE COMPLEX WITH THE CELL.

In experiments carried out at our laboratory it has been established that immune lipoprotein-antibody complex prepared in vitro
(human VLDL or LDL + rabbit serum against
apo B of human lipoproteins) and administered intravenously to a rabbit was eliminated
from the circulation quicker than a native
lipoprotein (Fig.1). The elimination rate
correlated with the amount of antibody ad -
ded.

In addition, in these experiments it was
found that at administration of the immune
complex the lipoprotein uptake in the spleen
was greater than the uptake following admi -
nistration of native lipoproteins. This
attests to a preferred uptake of immune com-
plexe by cells of the reticuloendothelial
system.
To understand the causes which lead to
increased elimination of lipoprotein-antibody complex from the circulation experiments
were performed to study the interaction of
the immune complex and free lipoproteins
with human fibroblasts and mouse macropha -
ges. The results are shown in Table 1.

It is seen from the Table 1 that addition
of specific serum against apo B to LDL, leading to formation of the immune complex,in -
hibited LDL uptake by fibroblasts and in -
creased LDL uptake by macrophages. Thus, the
experimental data suggest that formation of
the lipoprotein-antibody complex increases

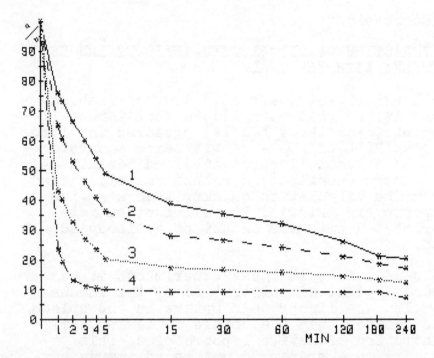

Fig.1 Elimination of LDL and LDL complexed
with antiapo B IgG from the circulation of
normal rabbits.

1. Native ^{125}I-LDL; 2,3,4. Immune complexes
^{125}I-LDL-IgG with Ag/Ab ratios 8,4 and 2

respectively.

lipoprotein elimination from the circulation.
    These results are not unexpected because
the physiological role of immune complex
formation is to remove the antigen from the
circulation as fast as possible.
    It is well known that uptake of immune
complexes by macrophages occurs via Fc-receptors to Fc-fragments of immunoglobulin.

Table 1

Uptake of native LDL and LDL complexed with antiapo B IgG by human lung fibroblasts and mouse peritoneal macrophages (in ng LDL protein/mg cell protein). Average data from 4 dishes.

Type of cells	^{125}I-LDL + normal rabbit serum (control)	^{125}I-LDL + antiserum to apo B	
		4:1	1:5
Fibroblasts	6747±132	4232±29	4231±121
P compared to control	–	<0.01	<0.01
Macrophages	3534±66	3850±26	6967±79
P compared to control	–	<0.01	<0.01

Notes: Isolation of IgG and its fragments was performed by the method of affinity chromatography on a column with LDL-Sepharose.

Splitting of IgG into fragments was carried out by standart methods (19). Provisionally the ratio of such quantities of lipoproteins and antiserum to apo B, which gave maximum precipitate formation, was taken for the equimolar ratio of Ag/Ab. In control experiments the volume of added normal serum corresponded to the volume of serum where Ag/Ab ratio was 1:5.

Cultured lung fibroblasts of a human embryo of the tenth passage and freshly-isolated peritoneal macrophages of mice were used in the experiments. The cells were incubated in an Eagle medium containing non-lipoprotein serum proteins in a concentration of 5 mg/ml during 4 h in a CO_2-incubator. The fibroblast culture was not subjected to preliminary preincubation in a medium not containing lipoproteins. In the rest, me - thods described in literature were used (20-23).

At the same time, it should be kept in mind that macrophages are capable to a certain degree of uptaking native lipoproteins also (24,25), but most actively they uptake some chemically modified LDL (methylated, ace - tylated, maleylated etc.), particularly if at modification they acquired an excessive negative charge (24-26).

Since the lipoprotein-antibody immune complex may be regarded as a peculiar modified form of lipoprotein particle, it is logical to assume that macrophages uptake such a complex both with the participation of Fc-receptors to the Fc-fragment of immunoglobulin and with the help of nonspecific endocytosis (scavenger pathway). In order to verify this assumption experiments in vitro were carried out to study the uptake by peritoneal macrophages of mice of native hu - man LDL, and LDL complexed with IgG against apo B of man, or with Fab- and $F(ab)_2$-fragments of a similar IgG (Table 2).

As seen from Table 2, immune complex LDL-IgG was uptaken by macrophages on the ave - rage by 23% more actively than native LDL. Immune complexes of LDL with Fab- and $F(ab)_2$-fragments of IgG (unrecognized by

Table 2

Uptake of native LDL and LDL complexed with IgG or with Fab-fragments of IgG by peritoneal macrophages of mice (ng LDL protein/ mg cell protein). Ratio of Ag/Ab in all cases was 4:1. Mean data from 4 dishes.

Index	^{125}I-LDL (control)	^{125}I-LDL complexed or mixed with			
		IgG against apo B	Fab-fragments of IgG	$F(ab)_2$-fragments of IgG	Nonspecific IgG
M	4488	5523	4975	5151	4669
m	43	135	75	20	69
Uptake in relation to control (in %)	-	+23	+11	+15	+4
P comared to control	-	<0.01	<0.01	<0.01	>0.05

Fc-receptors of macrophages) were uptaken approximately two fold less. These data can be considered as evidence that formation of lipoprotein-antibody complexes activates the uptake of lipoproteins not only via macro - phage Fc-receptors but also by means of non-specific uptake due to a change of superfi - cial properties of the lipoprotein particle. It is significant that addition of nonspecific IgG to LDL did not affect the rate of LDL uptake by macrophages.

Because the immune LDL-antibody complexes were taken up by macrophages more actively than native LDL, it is possible that uptake of these complexes may lead to an increased entry of cholesterol into macrophages and their transformation into foam cells. It is known that the appearance of foam cells in the intima of arteries is a characteristic morphological feature of a developing atherosclerotic process. It is namely these cells loaded with cholesteryl esters, when, undergoing destruction, form extracellular accumulations of cholesterol which serve as a basis for the formation of fatty streaks (the first morphological stage of an atherosclerotic process).

In experiments carried out in our laboratory it was shown that a 72-hour incubation of macrophages with LDL-IgG immune complex really did bring about a transformation of macrophages into foam cells. In ultraviolet light these cells after staining with 3,4-benzepyrene had a brightly gleaming cyto - plasm with an abundance of lipids in large and small vacuoles (Fig.2a). When the macrophages were incubated for this time only with native LDL, we observed the formation of few lipid vacuoles in the cell cytoplasm (Fig.2b). Electron microscopy of the macrophage cytoplasm, after incubation with an immune complex, showed the presence of a large number of lipid vacuoles. In separate cells besides lipid vacuoles one could see crystals of cholesterol (Fig.2c) and rem - nants of destroyed cell organelle. Some of the cells were completely filled with large and small vacuoles (a typical picture of a foam cell) and were in a state of destruction. At electron microscopy of macrophages

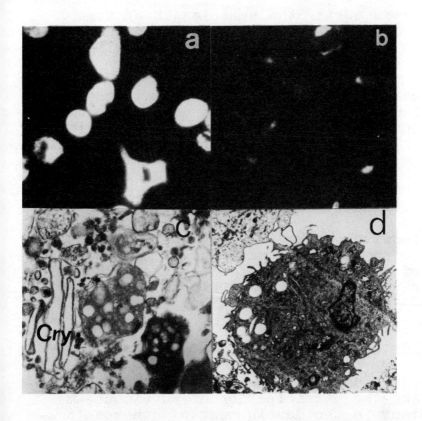

Figure 2. Transformation of macrophages into
foam cells after incubation with the LDL-IgG
immune complex for 72 h at 37°C.
a. Accumulation of lipids in macrophages after incubation with the immune complex. Staining with 3,4-benzepyrene, X 600; b. Incubation of macrophages with LDL (control). Staining with 3,4-benzepyrene, X 600; c. Trans -
formation of macrophage into foam cell after
incubation with the immune complex. Cry-crys-
tals of cholesterol, TEM, X 60 000; d. Macrophage after incubation with LDL (control),
TEM, X 40 000.

incubated during the same length of time
with native LDL, only single lipid vacuoles
were observed in the cytoplasm of cells
(Fig.2d).

Thus, the obtained data bears witness to
the fact that the formation of lipoprotein-
antibody complex may lead to a quick elimination of such a complex from the circulation due to its active uptake by cells of the
reticuloendothelial system, by macrophages
in particular, both with the help of Fc-receptors and by means of nonspecific endocytosis.
Excessive uptake of lipoprotein-antibody
immune complexes by macrophages leads to the
transformation of the latter into foam cells,
which play an important role in the formation of atherosclerotic lesions of the arteries.

CONCLUSION

In conclusion a scheme is presented, illustrating the participation of autoimmune me -
chanisms in the development of atherosclerosis (Fig.3).
Assessing the participation of immunological factors in atherogenesis, we may regard
this participation on a wider scale. Immune
complexes, containing non-lipoprotein auto-
antigens or heteroantigens of different origin, also produce a damaging effect upon the
endothelium of vessels (27). It may be antigens of the environment, including food antigens, and those that are administered into
the organism with vaccines, serums, tissue
preparations, to say nothing of haptens of
diverse chemical origin. It is quite possi -

ble that the high prevalence of atherosclerosis nowadays in highly developed countries may be partialy explained by the latter
circumstances also.

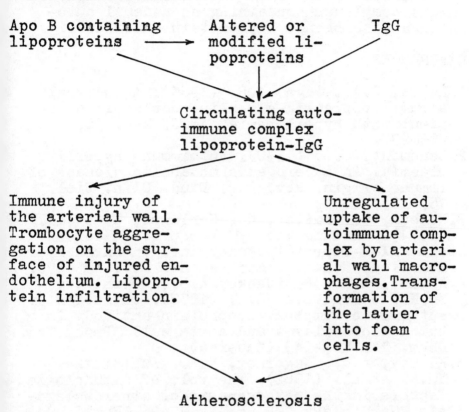

Figure 3. Scheme illustrating the autoimmune
theory of pathogenesis of atherosclerosis.

At the same time, the autoimmune theory of pathogenesis of atherosclerosis occupies a particular place. The peculiarity of the theory consists of the fact that the formation of immune complexes containing an unusual autoantigen-atherogenic lipoprotein underlies it.

REFERENCES

1.Lewis, L.A., Page, I.H. (1965). An unusual serum lipoprotein-globulin complex in a patient with hyperlipemia. Am.J. Med. 38, 286-297.
2.Beaumont, J.L. (1970). Autoimmune hyperlipidemia. An atherogenic metabolic disease of immune origin. Rev. Eur. Etud. Clin. Biol. 15, 1037-1041.
3.Noseda, G., Butler, R., Schlumpf, E. et al. (1971). Bindung von β-Lipoprotein durch ein IgA-Paraprotein: eine Antigen-Antikorper Reaction? Schweiz. med. Wschr. 101, 893-899.
4.Klimov, A.N., Denisenko, A.D., Zubzhitsky, Yu.N., Gerchikova, E.A. (1978). Detection of autoimmune complex lipoprotein-antibody in human blood plasma and aorta wall. Proc. Med. Chem. 24, 539-543 (Russian).
5.Klimov, A.N., Nagornev, V.A., Zubzhitsky, Yu.N. et al. (1982). The role of immunologic factors in the pathogenesis of atherosclerosis. Cardiology. 22, No12, 22-26 (Russian).
6.Szondy, E., Horvath, M., Mezey, Z. et al. (1983). Free and complexed anti-lipoprotein antibodies in vascular diseases. Atherosclerosis. 49, 69-77.
7.Ioffe, V.I., Zubzhitsky, Yu.N., Nagornev, V.A., Klimov, A,N. (1973). Immunological characteristics of experimental atherosclerosis. Bull. Exp. Biol. Med. 75, No6, 72-76 (Rus - sian).

8.Klimov, A.N., Petrova-Maslakova, L.G., Nagornev, V.A., Magracheva, E.Ya. (1975). Isolation and identification of autoimmune li -
poprotein-antibody complex from blood serum
of rabbits with experimental atherosclerosis.
Proc. Med. Chem. 21, 526-531 (Russian).
9.Klimov, A.N., Nagornev, V.A., Zubzhitsky,
Yu.N., Denisenko, A.D. (1980). Autoimmune
mechanisms in the development of atherosclerosis. In: Atherosclerosis V. Proc. of the
Fifth International Symposium, A.M. Gotto,
L.C. Smith and B. Allen (eds). Springer-Verlag, N.Y., pp. 348-350.
10.Klimov, A.N. (1974). Immunobiochemical mechanisms of atherosclerosis development.
Proc. Acad. Med. Sci. USSR. 2, 29-36 (Rus -
sian).
11.Klimov, A.N., Zubzhitsky, Yu.N., Nagornev,
V.A. (1979). Immunochemical aspects of atherosclerosis. Atherosclerosis Rev. 4, 119-156.
12.Zubzhitsky, Yu.N., Nagornev, V.A., Lovyagina,
T.N., Bankovskaya, E.B. (1971). Experience
in the prevention of experimental atherosclerosis by means of parenteral introduction to
newborn rabbits of atherogenic lipoproteins.
Bull. Exp. Biol. Med. 71, No2, 21-23 (Rus -
sian).
13.Bankovskaya, E.B., Dokusova, O.K., Zubzhitsky, Yu.N. et al. (1972). Peculiarities of
the lipid metabolism in rabbits with tole -
rance to experimental atherosclerosis induced by inroduction of homologous β -lipo -
proteins to newborn animals. Proc. Acad. Med.
Sci. USSR. 7, 78-85 (Russian).
14.Mahley, R.W., Weisgraber, K.H., Innerarity,
T. (1974). Canine lipoproteins and athero -
sclerosis. II. Characterization of the plasma lipoproteins associated with atherogenic

and nonatherogenic hyperlipidemia. Circulation Res. 35, 722-733.
15. Lovyagina, T.N. (1960). Alterations in
plasma lipoproteins and protein fractions
in animals with experimental hypercholesterolemia. Proc. Med. Chem. 6, 358-364.
16. Mahley, R.W. (1978). Alterations in plasma
lipoproteins induced by cholesterol feeding
in animals including man. In: Disturbances
in Lipid and Lipoprotein Metabolism, J.M.
Dietschy, A.M. Gotto, and J.A. Ontko (eds).
Amer. Physiol. Soc., Bethesda, pp. 181-197.
17. Seidel, D., Agostini, B., Müller, P. (1972).
Structure of an abnormal plasma lipoprotein
(LP-X) characterizing obstructive jaundice.
Biochim. Biophys. Acta. 260, 146-152.
18. Susaki, J., Okamura, T., Cottam, G.L.
(1983). Measurement of receptor-independent
metabolism of low-density lipoprotein. An
application of glycosylated low-density lipoprotein. Eur. J. Biochem. 131, 535-538.
19. Friemel, H. (1976). Immunologische Arbeits-
methoden. VEB Gustav Fischer Verlag, Jena.
20. Lindgren, F.T., Jensen, L.C., Hatch, R.T.
(1972). The isolation and quantitative analysis of serum lipoproteins. In: Blood Li -
pids and Lipoproteins, G.J. Nelson (ed).
Interscience, N.Y., pp. 181-274.
21. Helmkamp, R.W., Contreras, M.A., Izzo, M.J.
(1967). ^{131}I-labelling of proteins at high
activity level with ^{131}I-ICL produced by
oxidation of total iodine in Na^{131}I preparations. Int. J. Appl. Rad. Isotopes. 18, 747-
757.
22. Brown, M.S., Dana, S.E., Goldstein, J.L.
(1975). Receptor-dependent hydrolysis of
cholesteryl esters contained in plasma low

density lipoprotein. Proc. Natl. Acad. Sci. USA. 72, 2925-2929.

23. Goldstein, J.L., Ho, Y.K., Basu, S.K., Brown, N.S. (1979). Binding site on macro - phages that mediates uptake and degradation of acetylated low density lipoprotein, pro- ducing massive cholesterol deposition. Proc. Natl. Acad. Sci. USA. 76, 333-337.

24. Brown, M.S., Goldstein, J.L. (1983). Lipo- protein metabolism in the macrophage: impli- cations for cholesterol deposition in athe - rosclerosis. Ann. Rev. Biochem. 52, 223-261.

25. Mahley, R.W., Innerarity, T.L., Weisgraber, K.H., Oh, S.Y. (1979). Altered metabolism (in vivo and in vitro) of plasma lipopro - teins after selective chemical modification of lysine residues of the apoproteins. J. Clin. Invest. 64, 743-750.

26. Fogelman, A.M., Schechter, I., Seager, J. et al. (1980). Malondialdehyde alteration of low density lipoproteins leads to choles- teryl ester accumulation in human monocyte macrophages. Proc. Natl. Acad. Sci. USA. 77, 2214-2218.

27. Minick, C.R. (1980). The role of immunolo- gically induced arterial injury in athero - genesis. In: Immunity and Atherosclerosis, P. Constantinides, F. Pratesi, and C. Ca - vallero (eds). Academic Press, London, pp. 111-120.

MULTINUCLEAR MAGNETIC RESONANCE APPLICATIONS TO THE STUDY OF BRAIN METABOLISM

K. L. BEHAR and R. G. SHULMAN
Department of Molucular Biophysics and Biochemistry,
Yale University, New Haven, Connecticut 06511, USA

Our work at Yale University has involved the development of spectroscopic techniques that allow new kinds
of information to be obtained from the living brain.
One recently applied technique - high resolution
hydrogen-1 NMR - has been advanced to the stage where
proton studies of the rat and rabbit brain in vivo are
yielding consistent metabolic results. In this paper
I will concentrate on the kinds of information that is
available from the hydrogen-1 spectrum when combined
with phosphorus-31 and carbon-13 spectroscopy and the
methods we have developed to extract that information.
  A list of relevant properties of the three nuclei
(Table 1) - phosphorus-31, carbon-13 and hydrogen-1 -
in terms of their relative sensitivity, isotopic abundance, and their biological chemical shift range, allows
an assessment of the particular advantages and possible
disadvantages that each nucleus might have in the study
of biological tissues. The proton, while demonstrating
the greatest sensitivity of the three nuclei, has the
smallest chemical shift dispersion. Carbon-13 is the
least sensitive of the three, although its relative
sensitivity may be increased through an effect known
as the Nuclear Overhauser Enhancement. Because carbon-13
linewidths tend to be less than those of phosphorus-31
resonances at any given field strength, the combination
of these factors make the relative sensitivities of
carbon-13 and phosphorus-31 approximately equal.

THE PHOSPHORUS-31 NMR SPECTRUM

The phosphorus-31 spectrum records the state of high
energy phosphates, primarily phosphocreatine and
nucleoside triphosphates. Figure 1 shows the normal

Proceedings of the 16th FEBS Congress
Part A, pp. 251–262
© 1985 VNU Science Press

appearance of this spectrum for rat brain after the
broad component -- arising from bone phosphates -- is
removed by a convolution difference method. Intracellular pH is neasured from the chemical shift (pH sensitive) of inorganic orthophosphate by reference to
a suitable titration curve. Because of the importance
of these substances in energy metabolism, phosphorus-31
NMR is particularly useful in the study of ischemia,
hypoxia and seizure related encephalopathies. An example
of this is seen by the effect that bicuculine-induced
status epilepticus has upon the phosphorus-31 spectrum
of the rabbit brain (1). During 26 minutes of continuous seizure activity, phosphocreatine fell to a new
steady state level while inorganic phosphate rose;
intracellular pH decreasing concomitantly with these
changes. These changes were then compared to the magnitude and duration of seizure discharges on the electroencephalogram under various treatments.

THE CARBON-13 NMR SPECTRUM

Carbon-13 NMR can be used to detect the 1.1% natural
abundance signals of highly concentrated storage compounds (e.g., glycogen and fatty acids) in organs
other than the brain, or to detect small metabolites
in brain (e.g., amino acids and lactate) following
enrichment by an appropriately labeled precursor. In
contrast to muscle and hepatic tissues, glycogen levels
in the brain are extremely low (2-3 μmole/gm wet wt)
and cannot be detected by their natural abundance signals. The mobile fats, which given rise to NMR signals,
are relatively lower in brain and require longer signal averaging times to observe.
    The detection of carbon-13 signals from small metabo-
lites is accomplished by selective enrichment of the
molecule by administration of labeled substrate (e.g.,
$(1-^{13}C)$ glucose). The specific molecular site of the
label provides information about specific fluxes through
different metabolic pathways, label scrambling, and
flux cycling. In addition to providing the flux of
carbon-13 labels, carbon-13 NMR can be used in con-

junction with hydrogen-1 NMR to determine the amount
of unlabeled metabolite.

Carbon-13 NMR (1.9 Tesla; 20.2 MHz) was used recently
to detect cerebral amino acids and lactate in the rabbit
brain in vivo after a hypoxic stress (2). Following
an intravenous infusion of $(1-{}^{13}C)$ glucose, the cerebral amino acids glutamate and glutamine (unresolved)
were detected after about 15 minutes. A low oxygen gas
mixture was administrated shortly after an apparent
steady state was achieved in their levels. A prompt
rise was observed in the lactate C3 resonance at 21
parts-per-million (ppm) in the carbon-13 spectrum.
The resonances appearing after $(1-{}^{13}C)$ glucose administration are readily seen in the difference spectrum
obtained during the hypoxic period (Fig. 2).

Because resolution increases with field strength,
many overlapping resonances at the lower field of 1.9
Tesla are resolved at higher field (8.4 Tesla).
Increased resolution at higher field strengths, when
combined with more efficient hydrogen-1 decoupling
using single, double-tuned surface coils (3), allows
the separation of several amino acid resonances.

THE HYDROGEN-1 NMR SPECTRUM

Proton spectroscopy is a relatively new addition to
the techniques available for the study of organs and
tissues in vivo (4). When compared to carbon-13 or
phosphorus-31, the high sensitivity of hydrogen-1 NMR
allows metabolic transitions to be studied on the time
scale of seconds instead of minutes. For example;
recently we have followed the initial rate of rise
of lactate in rat brain following complete ischemia
with 12 sec time resolution (unpublished results).

Limited dynamic range and limited chemical shift
range are serious problems in obtaining high resolution
hydrogen-1 in vivo. The concentration of water protons
(110 molar) is between 2,000 to 200,000 times the intensity of metabolites that one wishes to observe.
The biological chemical shift range of the hydrogen-1
spectrum is 1/20 that of carbon-13 and 1/4 that of

phosphorus-31. The small spectral dispersion coupled with the numerous lines and multiplicities in the hydrogen-1 spectrum is discouraging at first sight.

The problems that must be overcome in order to obtain biochemically useful hydrogen-1 spectra can be grouped into two major categories: (i) water suppression and (ii) resolution improvement.

There are several methods now available to suppress or eliminate water selectively from the hydrogen-1 spectrum resulting in an icreased dynamic range. The methods that we employ (at the time of writing) consist either of presaturation, spin echo methods or both. The presaturation method consists of a gated selective radio frequency field applied on the water resonance frequency for several hundred milliseconds. This pulse, applied before the observation pulse, saturates the water resonance (Fig. 3A), so that the water intensity is reduced by several hundred times during observation (Fig. 3B). When these spectra are resolution enhanced (Fig. 3C), several sharp resonances are detected. These resonances were assigned by comparison to those detected in excised brain tissue and acid-methanol extracts of the rat brain frozen in situ (4).

The hydrogen-1 spectrum of the rat brain contains numerous resonances of metabolites that are present in the 1 to 10 millimolar range. These include glutamate, glutamine, aspartate, N-acetylaspartate, gamma--aminobutyric acid, creatine and phosphocreatine (unresolved) and choline containing molecules. Because the total creatine pool (consisting of creatine + phophocreatine) remains constant at about 10 to 11 millimolar in brain tissue, it can be used as an internal concentration standard.

The hydrogen-1 spectrum readily reveals dynamical processes in brain chemistry. Lactic acid formation during hypoxia is easily observed. The intensity of the lactic acid methyl protons is sensitive to the depth and duration of hypoxia (4).

Many factors may contribute to the rate of glycolysis during hypoxia or ischemia; one of importance is intracellular pH. Because intracellular pH regulation is a complex combination of physiochemical buf-

fering, metabolic reactions and transmembrane fluxes
of protons, it would be desirable to measure both lactate and intracellular pH "simultaneously" in vivo.
We have developed a method whereby phosphorus-31 and
hydrogen-1 spectra are collected alternately by using
a double-tuned surface coil that resonates at both the
hydrogen-1 and phosphorus-31 frequencies. This arrange-
ment allows correlations to be made between changes
in lactate, intracellular pH and high energy phosphate
with a time resolution that is limited by the sensitivity of detection of resonances in the phosphorus-31
spectrum. When physiological monitoring (e.g., the
electroencephalogram) is combined with the NMR measurements, insights may be gained into the relationships between metabolism and functional activity.

Lactic acid at high concentration (in excess of
16-20 millimolar) may be an important factor in the
development of irreversible brain damage during cerebral ischemia; its measurement in humans would therefore have diagnostic importance in clinical medicine.
Because the magnetic field strenghts of commercially
available magnets capable of supporting humans are
relatively low (1.9 Tesla), we have assessed the problems of lower chemical shift resolution encountered
at this field strenght in the rabbit brain (5). The
results of these experiments show that the spectral
resolution is adequate for hydrogen-1 NMR studies of
human brain metabolism in the large bore magnets now
available.

Many other resonances of metabolites are observed
in the hydrogen-1 spectrum in addition to lactate.
We have used a gated phosphorus-31 and hydrogen-1
approach to study the effects of profound insulin-
-induced hypoglycemia in the rat brain in vivo (6).
During the period of electrocerebral silence induced
by hypoglycemia, a large decrease in the proton resonance intensities of glutamate and glutamine occurred
concomitantly with an increase in aspartate. The reciprocal nature of the changes in glutamate and aspartate
probably reflect aminotransferase activity. Concurrently,
the phosphorus-31 spectrum shows large decreases in
phosphocreatine and nucleoside triphosphate and a large

255

increase in inorganic orthophosphate. Recovery from
hypoglycemia by glucose administration reverses most
of these changes. These experiments demonstrate the
ability of hydrogen-1 NMR to detect changes in the
concentrations of lactic acid and amino acids under
pathological conditions. They also show the kind of
information obtained by combining phosphorus-31 and
hydrogen-1 NMR measurements. Changes in the concentrations of cerebral metabolites generally occur in pathological processes. Metabolic regulation in non-patho-
logical states is accomplished by changes in the fluxes
of metabolites through specific pathways.

A recently developed technique for in vivo studies,
which we refer to as proton-observe carbon-decouple
spectroscopy, allows the measurement of fluxes from
hydrogen-1 spectra using carbon-13 labeled substrates
(7, 8). The presence of a directly bonded carbon-13
atom will induce a splitting of the spectral lines
of the proton resonance (the hydrogen-1 spectrum is
observed); allowing the measurement of both labeled
and unlabeled species. The method was applied to the
measurement of lactate (8) in the following
manner: during the course of a spin echo pulse sequence,
the tau-delay times are chosen such that the satelites
of the carbon-13 coupled protons invert in phase
(relative to carbon-12 bonded protons). At that instant,
the phase modulation is frozen by applying single-
-frequency irradiation to the C3 of lactate (a process
referred to as "decoupling") in the carbon-13 spectrum.
The spin echo pulse sequence is again repeated for
protons but now the C3 of lactate is continuously decoupled. When the two spectra are subtracted, only
those protons coupled to carbon-13 are retained. The
component spectrum that was obtained during continuous
carbon-13 decoupling gives the total metabolite resonance intensity ($^{12}C + ^{13}C$). In this way we obtain
the sensitivity of the proton and much of the resolution of the carbon-13 spectrum.

We have used this method to follow the incorporation
of carbon-13 label from intravenously administered
($1-^{13}C$) glucose to lactate C£ in the hydrogen-1 spectrum

of the rat brain during anoxia (8). During this experiment, the C3 of lactate is decoupled and the methyl
protons are observed. From these spectra, the rate of
carbon-13 labeled lactate formation, as well as the
total (^{12}C + ^{13}C) lactate produced, can be calculated.
If the fractional labeling of blood glucose is known
to be in a steady state, then it is possible to obtain
information about unlabeled glucose sources (e.g.,
glycogen release during anoxia).

The proton-observe carbon-decouple method was then
used to ,easure the turnover time of glutamate C4 in
the hydrogen-1 spectrum of the brain of a normoxic
rat (8); gated-carbon-13 decoupling was applied to the
C4 carbon atom.

A difficulty encountered with in vivo carbon-13 NMR
spectra using surface coils is determining the concentrations of the metabolites observed. The proton-observe
carbon-decouple method provides a means of determining
their concentrations in the carbon-13 spectrum (8).
The concentrations of the carbon-13 labeled metabolite
is first measured in the hydrogen-1 spectrum relative
to the total creatine resonance intensity. The concentration obtained will be equivalent to that of the same
species in the carbon-13 spectrum after corrections
for saturation and Nuclear Overhauser Effects.

One remaining obstacle to accurate quantitation is
the high degree of overlap that exists for several
resonances; particularly those of the animo acids.
How can this proble be delt with? Just as carbon-13
decoupling of proton coupled resonances provided selectivity in the hydrogen-1 spectrum, selective irradiation of certain proton-coupled resonances in the
hydrogen-1 spectrum can provide a resonance selection
method (9). The result is a hydrogen-1 spectrum containing only the desired resonance(s) -- all others
are eliminated. The method employs the phase modulation
properties of spin coupled protons during a spin echo
pulse sequence to select desired resonances.

For example, those resonances which exist as "doublets"
because of coupling to a single proton (e.g., the
methyl protons of alanine and lactate) may be selected

by single frequency decoupling of their alpha proton (3.7 and 4.1 ppm, respectively). The difference spectrum between the nondecoupled (time delay chosen that allows inversion of doublet) and decoupled spectrum (phase modulation inhibited) reveal the methyl protons no longer complicated by spectral overlap (9, 10). The "triplet" resonances of glutamate, taurine and gamma-aminobutyric acid may also be selected in a similar manner (10). To demonstrate the power of the method, in terms of resolving extensively overlapped resonances, we have measured the post mortem rise of gamma- aminobutyric acid during complete anoxia in the rat brain (10).

These methods should be compatible with the proton-observe carbon-decouple technique allowing the accurate quantitation of fluxes in vivo.

The proton double-resonance difference method should be also of general use in non-invasive studies of human brain where fatty tissues of the scalp would normally interfere with the hydrogen-1 spectrum (10).

REFERENCES

1. Petroff, O. A. C., Prichard, J. W., Behar, K. L., Alger, J. R. and Shulman, R. G. (1984). Annals Neurology 16, 169-177.
2. Behar, K. L., Petroff, O. A. C., Prichard, J. W., Alger, J. R. and Shulman, R. G. (1984). Proc. Natl. Acad. Sci., submitted.
3. den Hollander, J. A., Behar, K. L. and Shulman, R. G. (1984). J. Magn. Reson. 57, 311-313.
4. Behar, K. L., den Hollander, J. A., Stromski, M. E., Ogion, T., Shulman, R. G., Petroff, O. A. C. and Prichard, J. W. (1983). Proc. Natl. Acad. Sci. (USA) 80, 4945-4948.
5. Behar, K. L., Rothman, D. L., Shulman, R. G., Petroff, O. A. C. and Prichard, J. W. (1984). Proc. Natl. Acad. Sci. (USA) 81, 2517-2519.
6. Behar, K. L., den Hollander, J. A., Hetherington, H. P., Petroff, O. A. C., Prichard, J. W. and Shulman, R. G. (1984). J. Neurochem., in press,
7. Sillerud, L. O., Alger, J. R. and Shulman, R. G.

(1984). J. Magn. Reson. 45, 142-150.
8. Rothman, D. L., Behar, K. L., Hetherington, H. P.,
   den Hollander, J. A., Bendall, M. R. and Shulman,
   R. G. (1984). Proc. Natl. Acad. Sci., submitted.
9. Rothman, D. L., Arias Mendoza, F., Shulman, G. I.
   and Shulman, R. G. (1984). J. Magn. Reson., in
   press.
10. Rothman, D. L., Behar, K. L., Hetherington, H. P.
    and Shulman, R. G. (1984).
    Proc. Natl. Acad. Sci., in press.

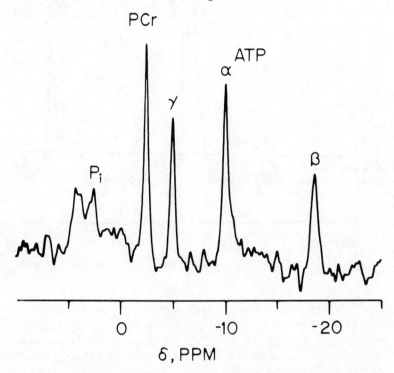

FIGURE 1. The phosphorus-31 spectrum (145.8 MHz) of
the rat brain. A surface coil was placed over the
exposed skull of a tracheotomized and paralyzed rat
breathing 30% oxygen in nitrous oxide. The spectrum
is the sum of 1000 scans recycled every 0.6 sec;
total time was 10 min. The peaks are labeled as follows:
P_i, inorganic orthophosphate; PCr, phosphocreatine;
$ATP_{\alpha, \beta, \gamma}$, adenosine triphosphate (αP, βP and γP).

259

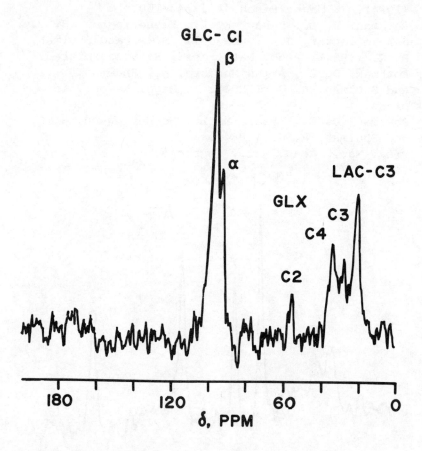

FIGURE 2. The proton decoupled carbon-13 difference spectrum (20.2 MHz) of a hypoxic rabbit brain during intravenous infusion of $(1-{}^{13}C)$-D-glucose. The resonances enriched by the labeled glucose include: Glx C4, C3 and C2; glutamate + glutamine (unresolved) carbons 4, 3 and 2 respectively; Lactate carbon 3; Glc Cl, ∝ and β; glucose carbons 1∝ and 1β, respectively.

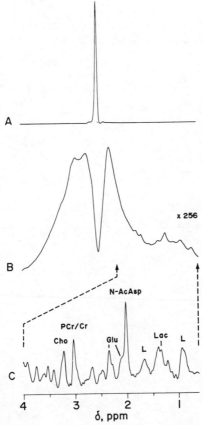

FIGURE 3. The hydrogen-1 spectrum (360.1 MHz) of the rat brain (30% oxygen; 70% nitrous oxide). A surface coil was placed over the exposed skull. (Spectrum A) Large resonance due to intra- and extracellular water. (Spectrum B) Saturation of the water resonance by an r.f. pulse brings other resonances into view. (Spectrum C) Resolution enhancement of the spectrum after water peak suppression reveals numerous metabolite resonances. Assignments are as follows: Cho, choline methyl containing compounds; PCr/Cr, phosphocreatine + creatine (unresolved); Glu, glutamate; N-AcAsp, N-acetylaspartate; Lac, lactate; L, lipids.

TABLE 1.

Nucleus	^{31}P	^{13}C	^{1}H
Frequency at 8.4 Tesla (MHz)	145.8	90.5	360.1
Frequency at 1.9 Tesla (MHz)	32.5	20.2	80.3
Relative Sensitivity	6.6	1.6	100
Isotopic Abundance (%)	100	1.1	100
Biological Chemical Shift Range (ppm)	25	200	10

ENERGETICS OF THE SARCOPLASMIC RETICULUM CALCIUM PUMP

WILHELM HASSELBACH
Max-Planck-Institut für Medizinische Forschung
Abt. Physiologie, Jahnstr. 29, 6900 Heidelberg

The most prominent structures in striated muscles
are the contractile proteins and the large membrane-
ous network of the sarcoplasmic reticulum (1,2).
Both structures are the main energy consuming elements in these muscles. Energy conversion in the sarcoplasmic reticulum membrane like that in the contractile
proteins is strictly controlled. The common determinant
is the level of ionised calcium in the myoplasma. Me-
chanic activity of the contractile apparatus as well as
the transport activity of the sarcoplasmic reticulum
calcium pump are turned on by the rapid release of calcium from the sarcoplasmic reticulum. Both activities
are switched off when the myoplasmic calcium level is
reduced and a steep calcium ion gradient is formed by
the activity of the calcium transport system in the reticulum. Concentrations and quantities of calcium which
are involved are well-known (3). These data allow to
discuss the energetics of muscular calcium turnover
under two viewpoints:
1) maintenance and the restitution of the calcium
   gradient and
2) transformation of chemical into osmotic energy.

The information given in Tab. 1 allows to estimate that
the resting muscle has to expend at least 13 % of its total resting metabolism for active calcium transport.
This fraction might even reach 40% since the steady
state calcium flux is approximately four times higher
than the unidirectional efflux used for the above calculations. Similar considerations show that the active
muscle consumes approximately 20-30% of its total energy
output, i.e. 1 mcal/g and twitch for calcium transport
during muscle relaxation.

Proceedings of the 16th FEBS Congress
Part A, pp. 263–270
© 1985 VNU Science Press

Tab. 1
Energy Requirement of the Calcium Pump
in the Resting Muscle

Calcium efflux	25 nmol/mg·min	
SR amount	6 mg/g	
Ca gradient or	10.000:1	0.13 cal/g·min
Transport ratio Ca/ATP	2	

Total resting energy output 1 cal/g·min

Hence, calcium transport during rest and activity considerably contributes to muscle metabolism. The energy requirement of the sarcoplasmic reticulum calcium transport system and thus its efficiency strictly depends on the stoichiometry of the pump on one hand and the size of the calcium leak of the membranes on the other hand. During ATP-driven calcium uptake as well as calcium efflux-driven ATP synthesis, the hydrolysis or the formation of 1 molecule of ATP is coupled to the translocation of 2 calcium ions, i.e. the system works at a coupling ratio of two. The overall reaction can thus be described by the following relation:

$$2\ Ca_o + ATP + H_2O \rightleftharpoons 2\ Ca_i + ADP + P_i$$

$$\frac{Ca_i^2}{Ca_o^2} = \frac{Keq \cdot ATP}{ADP \cdot P}$$

The calcium concentration ratios observed in the living muscle and in experiments with isolated membranes come quite near to the theoretical equilibrium. These findings indicate that energy transduction in the sarcoplasmic reticulum membranes is not or only very little affected by passive calcium efflux. The observed tight coupling supports the original concept that energy transduction occurs in a single cycle reaction sequence. Multi-cycle sequences permitting passive calcium leakage are not allowed (4).

264

A monocycle has originally been proposed by Makinose (5) and recently been renewed by Jencks (6). A more elaborate cycle has been proposed by de Meis (2) (Fig. 1).

Fig. 1

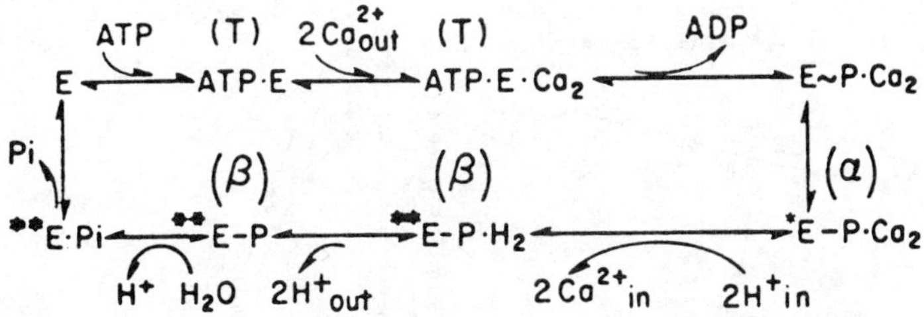

$$ATP \quad (T) \quad 2Ca^{2+}_{out} \quad (T) \qquad\qquad ADP$$

$$E \longrightarrow ATP \cdot E \longrightarrow ATP \cdot E \cdot Ca_2 \longleftarrow\!\!\!\!\!\longrightarrow E \sim P \cdot Ca_2$$

$$Pi \qquad\qquad (\beta) \qquad\qquad (\beta) \qquad\qquad\qquad (\alpha)$$

$$E \cdot Pi \longleftarrow E\text{-}P \longleftarrow E\text{-}P \cdot H_2 \longleftarrow E\text{-}P \cdot Ca_2$$

$$H^+ \quad H_2O \quad 2H^+_{out} \qquad\qquad 2Ca^{2+}_{in} \quad 2H^+_{in}$$

Diagram illustrating the catalytic and transport cycle of SR ATPase (7).

The isomerisation steps are connected with two phosphoryl transfer reactions. While the phosphoryl transfer reactions are soundly supported by experiments, the existence of the two isomerisation steps appear less well established. It is especially the assignment of calcium translocation to the transition between the so-called ADP-sensitive and the ADP-insensitive phosphoprotein intermediate which has not generally been accepted. Whatever the mechanism of calcium translocation might be, the protein's high affinity for calcium must be reduced in the reaction sequence, and calcium must be released from internally located sites. The simultaneous occurence of both events can be demonstrated if the experimental conditions are chosen in such a way that the low affinity intermediate has a long lifetime in the cycle. This appears to be the case at pH 6 in the presence of 5mM magnesium and at low temperature (Fig. 2).

Under these conditions, the phosphorylation of the protein by 2 equivalents of ATP occurs rapidly (8). Phosphoprotein formation is accompanied by a sudden release of 3-4 nmol of calcium/mg protein. When the phosphoprotein is hydrolytically cleaved, the high affinity calcium binding sites reappear with a definite time lag. Fig. 2 further shows that calcium release is related to

Fig. 2

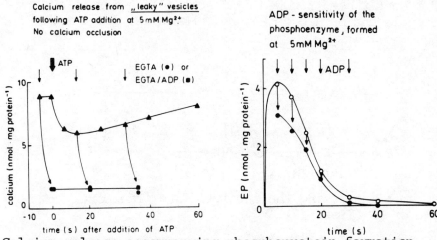

Calcium release from „leaky" vesicles
following ATP addition at 5 mM Mg^{2+}
No calcium occlusion

ADP - sensitivity of the
phosphoenzyme, formed
at 5 mM Mg^{2+}

Calcium release accompanying phosphoprotein formation.
Conditions: leaky vesicles, pH 6.0, Mg^{++} 5 mM, KCl 40 mM,
T = 4°C (8).

the formation of the ADP-insensitive phosphoprotein
species. This assignment has further been supported by
the finding that no calcium is released from the protein when it is phosphorylated at reduced magnesium
concentrations. Under this condition, phosphoprotein
is always ADP-sensitive (Fig. 3). Thus, in the foreward
running mode of the pump, the calcium translocation is
connected to the transition   from E $\sim PCa_2$ to
E - PCa_2. This assignment also holds when the pump runs
backward. After calcium has been removed from the external high affinity binding sites, an ADP-insensitive
phosphoprotein is formed by the incorporation of inorganic phosphate (Tab. 3). This ADP-insensitive phosphoprotein gains ADP-sensitivity when the calcium concentration is suddenly raised and low affinity calcium
sites   on the internal leaflet of the membrane are
occupied. These findings suggest that the phosphorylation by inorganic phosphate converts external high into
internal low affinity calcium binding sites. Conversely,
the occupation by calcium of the low affinity binding
sites of the ADP-insensitive phosphoprotein induces its

266

Fig. 3

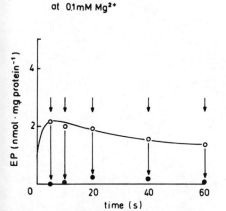

ADP - sensitivity of the phosphoenzyme, formed at 0.1mM Mg²⁺

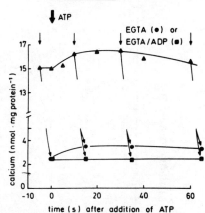

Additional binding and occlusion of calcium following ATP addition to „leaky" vesicles at 0.1 mM Mg²⁺

Calcium binding accompanying phosphoprotein formation. Conditions: leaky vesicles. pH 6.0, Mg^{++} 0.1 mM, KCl 40 mM, T = 4°C (8).

Tab. 2

Formation of ADP-Sensitive Phosphoprotein by Phosphorylation of SR ATPase with Inorganic Phosphate

$$E_o Ca_2 \rightleftharpoons E_o + 2Ca^o \qquad \mu M\ Ca^{++}$$

$$E_o \rightleftharpoons E_i$$

$$E_i + P_i \rightleftharpoons E_i - P \qquad mM\ P_i$$

$$E_i - P + 2Ca^i \rightleftharpoons (E_i-P) \sim Ca_2^i \qquad mM\ Ca$$

$$(E_i-P) \sim Ca_2^i \rightleftharpoons (E_o \sim P) - Ca_2^o$$

transition to the ADP-sensitive phosphoprotein. According to this concept, phosphorylation by inorganic phosphate should also result in a reduction of the enzyme's affinity for calcium. As shown in Fig. 4, the protein's

Fig. 4

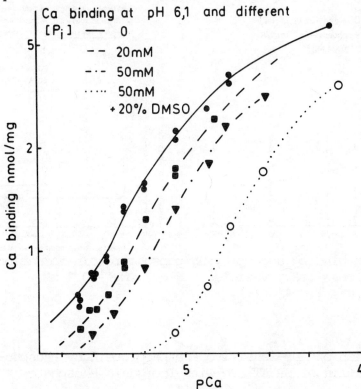

Ca binding at pH 6,1 and different
[Pᵢ]

Mutual interaction of calcium and phosphate with SR
transport ATPase.

affinity for calcium is in fact reduced when inorganic
phosphate is present. Yet the shifts of the calcium
binding curves are quite small and high concentrations
of phosphate were required. This mutual ligand interaction could be established more clearly by exchanging
phosphate with its high affinity analog vanadate.
0.1 mM vanadate abolishes nearly all high affinity
calcium binding sites. Simultaneously, a number of
new calcium binding sites of lower affinity emerge
(9,10). These low affinity calcium binding sites are
located on the luminal surface of the membrane. This
follows from the results showing that the displacement of vanadate from the protein at high concentration

Fig. 5

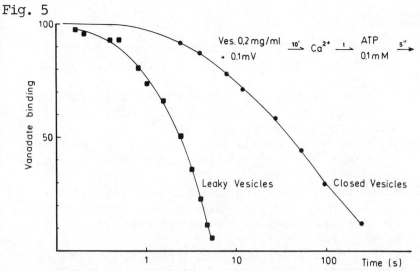

Displacement of vanadate by calcium from closed and Ca permeable vesicles.

of calcium occurs very slowly from closed vesicles. If, however, calcium is added to open membranes or together with an ionophore, vanadate is released in a few seconds. We must conclude that internal calcium binding sites must be accessible for calcium in order to expel vanadate. The consecutive occurence of external high affinity sites was detected by their phosphorylation with radioactive ATP (9). This transposition of sites is accompanied by a definite change in the structure of the sarcoplasmic reticulum membranes. On vanadate binding, the normally asymmetrically arranged electron dense protein particles become symmetrically distributed. Thus, with vanadate, it is possible to follow, like in slow motion pictures, what happens when calcium is translocated from one to the other site of the membrane (10).

References:

1) Hasselbach, W. (1964). Relaxing factor and the relaxation of muscle. Progr. Biophys. Mol. Biol. 14, 167–222.

2) de Meis, L. (1981). The sarcoplasmic reticulum in transport. In: Life Science, E.E. Bittar (ed.). John Wiley Sons, New York, pp. 1–163.

3) Hasselbach, W. and Oetliker, H. (1983). Energetics and electrogenicity of the sarcoplasmic reticulum calcium pump. Ann. Rev. Physiol. 45, 325–339.

4) Tanford, Ch. (1984). The sarcoplasmic reticulum calcium pump. Localization of free energy transfer to discrete steps of the reaction cycle. FEBS Letters 166, 1–7.

5) Makinose, M. (1973). Possible functional states of the enzyme of the sarcoplasmic calcium pump. FEBS Letters 37, 140–143.

6) Pickart, C.M. and Jencks, W.P. (1984). Energetics of the calcium-transporting ATPase. J. Biol. Chem. 259, 1629–1643.

7) Inesi, G. and Hill, T.L. (1983). Calcium and proton dependence of sarcoplasmic reticulum ATPase. Biophys. J. 44, 271–280.

8) Hasselbach, W., Agostini, B., Medda, P., Migala, A. and Waas, W. (1983). The sarcoplasmic reticulum calcium pump. Early and recent developments critically overviewed. In: Structure and Function of Sarcoplasmic Reticulum, Y. Tonomura and S. Fleischer (eds.). Academic Press, New York.

9) Medda, P. and Hasselbach, W. (1983). The vanadate complex of the calcium-transport ATPase of the sarcoplasmic reticulum, its formation and dissociation. Eur. J. Biochem. 137, 7–14.

10) Hasselbach, W., Medda, P., Migala, A. and Agostini, B. (1983). A conformational transition of the sarcoplasmic reticulum calcium transport ATPase induced by vanadate. Z. Naturforsch. 38c, 1015–1022.

PHOSPHORYLATION OF THE CONTRACTILE PROTEINS AND THE REGULATION OF CONTRACTION.

PERRY, Samuel Victor
Department of Biochemistry, University of Birmingham
P O Box 363, Birmingham B15 2TT. U.K.

Evidence now exists for the phosphorylation of all the major protein components of the A and I filaments of the myofibril of striated muscle apart from troponin C. In the cases of the P light chain of myosin, C protein and troponin I of cardiac muscle it has been shown that the covalently bound phosphate is in rapid dynamic equilibrium with the intracellular pools of phosphate and that the levels change according to the activity state of the muscle. Sites have been identified in tropomyosin and troponin T from skeletal muscle that are partially phosphorylated when the protein is isolated from fresh tissue with precautions to prevent the action of endogenous enzymes. The phosphate contents of these I filament proteins remain relatively constant, and there is no evidence that they rapidly change in response to activity or hormones.

I FILAMENT PHOSPHORYLATION

Tropomyosin

α-Tropomyosin is phosphorylated in the penultimate residue, serine 283 (1). Four isoforms of the tropomyosin subunit have been identified in adult skeletal muscle, namely α, β, γ and δ, by two-dimensional electrophoresis. In normal adult muscle the α, β, γ forms and probably also the δ form are partially phosphorylated Usually 10-20% of the total tropomyosin is phosphorylated of which the largest fraction is α-tropomyosin (2). Before birth, the level of phosphorylation is much increased, rising to over 70% in the rat foetal heart. This observation supports the view that phosphorylation of tropomyosin may regulate the head-to-tail aggregation involved in filament formation and hence play a role in

Proceedings of the 16th FEBS Congress
Part A, pp. 271–279

myofibrillogenesis. Not all the experimental findings support this hypothesis for little significant increase in phosphorylation of the tropomyosin subunits could be observed in muscles regenerating after injury where myofibrillogensis would be expected to be very active (3), nor was it consistently observed after cross-innervation when changes in gene expression were occurring.

Troponin I

Troponin I from rabbit fast twitch muscle possesses two major sites, threonine 11 and serine 117, that can be phosphorylated by phosphorylase kinase and by cAMP-dependent protein kinase respectively (4,5). These sites are close to regions of troponin I that are involved in interaction with troponin C. When isolated by affinity chromatography from fresh skeletal muscle troponin I is partially phosphorylated but the precise location of the phosphate is not known. There is, however, no evidence of the phosphorylation of skeletal troponin I changing in response to activity (6). Sites homologous to the major phosphorylation sites of the fast skeletal muscle isoform are present in troponin I from slow skeletal and cardiac muscles (7). The cardiac isoform possesses an additional N-terminal peptide of 26 amino acid residues that contains a serine in position 20 which is the preferred site of phosphorylation by cAMP-dependent protein kinase. In the normal beating rabbit heart this site is about 30% phosphorylated and after intervention with adrenaline phosphorylation increases up to 100% (8,9). After the inotropic response disappears the phosphate content of cardiac troponin I returns to the normal level. Phosphorylation of cardiac troponin I causes a change in the Ca^{2+}-binding properties of the troponin C with which it is associated in the troponin complex (10,11). In consequence the actomyosin ATPase requires a higher Ca^{2+} concentration for 50% activation. Thus phosphorylation of cardiac troponin I produces a fall in the Ca^{2+} sensitivity of the myofibrillar ATPase and hence is responsible for the decrease in relaxation time that is associated with the inotropic response in the heart.

Acting as a negative feed-back process it is a special modulating mechanism evolved for cardiac muscle. In skeletal muscle the Ca^{2+} flux is relatively constant for each cell type and increase in force is obtained by recruitment of fibres. There is no evidence that phosphorylation of troponin I in skeletal muscle modulates the Ca^{2+} sensitivity of the actomyosin ATPase. Every myocardial cell contracts, however, and the heart is able to vary its contractile response by changing the Ca^{2+} flux over a wide range. To accommodate this the contractile system has a specialised mechanism of changing its response to Ca^{2+} at the myofibrillar level.

A FILAMENT PHOSPHORYLATION

C-protein
C protein is a component of the A filament located at a periodicity of 430 A° (12). It is associated with at least seven of the eleven transverse stripes observed in each half of the A band. The protein in cardiac muscle appears to differ from the skeletal forms in that it is partially phosphorylated and contains approximately 1 mole phosphate per mole of C protein in the normal beating heart. After treatment with adrenaline, the covalently bound phosphate of C protein increased to approximately 5 mole P/mole (13). As the function of C protein is uncertain, the physiological function of its phosphorylation is likewise unknown. When fully phosphorylated in vivo there will be 12-15 phosphate groups highly localized on the A filament at a 430 A° period periodicity.

Myosin
Phosphorylation and dephosphorylation of the P light chain of myosin is catalysed by specific enzymes, myosin light chain kinase and phosphatase respectively. Apart from troponin T (14,15) it is the only myofibrillar protein so far shown to be phosphorylated by a specific enzyme. Myosin light chain kinase is present in all muscles, with the exception of molluscan adductor and represents the most active myofibrillar protein phos-

273

phorylation system in fast skeletal and smooth muscles.
Requiring calmodulin as a cofactor, the kinase is
activated at similar concentrations of Ca^{2+} to those
which activate the myofibrillar ATPase in striated muscle
Thus, as would be expected, phosphorylation of the P
light chain increases on stimulation of both skeletal and
smooth muscles (see 16 for review). Although the enzyme
and substrate and the actomyosin systems are very similar
in striated and smooth muscles, the role of the enzyme
appears to be different in these two tissues, which will
therefore, be discussed separately.

Striated muscle. In resting striated muscle the P light
chain of myosin is, according to most reports, partially
phosphorylated and values usually range from 10-50%
phosphorylation in resting muscle. On stimulation
phosphorylation increases particularly in fast twitch
muscle where values of 100% have been reported after a
short tetanus. It can be concluded, however, that
phosphorylation is not essential for contraction and is
probably not synchronous with the crossbridge cycle.
Indeed the general impression is that the increase in
phosphorylation is relatively sluggish compared to the
mechanical response. During tetanus the extent of phosphorylation depends on the frequency of stimulation. At
higher levels of phosphorylation of the P light chain
in vivo there is some correlation with post-tetanic
potentiation (17,18). Nevertheless the latter effect
disappears before phosphorylation returns to the resting
level. Also P light chain phosphorylation occurs in slow
twitch muscle which does not exhibit post-tetanic
potentiation. It seems likely that P light chain phosphorylation modulates the contractile response but the
manner is not understood. An obvious mechanism would
involve changing the enzymic activity of the myosin but
the results of in vitro studies on the effect of phosphorylation on the MgATPase of actomyosin systems are
somewhat unequivocal. Phosphorylation of myosin is not
essential for actin-activation of the ATPase. Although
reports in general suggest that after phosphorylation
there is little change in the MgATPase of actomyosin of

274

the extracted proteins, activity may be lowered if the actomyosin is maintained in the myofibrillar form by crosslinking (18,19).

Smooth muscle. Smooth muscle possesses myosin light chain kinase activity comparable to that of fast twitch muscle but the catalytic component of the enzyme system has a higher molecular weight and differs in that its activity can be modulated by the phosphorylation of sites on it by cAMP-dependent kinase (20). It is now widely established that actin-activation of MgATPase of smooth muscle myosin requires phosphorylation of the P light chain. Activation is complete when both heads are fully phosphorylated but the increase in activity is not linearly related to the extent of phosphorylation. These results have been interpreted as indicating that only myosin with two heads phosphorylated is enzymically active and that the two heads are not randomly phosphorylated by the kinase (21,22). Once fully phosphorylated the MgATPase of actomyosin is calcium insensitive, but there is evidence that the enzymic activity of partially phosphorylated actomyosin is calcium sensitive (23). Although it is clear that smooth myosin requires to be phosphorylated for actin activation of the MgATPase it is probable that other systems exist in smooth muscle for the regulation of the actomyosin ATPase (see 24 for review).

GENERAL COMMENTS

Differences in function exist in the two types of systems for phosphorylating proteins of the myofibril. The first system involves those phosphate groups on proteins such as tropomyosin and troponin T that are not in rapid dynamic equilibrium with the intracellular phosphate pool and in which the level of phosphorylation does not change rapidly with contractile activity. The relative inertness of the phosphate groups, both metabolically and during isolation suggests a structural role. It is of interest that the sites phosphorylated in both proteins are at the termini of the polypeptide chains and which are conceivably regions of interaction with other proteins. Another explanation could be that these are simply exposed regions of molecules that have serine residues in sites appropriate for covalent modification by the kinases present in the sarcoplasm and have no specific functional role. This seems unlikely in both cases for there exists a specific kinase for troponin T and the phosphorylation level of tropomyosin changes markedly during development. It can be concluded however, that in vivo there will not be marked changes in charge density due to the short term reversible changes in phosphorylation of these proteins.

The situation with the phosphorylation of C protein, troponin I and the P light chain of myosin is markedly different. During a relative short-time interval, but probably not synchronous with the cross-bridge cycle, marked changes in charge can occur particularly along the A filament. Assuming the covalently bound phosphate is fully ionised in intracellular conditions the phosphorylation of the P light chain of myosin associated with the change from the resting to the tetanised state in fast skeletal muscle phosphorylation of the P light chain of myosin would result in an increase in about 9 negative charges per 143 A° in the cross-bridge region of the A filament, i.e. about 900 negative charges per A filament. This is assuming phosphorylation changes from 25% to 100% during activity. This must clearly have a profound effect on the interaction between the A and I filaments. It may be of significance in cardiac muscle, where little change occurs in P light chain phosphorylation during increased activity, that a similar increase in negative charge density is produced by phosphorylation of the C protein (13).

The phosphorylation of cardiac troponin I provides the the best documented example of a role for phosphorylation which brings about a change in the binding properties of a calcium binding protein, troponin C. This protein interacts with specific regions of troponin I and unlike troponin C from fast twitch muscle which has two sites, possesses only one effective Ca^{2+} specific binding site. This corresponds to site II of fast skeletal muscle

276

troponin C. Thus in some way phosphorylation at serine 20 on troponin I produces effects that are transmitted to the region of site II on the adjacent troponin C resulting in a change in its calcium-binding characteristics.

Similar changes in calcium binding properties caused by phosphorylation can be demonstrated in a number of other muscle systems. Phosphorylation of the smooth muscle myosin light chain kinase catalytic unit leads to a higher Ca^{2+} requirement for activation (20). Phosphorylation of the β-subunit of phosphorylase much reduces the Ca^{2+} concentration required to activate this enzyme, the δ-subunit of which is calmodulin (25). These are three clear examples of systems consisting of a calcium binding protein and an associated protein, the phosphorylation of which leads to a change in affinity of the calcium binding protein. Less clear cut, but suggestive, is the change in calcium sensitivity of the MgATPase of smooth muscle actomyosin when the P light chain is phosphorylated (23). Thus it would appear that a major role of protein phosphorylation in muscle is to modulate the response of the contractile system to the calcium flux.

REFERENCES

1. Mak, A, Smillie L.B. & Barany, M. (1978) Specific phosphorylation at serine 283 of α-tropomyosin from frog skeletal and rabbit skeletal and cardiac muscle. Proc.Natl.Acad.Sci. (USA), 75, 3588-3592
2. Heeley, D.H., Moir, A.J.G. & Perry, S.V. (1982) Phosphorylation of tropomyosin during development. FEBS Lett. 146, 115-118
3. Heeley, D.H., Dhoot, G.K. & Perry, S.V. Factors determining the subunit composition of tropomyosin in mammalian skeletal muscle. Biochem.J. Submitted for publication.
4. Moir A.J.G., Wilkinson, J.M. & Perry, S.V. (1974) The phosphorylation sites of troponin I from white skeletal muscle of the rabbit. FEBS Lett. 42, 253-256

5. Huang, T.S., Byland, D.B., Stull, J.T. & Krebs, E.G. (1974) The amino acid sequences of the phosphorylated sites in troponin I from rabbit skeletal muscle. FEBS Lett. 42, 249-252

6. Ribolow, H., Barany, K., Steinschneider, A. & Barany, M. (1977) Lack of phosphate incorporation into troponin I in live frog muscle. Arch.Biochem. Biophys. 179, 81-88

7. Wilkinson, J.M. & Grand, R.J.A. (1978) Comparison of amino acid sequence of troponin I from different striated muscles. Nature, 271, 31-35

8. England, P.J. (1975) Correlation between contraction and phosphorylation of the inhibitory subunit of troponin in perfused rat heart. FEBS Lett. 50, 57-60

9. Moir, A.J.G., Solaro, R.J. & Perry, S.V. (1980) The site of phosphorylation of troponin I in the perfused heart: the effect of adrenaline. Biochem.J 185, 505-513

10. Solaro, R.J., Moir, A.J.G. & Perry, S.V. (1976) Phosphorylation of troponin I and the inotropic effect of adrenaline in the perfused rabbit heart. Nature (Lond.) 262, 615-617

11. Ray, K.P. & England, P.J. (1976) Phosphorylation of inhibitory subunit of troponin and its effect on the calcium dependence of cardiac myofibril adenosine triphosphatase. FEBS Lett. 70, 11-16

12. Offer, G., Moos, C. & Starr, R. (1973) A new protein of the thick filaments of vertebrate skeletal myofibrils. J.Mol.Biol. 74, 653-676

13. England, P.J. (1983) Cardiac function and phosphorylation of contractile proteins. Phil.Trans.R.Soc. B302, 83-90

14. Kumon, A. & Villar-Pallasi, C. (1978) Purification and properties of troponin T kinase from rabbit skeletal muscle. Biochem.Biophys.Acta, 566, 305-320

15. Gusev, N.B., Dobrovolskii & Severin, S.E. (1980) Isolation and some properties of troponin T kinase from rabbit skeletal muscle. Biochem.J. 189, 219-226

16. Perry, S.V., Cole, H.A., Hudlicka, O., Patchell, V.B. & Westwood, S.A. (1984) The role of myosin light chain kinase in muscle contraction. Fed.Proc. In the press.

17. Stull, J.T., Silver, P.J., Miller, J.R., Blumenthal, D.R. Botterman, B.R., & Klug, G.A. (1983) Phosphorylation of myosin light chains in skeletal and smooth muscle. Fed.Proc. 42, 21-26

18. Westwood, S.A., Hudlicka, O. & Perry, S.V. (1984) The effect of contractile activity on the phosphorylation of the P light chain of myosin of rabbit skeletal muscle. Biochem.J. 218, 841-847

19. Cooke, R., Franks, K. & Stull, J.T. (1982) Myosin phosphorylation regulates the ATPase activity of permeable skeletal muscle fibres. FEBS Lett. 144, 33-37

20. Adelstein, R.S., Conti, M.A. & Pato, M.D. (1980) Regulation of myosin light chain kinase by reversible phosphorylation and calcium calmodulin. Annals.New York, Acad.Sci. 356, 142-150

21. Persechini, A. & Hartshorne, D.J. (1981) Phosphorylation of smooth muscle myosin. Evidence for cooperativity between the myosin heads. Science, 213, 1383-1385

22. Sellers, J.R., Chock, B.P. & Adelstein, R.S. (1983) apparently negatively cooperative phosphorylation of smooth muscle myosin at low ionic strength is related to its filamentous state. J. Biol.Chem. 258, 14181-14188

23. Cole, H.A., Patchell, V.B. & Perry, S.V. (1983) Phosphorylation of chicken gizzard myosin and the Ca^{2+}-sensitivity of the actin-activated Mg^{2+}ATPase. FEBS Lett. 158, 17-20

24. Marston, S.B. (1982) The regulation of smooth muscle contractile proteins. Prog.Biophys.Mol.Biol. 41, 1-41

25. Cohen, P. (1983) Protein phosphorylation and the control of glycogen metabolism in skeletal muscle. Phil.Trans.Roy.Soc.B. 302, 13-25

MECHANISM OF ENERGY SUPPLY FOR CONTRACTION - BIOCHEMICAL AND NMR STUDIES

V.A.SAKS, V.V.KUPRIYANOV and R.VENTURA-CLAPIER*

Laboratory of Cardiac Bioenergetics, USSR Research Center for Cardiology, Moscow,USSR;

*Unite de Recherches de Physiologie Cellulaire Cardiaque, Centre Universitaire Paris-Sud, France

1.INTRODUCTION

In muscle cells, when they are actively contracting, energy is channelled from mitochondria where ATP is aerobically produced, to myofibrils mostly via phosphocreatine shuttle (1-3). The function of this shuttle may be considered to be to overcome some specific difficulties for ATP movements apparently existing in intact muscle cells, for which the adenine nucleotide compartmentation has been proposed on the basis of biochemical and functional studies of normal and ischemic myocardium (4), and to integrate the processes of energy production and utilization into a efficiently regulated system. In spite of the results of many experimental works convincingly showing the existence of this shuttle (see ref. 1-13), there are numerous conflicting reports in which the authors have failed to find evidence for the existence of phosphocreatine shuttle (14-17). The purpose of this report is to consider several central points of this problem and to demonstrate some new data which additionally point to the physiological role of phosphocreatine in cardiomyocytes.

2. MITOCHONDRIAL CREATINE KINASE

The first key enzyme in the phospho-

Proceedings of the 16th FEBS Congress
Part A, pp. 281-290

creatine shuttle is the mitochondrial creatine kinase. This specific isoenzyme, CK mit., is localized on the outer surface of the inner mitochondrial membrane (5) apparently in very exact position which allows its efficient interaction with the adenine nucleotide translocase (6-9). The latter is in position of kinetic control of mitochondrial oxidative phosphorylation and is the first step of intracellular energy transport. When the creatine kinase reaction is coupled to oxidative phosphorylation via adenine nucleotide translocase, the apparent dissociation constant for MgATP from the central complex, CK mit·MgATP·creatine, is decreased by an order of magnitude (6,7). This clear kinetic effect may be considered as an evidence of direct and efficient channelling of ATP from translocase to creatine kinase that accelerates the reaction of phosphocreatine (PCr) production (6,7). Simultaneously ADP movement back from CK_{mit} to translocase without significant release into the medium has been also clearly evidenced by atractyloside inhibition (8) and competitive enzyme studies (9). All these effects are observed for mitochondria as well as for mitoplasts with removed outer membrane that showing that this effect is inherent to the inner membrane system (data in preparation for publication). Such a coupling between CK_{mit} and translocase has several important consequences: 1) CK_{mit} is rapidly saturated by mitochondrial ATP and PCr is produced aerobically with high rate; 2) rapid utilization of ATP at outer side of mitochondrial membrane releases translocase from inhibition by this substance; 3) rapid removal of ADP from the vicinity of CK_{mit} by translocase significantly decreases the possibility of the reverse creatine kinase reaction

(ATP production from PCr) in mitochondria and thus the inhibition of PCr production; 4) ADP is made directly available for translocase in the intermembrane space without necessity of adenine nucleotide diffusion between mitochondria and cytoplasm; that also points to the importance of CK_{mit} in the control of oxidative phosphorylation. As a result, in the intact muscle cells high level of PCr is maintained in spite of its rapid utilization in myofibrils to support contraction, since the coupling described above releases the CK_{mit} reaction from inhibition by phosphocreatine and therefore ensures its synthesis with high rate from mitochondrial ATP at high physiological concentrations of PCr in cytoplasm (6-9). Some authors have managed to completely omit this mostly important consequence of coupling between CK_{mit} and translocase from their consideration of the CK_{mit} reaction (15) and in this way have arrived at the conclusion of nonsignificance of the membrane-bound CK_{mit} reaction and simultaneously, from our point of view, have created logical difficulties in explaining the events in intact muscle cells.

3. MYOFIBRILLAR CREATINE KINASE

Several recent experimental investigations have elegantly shown that particulate MM creatine kinase isoenzyme, CK_{mm}, bound to cardiac or skeletal muscle myofibrils (10) ensures very efficient replenishment of myofibrillar ATP at the expense of PCr and very clearly is able to overcome the difficulties of utilization of external, or cytoplasmic, ATP for relaxation of the muscle from its rigor state (11-13). All these data allow us to suggest

that there is a very close functional cooperation between CK_{mm} and the actine-activated
myosin ATPase reaction which involves preferential movement of adenine nucleotides
between the ATPase and CK_{mm} active centers.
Good illustration of this phenomenon is
given in Fig.1. This figure shows the results of the experiments in which we used
the Triton-treated skinned fibers prepared
from rat papillary muscle. These skinned
fibers have good contractile properties and
intact myofibrils but are almost completely
deprived of the membranes. In the presence
of ATP these fibers produce ADP due to the
ATPase reaction. In our experiments the
ADP release was recorded by the added pyruvate kinase system coupled with lactate
dehydrogenase. In this system a decrease
in NADH concentration is stoichiometrically
related to ADP production by myofibrils. All
these coupled reactions were completely stopped when PCr was added to activate CK_{mm} in
myofibrils (Fig.1). In this case, no ADP was
released from myofibrils but all ADP was
trapped and rephosphorylated in situ by
CK_{mm}. Inhibition of this enzyme by 10 μM
FDNB entirely restored the rate of the
coupled reactions, this showing that ADP
was again released into the medium. This
effect shows that if CK_{mm} is activated by
PCr, adenine nucleotides are functionally
completely compartmentalized in myofibrils
due to close interaction, or coupling, between CK_{mm} and ATPase. Additionally, Fig.1 shows
an interesting phenomenon of CK rebinding
to myofibrils.

4. ^{31}P-NMR DATA

^{31}P-NMR saturation transfer method has
been sucessfully used to measure the meta-

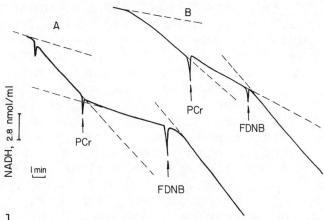

Fig.1.

Recording of MgATPase activity by a fluo-
rimetric method.
Triton-treated rat papillary muscles were
used (~ 0.1-0.5 mg). The medium (2 ml)
contained pyruvate kinase (2 IU/ml), lactate dehydrogenase (2 IU/ml), 2 mM phosph-
enolpyruvate, 50 μM NADH, 1 mM MgATP. PCr
was added to 5 mM, fluoro-2,4-dinitroben-
zen (FDNB) was added to 10 μM. A. Freshly
prepared fibers were used. B. FDNB-inhibited
fibers were additionally incubated with
0.5 mg/ml MM creatine kinase and washed for
30 min. This recording shows the rebinding
of soluble MM creatine kinase to myofibrils
with partial recovery of the effect of PCr.

bolic fluxes in intact cells (18,19). This
method has also been applied to study isolated perfused heart in attempt to find an
evidence of the existence of PCr shuttle for
energy channelling, and the results have
been sometimes conflicting and confusing
(16,17). Some authors have recorded only
slight changes in the fluxes through the
creatine kinase system, the rate of oxygen

uptake and ATP turnover being increased (16).
Recently it was reported that when PCr was
replaced by phospho-β-guanidinopropionate
(PGPA) by a diet procedure (17), no changes
in the fluxes through CK were observed in-
spite of the fact that PGPA is not an effective substrate for CK. From our point
of view, these experiments are open to serious critisism mostly on their physiological part: in these experiments due to
very low workload contraction and O_2 uptake
were not significantly stimulated and therefore the PCr shuttle was not enough activated to be observed or studied by a method of substrate replacement. In fact,
in ref. 17 O_2 uptake was changed in very
narrow range from 15 to 30 μmole O_2 per
min per g d.w. (recalculated from 17) while
in the contracting perfused heart the rate
of oxygen uptake reaches values up to
150 μmoles per min per g d.w. at high work-
loads (20). Figure 2, which reproduces the
results of our experiments by using [31]P-
NMR saturation transfer method to study
the rates of metabolic processes in isolated perfused rat heart shows that if the
rate of O_2 uptake (and ATP turnover) is
increased significantly enough, e.g. to
values of 60 μmol/min·g d.w. from 8 μmol/
min·g d.w. in the resting state, linear
increase in the flux through the CK system
is observed with the ratio $\Delta F_{CK}/\Delta V_{ATP} > 1$.
Thus, an increase in the ATP turnover rate
results in activation of flux through the
CK system with molar ratio higher than one
that is consistent with the concept of PCr
shuttle which predicts this ratio to be at
least 1. An experimental approach described
in Fig.2 represents, from our point of view,
the way of revealing PCr shuttle by ^{31}P-NMR
technique. We doubt that in experiments with

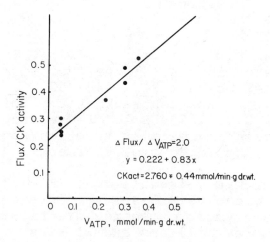

Fig.2.

Correlation between the flux through creatine kinase (PCr →ATP) and the rate of
ATP turnover in perfused rat hearts.
Fluxes (PCr → ATP) were determined by
^{31}P-NMR saturation transfer from dependences
of PCr signal intensity on time of γ-P(ATP)
saturation as described previously. Flux is
reffered to total CK activity of the heart
determined after perfusion in heart homogenate at 37°C and pH 7.4. Average value
of CK activity in this hearts was 2.76+0.44
mmol/min·g d.w. The rate of ATP turnover
was calculated from the oxygen consumption
rate, $V_{ATP}=6Vo_2$.

PGPA (17) high Vo_2 values could be reached
at all. On the basis of the concept of
PCr-shuttle it seems to be difficult to
imagine, since the inability of PCr shuttle
to function in the presence of PGPA should

put a low   range limit to the rate of integrated reactions of ATP utilization and production.

REFERENCES

1. Bessman S.P., Geiger P.J. 1981. Transport of energy in muscle: the phosphocreatine shuttle. Science 211, 448-452.
2. Saks V.A., Rosenshtraukh L.V., Smirnov V.N., Chazov E.I. 1978. Role of creatine phosphokinase in cellular function and metabolism. Can.J.Physiol.Pharmacol. 56, 691-706.
3. Jacobus W.E., Ingwall J.S. (Eds) 1980. Heart creatine kinase: the integration of isoenzymes for energy distribution. Baltimore, Williams and Wilkins.
4. Gudbjarnason S., Mathes P., Ravens K.G. 1970. Functional compartmentation of ATP and creatine phosphate in heart muscle. J.Molec.Cell.Cardiol. 1, 325-339.
5. Jacobus W.E., Lehninger A.L. 1977. Creatine kinase of rat heart mitochondria. Coupling of creatine phosphorylation to electron transport. J.Biol.Chem. 248, 483(-4810.
6. Saks V.A., Kupriyanov V.V., Elizarova G.V., Jacobus W.E. 1980. Studies of energy transport in heart cells. J.Biol. Chem. 255, 755-763.
7. Jacobus W.E., Saks V.A. 1982. Creatine kinase of heart mitochondria: changes in its kinetic properties induced by coupling to oxidative phosphorylation. Arch.Biochem.Biophys. 219, 167-178.
8. Moreadith R.W., Jacobus W.E. 1982. Creatine kinase of heart mitochondria. Functional coupling of ADP transfer to the adenine nucleotide translocase. J.Biol. Chem. 257, 899-905.

9. Gellerich F., Saks V.A. 1982. Control of heart mitochondrial oxygen consumption by creatine kinase: the importance of emzyme localization. Biochem.Biophys.Res. Comm. 105, 1473-1481.

10. Wallimann T., Schlosser T., Eppenberger H.H. 1984. Function of M-line bound creatine kinase as intramyofibrillar ATP regulator at the receiving end of the phosphocreatine shuttle in muscle. J.Biol. Chem. 259, 5238-5246.

11. McClellan G., Weisberg A., Winegrad S. 1983. Energy transport from mitochondria to myofibrils by a creatine phosphate shuttle in cardiac cells. Am.J.Physiol. 245, C423-C427.

12. Sarabi F., Geiger P.J., Bessman S.P. 1983. Kinetic properties and functional role of creatine phosphokinase in glycerinated muscle fibers - further evidence for compartmentation. Biochem.Biophys. Res.Comm. 114, 785-790.

13. Veksler V.I., Kapelko V.I. Creatine kinase in regulation of heart function and metabolism. Biochim.Biophys.Acta 803, 265-270.

14. Lipskaya T.Yu., Temple V.D., Belousova L.V., Molokova E.V., Rybina I.V. 1980. (Study of the interaction between mitochondrial creatine kinase and mitochondrial membranes) Biokhimiia 45, 1155-1166.

15. Hird F.J., McLean R.M. 1983. Synthesis of phosphocreatine and phosphoarginine by mitochondria from various sources. Comp.Biochem.Biophys. 76, 41-46.

16. Mathews P.M., Bland J.L., Gadian D.G., Radda G.K. 1982. A ^{31}P-NMR saturation transfer study of the regulation of creatine kinase in the rat heart. Biochim. Biophys.Acta 721, 312-320.

17. Meyer Ronald A., Brown T.R., Kushmerick
    M.J. 1984. CK kinetics in phosphocreatine
    depleted rat hearts. Biophysical Jour-
    nal 45, 91a.
18. Brown T.R., Gadian D.G., Garlick P.B.,
    Radda G.K., Seely J.P., Styles P. 1978.
    Creatine kinase activities in skeletal
    and cardiac muscle measured by satura-
    tion transfer NMR. Frontiers of Biolo-
    gical Energetics, vol.2, pp.1341-1349,
    Acad.Press, New York.
19. Gadian D.G. and Radda G.K. 1979. NMR
    studies of tissue metabolism. Ann.Rev.
    Biochem., 50, 69-83.
20. Williamson J.R., Ford G., Illingworth J.,
    Safer B. 1976. Coordination of atric
    acid cycle activity with electron trans-
    port flux. Circ.Res. 38, suppl. 1, 39-
    48.
21. Kupriyanov V.V., Steinschneider A.Ya.,
    Ruuge E.K., Zueva M.Yu., Lakomkin V.L.,
    Smirnov V.N., Saks V.A. 1984. Regulation
    of energy flux through the creatine
    kinase reaction in vitro and in per-
    fused rat heart: ^{31}P-NMR studies. Bio-
    chim.Biophys.Acta, in press.

THE EFFECT OF REPEATED EPISODES OF EXERCISE ON BLOOD FLOW AND METABOLISM OF RAT SKELETAL MUSCLE

R. WILKE and D. ANGERSBACH
R & D Laboratories, Beecham-Wülfing, D-3212 Gronau, FRG

INTRODUCTION

Muscle exercise is accompanied by marked metabolic changes and an increase in blood flow. During isometric contractions, muscle blood flow depends on the balance between locally released vasodilating metabolites, the degree of increase in muscle tone and the increase in perfusion pressure (1).

The breakdown of metabolites is mainly due to the workload, or muscle developed tension and fibre type distribution, while the accumulation of pathway products and the recovery of metabolite stores is mainly dependent on blood flow and oxygen supply.

Our experiments were performed to study the interdependence of muscle contraction force, blood flow, pH and metabolite concentrations before, during and after repeated periods of isometric contractions and under various degrees of blood supply.

METHODS

All experiments were performed on male Wistar rats (280-320 g body weight) anaesthetized with thiopentone (Thiopental Lentia^R), 100 mg/kg body mass, injected intraperitoneally. The tendon of the calf muscles was cut and connected with an isometric force-displacement transducer under a resting tension of ca. 1N. Muscle contraction was induced by stimulation of the sciatic nerve with square wave pulses (duration 4 msec, frequency 2.5 Hz, stimulus 2.5 V). Muscle blood flow, pH, metabolites and muscle contraction force were recorded during five successive 2 min periods of exercise, interspaced with 30 min intervals of rest. Blood flow was determined by use of the xenon-133 clearance method.

Proceedings of the 16th FEBS Congress
Part A, pp. 291–297
© 1985 VNU Science Press

Measurement of pH was performed in a separate group of
rats using glass-microelectrodes (tip diameter ca. 5 μm),
inserted to a depth of 3-4 mm into the gastrocnemius
muscle.

Tissue samples were taken prior to and at the end of
exercise by freeze-clamping the calf muscle. Metabolites
were determined using standard methods (2).

In experiments performed on femoral artery ligated
animals, one femoral artery was ligated in the vicinity
of the superior circumflex iliac artery, whilst the rat
was anaesthetized with ether, acutely (1 week) or chronically (6-10 weeks), prior to the experimental period.

RESULTS

In normally perfused gastrocnemius muscle, the profile
of muscle developed tension showed a decrease of 20 to
30 percent between the first and fifth period of exercise. In contrast to the muscle contractile force, exercise hyperaemia declined more markedly between successive
periods of exercise (Fig. 1). The peak flow showed a
significant decrease from 17.0 ml to 6.0 ml during such
a sequential exercise programme. This is in good agreement with the behaviour of proton activity, represented
as pH-profiles (Fig. 2). The pH showed a decrease to
6.99 at the end of the first working period, this decline
was diminished to 7.21 after the fifth working period.

At the onset of exercise, the muscle pH increased
transiently, this increase was reduced in magnitude, but
prolonged in duration with successive periods of exercise. The transient pH-increase with the start of
contractions is explained by the rapid hydrolysis of
creatine phosphate (3,4).

The progressive decline of hyperaemic response and
proton activity profiles during successive periods of
exercise is paralleled by a diminution of glycogen stores
and glycogen breakdown and vice versa by a decrease of
lactate formation. Energy-rich phosphate stores showed
a constant reduction during repeated exercise periods,
and were largely restored within the rest intervals.

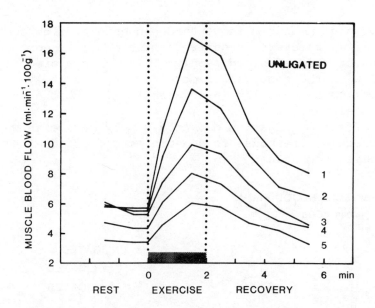

Fig. 1 Muscle blood flow before, during and after five successive (1-5) periods of 2 min isometric exercise interspaced with 30 min intervals of rest.

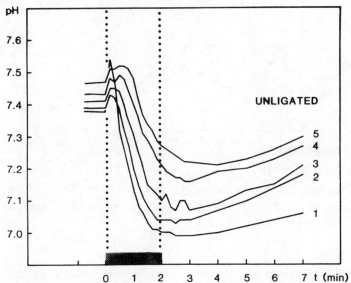

Fig. 2 Muscle pH-profiles before, during and after five successive (1-5) periods of 2 min isometric exercise (rest intervals 30 min).

We have also measured the interdependence of flow and metabolic parameters in gastrocnemius muscle under conditions of reduced blood supply. This was performed by ligation of the supplying femoral artery - acutely (1 week) or chronically (6-10 weeks) prior to the experimental period.

The effect of ligation on blood supply can be shown by the hyperaemic response to a 5 min period of total ischaemia (tourniquet, Fig. 3).

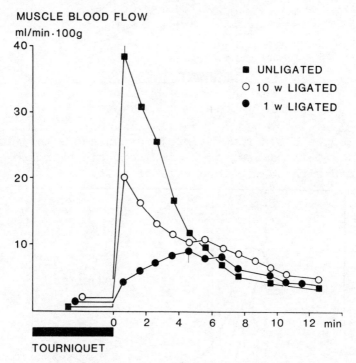

Fig. 3 Muscle blood flow following a 5 min tourniquet of non-ligated (■), acutely ligated (●) and chronically ligated (○) rats (n=5).

The ligation produces a reduction and a delay in the hyperaemic response. This reduction and the delay are more pronounced in the acutely ligated rat than in the chronically ligated animal.

Exercise hyperaemia in 1 week ligated animals was also markedly reduced and delayed in comparison to unligated animals. The hyperaemia was further reduced with successive periods of exercise (Fig. 4).

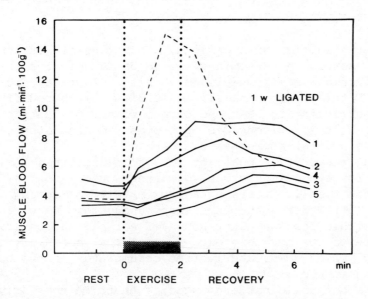

Fig. 4 Five sequential blood flow profiles of five (1-5) successive exercise periods in acutely ligated rats. Broken line illustrates the first hyperaemic response in non-ligated animals.

Muscle pH-profiles were markedly decreased, and the time taken, post exercise, to reach the pH minimum was greatly delayed, compared to unligated animals. The main difference of metabolite pattern in comparison to normally perfused gastrocnemius muscle was the stronger decline of the creatine phosphate levels and the marked accumulation of lactate. Initial contraction force was not significantly different in non-ligated and acutely ligated animals. However the muscle fatigue developed within each period of stimulation was greater in the ligated animals and additionally these animals were less able to sustain contraction force upon repeated periods of exercise.

295

When the animals have been ligated chronically for
6-10 weeks, the muscle supply situation has improved, as
all the parameters measured and determined are substantially normalized.

DISCUSSION

During the initial work periods, a substantial portion
of the exercise hyperaemia seems to be induced for the
removal of anaerobic muscle metabolites (lactate, protons). A relatively small increase of muscle blood flow
seems sufficient to meet the oxygen demand of contracting
muscle. This is evidenced by pO_2-measurements before,
during and after isometric exercise.

During the initial phase of isometric exercise, the
muscle force declines steeply, whereas muscle pO_2, after
a transient fall, increases approximately to resting
levels (5). Under such conditions, enough oxygen would
be available for the maintenance of aerobic metabolism.
In spite of the adequate oxygen supply, glycogen is
rapidly broken down, and lactate accumulates in the contracting muscle.

Such a metabolic pattern suggests that, in the early
phase, white muscle fibres, with a mainly anaerobic metabolism, contribute substantially to muscle contraction.
Owing to the rapid exhaustion of white muscle fibres,
contraction force decreases markedly within this period.

The decrease of muscle contraction force during repeated periods of exercise is accompanied by progressively
reduced muscle glycogen stores.

In the femoral artery ligated animals - though there
is a full restoration of high energy phosphate stores -
the decline of contraction force and the muscle fatigue,
following repeated periods of exercise, are greater than
in normally perfused gastrocnemius muscle. We believe
that this can be attributed mainly to the greater lactate
accumulation and pH-decrease in the acutely ligated animals. The background for this increased accumulation is
the strong decrease (60%) of muscle blood flow and the
attenuated and delayed hyperaemic response during exercise. The decreased blood flow and muscle pH leads to a
reduction in the amount of energy available for electro-

mechanical processes and causes fatigue (6). In chronically ligated animals, the restored vascular capacity is accompanied by a reduction in muscular fatigue, which can presumably be explained by the improved nutrient supply and enhanced waste product removal.

REFERENCES

1. Shepherd, J.T., Blomquist, C.G., Lind, A.R., Mitchell, J.H. and Saltin, B. (1981). Static (isometric) exercise. Circ. Res. 48 (Suppl. I), 179-188.

2. Faupel, R.P., Seitz, H.J., Tarnowski, W., Thiemann, V. and Weiss, C. (1972). The problem of tissue sampling from experimental animals with respect to freezing technique, anoxia, stress and narcosis. Arch. Biochem. Biophys. 148, 509-522.

3. Sahlin, K. (1978). Intracellular pH and energy metabolism in skeletal muscle of man. Acta Physiol. Scand., Suppl. 455.

4. Steinhagen, C., Hirche, H.J., Nestle, H.W., Bovenkamp, U. and Hosselmann, J. (1976). The interstitial pH of working gastrocnemius muscle of the dog. Pflügers Arch. 367, 151-156.

5. Wilke, R., Angersbach, D. and Ochlich, P. (1983). Metabolic pattern and blood flow of the contracting rat calf muscle. In: Biochemistry of exercise, Vol. 13, Knuttgen, H.G., Vogel, J.A. and Poortmans, J. (eds). Human Kinetics Publishers, Inc., Champaign, Il 61820, pp. 264-268.

6. Edwards, R.H.T. (1981). Human muscle function and fatigue. Ciba Found. Symp. 82, 1-18.

METHIONINE SULFOXIDE FORMATION - THE CAUSE OF SELF-INACTIVATION OF LIPOXYGENASES

B. HÄRTEL, H. KÜHN and S. M. RAPOPORT

Institute of Physiological and Biological
Chemistry, Humboldt University, DDR - 104
Berlin, GDR

The discovery of the lipoxygenase pathway in various animal cells as well as the identification of the SRS-A lipoxygenase products has stimulated greatly lipoxygenase research in recent years. In 1975 Rapoport et al (1) discovered in reticulocytes, an immature red blood cell, a lipoxygenase which disappears during maturation of the red cell. This enzyme plays a crucial role by breaking down of mitochondrial membranes. It has been purified to homogenity (2). The reticulocyte lipoxygenase contains one mole non-haem iron per mole enzyme as also described for the lipoxygenase from soybeans. The iron is involved in a catalytic cycle (3). The reticulocyte lipoxygenase also catalyzes under anaerobic conditions the lipohydroperoxidase reaction by which the primary oxygenation products are decomposed. Here also the iron undergoes a catalytic cycle. In contrast to other lipoxygenases the reticulocyte enzyme does not only oxygenate free poly-cis-unsaturated fatty acids but also corresponding phospholipids and even biological membranes.

A remarkable feature of this enzyme is the suicidal character of the oxygenase reaction at temperatures above 20°C (4).

In further work it was demonstrated that under anaerobic conditions at 37°C the

Proceedings of the 16th FEBS Congress
Part A, pp. 299–304

reticulocyte enzyme was completely inactivated
with the conversion of one single methionine
out of 14 to methionine sulfoxide (5). It was
concluded that the susceptible methionine is
located at the active center of the enzyme or
close-by. One mole methionine sulfoxide per
mole enzyme was also formed during the inactivation of soybean lipoxygenase by the
commonly used lipoxygenase inhibitor 5,8,11,
14-eicosatetraynoic acid (ETYA) (6). We postulate that the acetylenic fatty acid undergoes
a lipoxygenase reaction with the formation of
an allene hydroperoxide which may act as
oxidant for a distinct methionine.

There remained the question whether the inactivation of the enzyme is related to the hydroperoxidase reaction, during the course of
which aggressive radical intermediates are
formed or is caused by a direct attack of the
hydroperoxy-fatty acid. To answer this question comparative studies were performed with
13- and 9-hydroperoxy linoleic acid. With soybean lipoxygenase it has been shown that the
13-hydroperoxy compound is practically inert
by itself, whereas the 9-hydroperoxy linoleic
acid is attacked at about a twenty-fold rate.
On the other hand, the addition of linoleic
acid, which permits the hydroperoxidase reaction to proceed, stimulated the breakdown
of the 13-hydroperoxide 1500fold, but had no
effect on the reaction rate with 9-hydro-
peroxide (7). If the inactivation of the reticulocyte enzyme were related to the hydroperoxidase reaction, one should expect large
differences in the inactivation rate between
the 2 hydroperoxides and a strong influence of
the addition of linoleic acid.

Fig. 1 demonstrates that both 13- and 9-
hydroperoxy linoleic acids completely inactivate the enzyme under both aerobic and anaerobic
conditions.

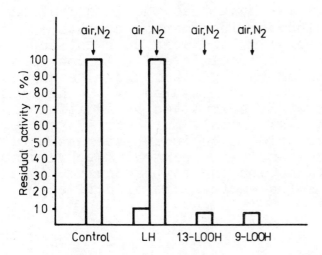

Fig. 1   Inactivation of the reticulocyte lipoxygenase by linoleic acid (LH) and 13- and 9-hydroperoxylinoleic acid (13-LOOH, 9-LOOH) at 37°C

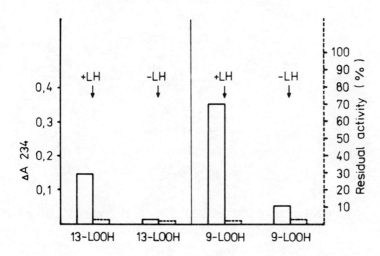

Fig. 2   Anaerobic conversion of 13- and 9-LOOH in presence and absence of LH and self-inactivation at 25°C

In fig. 2 it is shown that the inactivation
of the reticulocyte lipoxygenase by both 13-
and 9-hydroperoxylinoleic acid does not depend
on the presence of linoleic acid. In contrast
the conversion of the hydroperoxides catalyzed
by the lipoxygenase as measured by the decrease
of A_{234} is strongly stimulated by addition of
linoleic acid (not shown). Moreover, 9-hydro-
peroxylinoleic acid which is a better substrate
for the linoleic acid-independent lipohydroperoxidase reaction with the soybean enzyme does
not inactivate the enzyme more effectively.

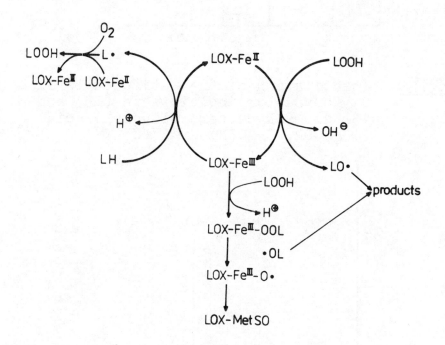

<u>Fig. 3</u> Postulated mechanism of reactions of
reticulocyte lipoxygenase

Fig. 3 summarizes the mechanism which is proposed for the inactivation of the reticulocyte
lipoxygenase during the oxygenation of linoleic

302

acid. It is proposed that the methionine sulfoxide is formed during a haemlike hydroperoxidase reaction in which the enzyme-bound
iron takes part without a valence change (8).
   The phenomenon of the self-inactivation is
not restricted to the reticulocyte lipoxygenase. Other lipoxygenases, e.g. that from
blood platelets, green pea seeds, and the
cyclooxygenase, the initial enzyme of the
prostaglandin synthesis, are rapidly inactivated during their enzymatic reactions. It remains to ascertain whether the inactivation
of these enzymes is also caused by selective
methionine sulfoxide formation.

REFERENCES

1. Schewe, T., Halangk, W., Hiebsch, C. &
      Rapoport, S.M. (1975). A lipoxygenase
      in rabbit reticulocytes which attacks
      phospholipids and intact mitochondria.
      FEBS Lett. 60, 149-152
2. Rapoport, S.M., Schewe, T., Wiesner, R.,
      Halangk, W., Ludwig, P., Janicke-Höhne,
      M., Tannert, Ch., Hiebsch, Ch. & Klatt,
      D. (1979). The lipoxygenase of reti-
      culocytes. Eur. J. Biochem. 96, 545-
      561
3. De Groot, J.J.M.C., Veldink, G.A.,
      Vliegenthart, J.F.G., Boldingh, J.,
      Wever, R. & Van Gelder, B.F. (1975).
      Demonstration by EPR spectroscopy of
      the functional role of iron in soybean
      lipoxygenase-1. Biochim. Biophys. Acta
      377, 71-79
4. Härtel, B., Ludwig, P., Schewe, T. &
      Rapoport, S.M. (1982). Self-inactivat-
      ion by 13-hydroperoxylinoleic acid
      and lipohydroperoxidase activity of
      the reticulocyte lipoxygenase. Eur. J.
      Biochem. 126, 353-357

5. Rapoport, S.M., Härtel, B. & Hausdorf, G. (1984). Methionine sulfoxide formation: the cause of self-inactivation of reticulocyte lipoxygenase. Eur. J. Biochem. 139, 573-576
6. Kühn, H., Holzhütter, H.-G., Schewe, T., Hiebsch, Ch. & Rapoport, S.M. (1984). The mechanism of inactivation of lipoxygenases by acetylenic fatty acids. Eur. J. Biochem. 139, 577-583
7. Verhagen, J., Bouman, A.A., Vliegenthart, J.F.G. & Boldingh, J. (1977). Conversion of 9-D- and 13-L-hydroperoxy-linoleic acids by soybean lipoxygenase-1 under anaerobic conditions. Biochim. Biophys. Acta 486, 114-120
8. Kühn, H., Götze, R., Schewe, T. & Rapoport, S.M. (1981). The quasi-lipoxygenase activity of hemoglobin: A model for lipoxygenases. Eur. J. Biochem. 120, 161-168

RENAL ARACHIDONIC ACID METABOLISM

JOHN C. McGIFF and MARK J.S. MILLER
Departments of Pharmacology and Medicine
New York Medical College, Valhalla, New York 10595

Metabolism of arachidonic acid (AA) involves two main pathways initiated by the cyclo-oxygenase and lipoxygenase enzymes. Cyclo-oxygenase products - prostaglandins, thromboxane and prostacyclin - can be released intra-renally by hormones and neurotransmitters and act locally to affect renal function (1,2). Lipoxygenase pathways leading to the formation of hydroperoxy- and hydroxyeico-satetraenoic acids (HPETEs and HETEs) and leukotrienes have been well characterized in leukocytes (3) and plate-lets (4). Winokur and Morrison (5) described several li-poxygenase-derived products using subcellular fractions from medullae of hydronephrotic kidneys. Jim et al. (6) have demonstrated lipoxygenase activity in rat kidney glomeruli, glomerular epithelial cells and in homogenized cortical tubules. AA may also be oxygenated by microsomal cytochrome P450-dependent mono-oxygenases, a mixed function oxidase system (7,8). This system can metabolize AA by three types of reactions: 1. lipoxygenase-like, 2. epoxidation, 3. ω- and $\omega-1$ hydroxylation. Thus, the oc-currence of cytochrome P450 in various renal cell types may influence the profile of products formed within the kidney. For example, within the cells of the thick as-cending limb of the loop of Henle (TALH), AA is metabo-lized primarily by a cytochrome P450-dependent mono-oxy-genase (9). As these pathways of AA metabolism are not inhibited by aspirin-like drugs, those effects of vaso-active hormones evoked after indomethacin treatment may result from liberation of AA by the hormones and subse-quent transformation to lipoxygenase or cytochrome P450-dependent pathway products.

One of these alternative pathways of AA metabolism within the endothelium may provide mediators for the vaso-dilatation evoked by acetylcholine and bradykinin (10). This interpretation is supported by the finding that

Proceedings of the 16th FEBS Congress
Part A, pp. 305–312
© 1985 VNU Science Press

acetylcholine-induced relaxation of rabbit aorta was inhibited by either removal of the endothelium or by eicosatetraynoic acid (ETYA), but not by indomethacin. ETYA inhibits transformation of AA by all the known major pathways: cyclo-oxygenase, lipoxygenase and cytochrome P450-dependent pathways. In the dog, bradykinin-induced relaxation of isolated blood vessels, including renal arteries, was also shown to be dependent upon an intact endothelium and independent of the cyclo-oxygenase pathway (11).

TRANSFORMATION OF PGE$_2$

As thromboxane A$_2$ (TxA$_2$), PGI$_2$, PGE$_2$ and PGF$_{2\alpha}$ differ greatly in their biological properties, the principal product of AA is of great functional importance. For example, PGE$_2$ causes renal vasodilatation and diuresis whereas PGF$_{2\alpha}$ affects renal function only at very high doses. PGE$_2$ may be transformed by PGE-9 ketoreductase to PGF$_{2\alpha}$ at PGE$_2$ concentrations of 10^{-10} to 10^{-7}M in rabbit isolated perfused kidneys (12). Most PGE-9 ketoreductase activity was in conjunction with β-oxidation with intact PGF$_{2\alpha}$ accounting for only 25% of this activity. These results are consistent with those of Granstrom and Kindahl (13) and Rosenkranz et al (14) who examined in vivo metabolism of PGE$_2$ and PGE$_1$, respectively. Recovered metabolites were predominantly products of β-oxidation in an F-type configuration. Urinary prostaglandins are thought to originate primarily from medullary sites such as the interstitial cells (15) and collecting tubules (16). Prostaglandins synthesized in the medulla and papilla can enter the luminal fluid at the thin limb of the loop of Henle (17) and are subsequently transported to the cortex and ultimately exit via the urine. The major prostaglandins in urine are PGE$_2$ and PGF$_{2\alpha}$ and, while the sources of urinary PGE$_2$ have been well defined (18,19), the source of urinary PGF$_{2\alpha}$ is uncertain. One possibility is transformation of PGE$_2$ to PGF$_{2\alpha}$ by PGE - 9 ketoreductase. PGE$_2$ metabolism has been studied in rabbit renal slices and cell suspensions from the outer medulla, before and after enrichment of the TALH (20). Metabolism was negligible in intact cell preparations. However, in

306

outer medullary cell homogenates, transformation of PGE_2 to $PGF_{2\alpha}$ by NADPH-dependent PGE-9 ketoreductase was observed at a PGE_2 concentration of $4 \times 10^{-9}M$. This activity was enriched tenfold in the thick ascending limb cells. However, $PGF_{2\alpha}$ formation could not be detected in homogenates of cortex, medulla or papilla. PGE_2 metabolism in the medullary portion of the TALH is of particular interest as it is an important site of action of PGE_2 on NaCl reabsorption (21), in addition to its close anatomical relationship to newly-synthesized PGE_2. In view of the high activity of PGE-9 ketoreductase in the TALH and its strategic location relative to newly-synthesized PGE_2, PGE-9 ketoreductase may constitute an important regulatory mechanism, terminating the tubular effects of PGE_2 as well as being a hitherto unrecognized source of $PGF_{2\alpha}$ in urine.

RENAL COMPARTMENTATION OF EICOSANOIDS

Renal prostaglandins are selectively released into urinary and venous compartments (22). The sites and magnitude of prostaglandin release is stimulus-dependent. Bradykinin, infused into the renal artery, caused a surge of immunoreactive PGE_2 (iPGE) into the urine, whereas i6-keto-$PGF_{1\alpha}$ appeared in greatest quantities in the venous effluent. Differences in the profile of prostaglandins recovered from effluents of the vascular and tubular compartments are reflected in zonal and structural variations in prostaglandin synthesis. Renal arteries, large and small, generate primarily PGI_2, although large amounts of PGE_2 and $PGF_{2\alpha}$ are also synthesized (23). In contrast, isolated convoluted tubules obtained from the outer cortex have a low capacity to convert ^{14}C-AA to prostaglandins. The medulla is able to form large amounts of PGE_2 and $PGF_{2\alpha}$, presumably originating from collecting ducts, interstitial cells, and small blood vessels (24). These differences are evident in the profile of prostaglandins excreted into the urine, reflecting primarily the contribution of the renal medullary interstitium and nephron, whereas those exiting in the renal vein originate mainly from blood vessels. The principal products of AA metabolism also vary segmentally along the nephron and probably

longitudinally within the renal vasculature. Such differences are manifest when comparing the TALH with the collecting ducts (25). The cytochrome P450-related pathway
predominates in the TALH (26), whereas PGE_2 is the principal product of AA metabolism in the collecting ducts (27).

AA METABOLISM IN THE NEPHRON

The concept introduced above is central to understanding
the role of prostaglandins and other AA metabolites in
regulating salt and water excretion; viz, that in addition
to differences in the profile of eicosanoids generated by
zones and structures within the kidney, prostaglandin synthesizing capacity and AA metabolism varies longitudinally
within the nephron. For example, the convoluted tubules
demonstrated a low capacity to generate prostaglandins
(23) in contrast to the collecting ducts which had a high
density of cyclo-oxygenase. The nephron has been profiled
in terms of distribution of prostaglandin synthesizing capacity, based on immunohistofluorescence techniques for
detecting cyclo-oxygenase (24). Of particular note was
the reduced cyclo-oxygenase antigenicity in the TALH, suggesting low prostaglandin-forming capacity in this portion
of the nephron. This region has been identified, at least
in the medulla, as a principal site of the inhibitory action of PGE_2 on sodium chloride absorption (28). However,
as will be shown, the fact that the TALH is not well en-
dowed with cyclo-oxygenase does not mean that it has a
limited ability to metabolize AA as other pathways of
arachidonate metabolism may predominate in a particular
tissue. Further, the thin limb of Henle may be a source
of PGE_2 (29).
Because of the importance of prostaglandin-dependent
mechanisms to renal function and the heterogeneous nature
of the nephron with respect to ion transport and hormonal
responsiveness, the pattern of AA metabolism should be related to specific cells within the nephron (26). The TALH
was of particular concern because of its pivotal role in
the regulation of extracellular fluid volume, as well as
its containing the principal target cells for the most
potent diuretics: the "loop diuretics" furosemide, etha-
crynic acid and bumetanide. A cell suspension containing

308

principally cells of the TALH was obtained from the excised inner stripe of the outer medulla of the rabbit kidney (26). Based on comparison of specific activities of
enzymes before and after separation - alkaline phosphatase, Na^+-K^+ ATPase as well as Tamm-Horsfall glycoprotein
and electron microscopic appearance - 80% of these cells
were estimated to be TALH in origin. TALH cells, as
noted, have low cyclo-oxygenase activity. However, TALH
cells selectively converted exogenous AA to oxygenated
metabolites by cytochrome P450-related mechanisms. AA
metabolites were produced in large quantities, representing 30-40% conversion of ^{14}C-AA, that is 1 to 5 µg per mg
of protein per hour, and were increased fivefold after
separation of TALH cells from a suspension of outer medullary cells. Preliminary gas chromatographic-mass spectroscopic analysis indicated that one of the metabolites
was an epoxide of AA with three unconjugated double bonds.
Jacobson et al. (30) have recently reported that the same
or a similar compound, the 5,6 epoxide of AA, when injected into perfused rabbit cortical collecting tubules
inhibited sodium transport. AA metabolites arising from
the cytochrome P450-dependent pathway in the TALH may perform an essential function in the regulation of salt and
water transport and, thereby, extracellular fluid volume.

PROSTAGLANDIN-RELATED RENIN RELEASE

Prostaglandins are not only involved in determining the
final effects of the renin-angiotensin system by modulating the actions of the peptide (1), but, in addition,
prostaglandin-related mechanisms are also involved in controlling release of renin. The importance of a prostaglandin-dependent mechanism to the regulation of renin
release has been recognized since the initial report in
1974 by Larsson et al. (31). However, it is uncertain
that all of the known signals that can release renin must
operate through a prostaglandin-related mechanism. There
are studies which do not support this view and which suggest that such a mechanism serves only to amplify some of
the signals. Which of the known prostaglandins acts as
the mediator of prostaglandin-related renin release is
also unsettled.

309

The proposal that prostacyclin is a mediator (32) of renin secretion has been supported by the in vitro experiments of Whorton et al. (33) who have shown that prostacyclin-induced stimulation of renin release from the rabbit kidney was time dependent. Renin release from the cortical slices proceeded in a linear fashion after PGI_2 addition and continued unabated for 30 minutes. The prolonged response was unexpected, as PGI_2 is rapidly hydrolyzed to 6-keto-$PGF_{1\alpha}$ at physiological pH and temperature. Wong et al. (34) have provided evidence that PGI_2 can be transformed to an active metabolite with biological activity similar to that of prostacyclin. The active metabolite, a stable substance at physiological pH, has been identified as having the properties of 6-keto-PGE_1 based on chemical, chromatographic and biochemical criteria. The discovery of enzymatic activity in the liver capable of generating 6-keto-PGE_1 was soon followed by reports that this prostaglandin, like PGI_2, inhibited platelet aggregation (35) and produced hypotension and vasodilatation (36); in addition, it was a potent renin secretagogue (37). Moreover, interest in 6-keto-PGE_1 has been heightened by increasing evidence that PGI_2 may be transformed to biologically-active metabolites.

It remains an open question, however, as to whether some of the effects ascribed to PGI_2 may be dependent upon transformation of prostacyclin to 6-keto-PGE_1. Only a few studies have explored this possibility, and the results are, thus far, inclusive. In platelets, in the juxtaglomerular apparatus and in blood vessels, there is evidence suggesting that conversion of prostacyclin to 6-keto-PGE_1 is a distinct possibility and that the enzyme involved in this step constitutes an additional mechanism for containing or amplifying the actions of PGI_2.

REFERENCES

1. McGiff, J.C., Crowshaw, K., Terragno, N.A. and Lonigro, A.J. (1970). Circ. Res. 27 (suppl. 1), 121-130.
2. McGiff, J.C., Crowshaw, K., Terragno, N.A. and Lonigro, A.J. (1970). Nature (Lond.) 227, 1255-1257.

3. Borgeat, P. and Samuelsson, B. (1979). Proc. Natl. Acad. Sci. 76, 2148-2152.
4. Farlardeau, P., Hamberg, M. and Samuelson, B. (1976). Biochim. Biophys. Acta 441, 193-200.
5. Winokur, T.S. and Morrison, A.R. (1981). J. Biol. Chem. 256, 10221-10223.
6. Jim, K., Hassid, A., Sun, F. and Dunn, M.J. (1982). J. Biol. Chem. 257, 10294-10299.
7. Oliw, E.H., Guengerich, F.P. and Oates, J.A. (1982). J. Biol. Chem. 257, 3771-3781.
8. Capdevila, J., Marnett, L.J., Chacos, N., Prough, R.A. and Estabrook, R.W. (1982). Proc. Natl. Acad. Sci. 79, 767-770.
9. Ferreri, N.R., Schwartzman, M., Ibraham, N., Chander, P.N., and McGiff, J.C. (in press). J. Pharmacol. Exp. Ther.
10. Furchgott, R.F. and Zadwadski, J.V. (1980). Nature 288, 373-376.
11. Altura, B.M. and Chand, N. (1981). Br. J. Pharmacol. 74, 10-11.
12. Miller, M.J.S., Spokas, E.G. and McGiff, J.C. (1982). Biochem. Pharmacol. 31, 2955-2960.
13. Granstrom, E. and Kindahl, H. (1982). Biochim. Biophys. Acta 713, 555-569.
14. Rosenkranz, B., Fischer, C., Boeynaems, J-M and Frolich, J.C. (1983). Biochim. Biophys. Acta 750, 231-236.
15. Zusman, R.M. and Keiser, H.R. (1977). J. Clin. Invest. 60, 215-223.
16. Smith, W.L. and Wilkin, G.P. (1977). Prostaglandins 13, 873-893.
17. Williams, W.M., Frolich, J.C., Nies, A.S. and Oates, J.A. (1977). Kidney Int. 11, 256-260.
18. Cagen, L.M. and Kauker, M.L. (1983). Biochem. Pharmacol. 32, 3665-3668.
19. Sun, F.F., Taylor, B.M., McGuire, J.C. and Wong, P.Y-K (1981). Kidney Int. 19, 760-770.
20. Miller, M.J.S., Carroll, M.A., Schwartzman, M., Ferreri, N.R. and McGiff, J.C. (submitted for publication). Biochem. Biophys. Res. Commun.
21. Stokes, J.B. (1981). Am. J. Physiol. 240, F471-F480.

22. Miller, M.J.S., Bednar, M.M. and McGiff, J.C. (1983). Renal metabolism of sulindac; a novel non-steroidal and antiinflammatory agent. In: Advances in Prostaglandin, Thromboxane and Leukotriene Research (Vol. 11), B. Samuelsson, R. Paoletti and P. Ramwell (Eds). Raven Press, New York, pp. 487-491.

23. Terragno, N.A., Terragno, A., Early, J.A., Roberts, M.A. and McGiff, J.C. (1978). Clin. Sci. Mol. Med. 55, 199s-202s.

24. Smith, W.L. and Bell, T.G. (1978). Am. J. Physiol. 235, F451-F457.

25. Garcia-Perez, A. and Smith, W.L. (1984). J. Clin. Invest. 74, 63-74.

26. Schwartzman, M., Ferreri, N.R., Carroll, M.A., Songu-Mize, E. and McGiff, J.C. (submitted for publication). Nature.

27. Grenier, F.C., Rollins, T.E. and Smith, W.L. (1981). Am. J. Physiol. 241, F94-F104.

28. Stokes, J.B. (1979). J. Clin. Invest. 64, 495-502.

29. Currie, M.G. and Needleman, P. (1984). Ann. Rev. Physiol. 46, 327-341.

30. Jacobson, H.R., Corona, S., Capdevila, J., Chacos, N., Manna, S., Womack, A. and Falck, J.R. (1984). Kidney Int. 25, 330 (abstract).

31. Larsson, C., Weber, P. and Anggard, E. (1974). Eur. J. Pharmacol. 28, 391-394.

32. Oates, J.A., Whorton, A.R., Gerkens, J.F., Branch, R.A. Hollifield, J.W. and Frolich, J.C. Fed. Proc. (1979) 38, 72-74.

33. Whorton, A.R., Misono, K., Hollifield, J., Frolich, J., Inagami, T. and Oates, J.A. (1977). Prostaglandins 14, 1095-1104.

34. Wong, P.Y-K, Malik, K.U., Desiderio, D.M., McGiff, J.C Sun, F.F. (1980). Biochem. Biophys. Res. Commun. 93, 486-494.

35. Quilley, C.P., McGiff, J.C., Lee, W.H., Sun, F.F. and Wong, P.Y-K. (1980). Hypertension 2, 524-528.

36. Quilley, C.P., Wong, P.Y-K and McGiff, J.C. (1979). Eur. J. Pharmacol. 57, 273-276.

37. McGiff, J.C., Spokas, E.G. and Wong, P.Y-K. (1982). Br. J. Pharmacol. 75, 137-144.

ENZYMATIC SYNTHESIS OF PROSTAGLANDINS AND MECHANISMS OF ITS REGULATION

SERGEY D. VARFOLOMEEV

Department of Biokinetics, Laboratory of
Molecular Biology and Bioorganic Chemistry,
Moscow State University, Moscow 119899,
USSR

The prostanoid synthesis requires a large
number of enzymes, but the first stage of
any prostanoid synthesis is determined by
the functioning of PGH synthetase. This
enzyme realized the conversion of arachidonic acid into PGH_2 /1/. PGH synthetase
appears to be the limiting enzyme of
prostaglandin and thromboxane synthesis.

Kinetics and mechanisms of PGH synthetase action

We have studied PGH synthetases from
different sources. In particular, PGH synthetase from human platelets has been
compared in detail with PGH synthetase
from sheep vesicular glands /2-4/. This
comparative study has showed that by all
the kinetic characteristics the both enzymes
look extremely similar. PGH synthetases
catalyse a rather complex reaction,

$$AA \xrightarrow{2O_2} PGG_2 \xrightarrow[DH]{D} PGH_2 \quad (1)$$

in which at least four molecules of substrate
take part, i.e. one molecule of fatty acid,
two molecules of oxygen and reducer --
electron donor - take place. PGH synthetases
are heme-dependent enzymes.

The method that enables to obtain the
almost homogeneous protein, retaining 100%

Proceedings of the 16th FEBS Congress
Part A, pp. 313–320
© 1985 VNU Science Press

of its activity was developed. The method
includes chromatography on DEAE-Toypearl-650
with separation in continuous pH gradient.

We have made a detailed kinetic analysis
of the action of PGH synthetase from vesicular
glands /5/. In particular, we have studied
the dependences of the velocity of PGH
synthetase action on the concentration of
each reaction component, i.e. arachidonic
acid, oxygen, various electron donors.

We have developed a theory of multisubstrate
enzymic reactions that has enabled to
elucidate to a great extent the mechanism of
PGH synthetase reaction and the sequences of
interaction between the enzyme active site
and four molecules of substrates /5/.

On the basis of the results obtained and
published data a detailed kinetic scheme has
been developed. According to the kinetic data,
the reaction mechanism involves at least 7
intermediates /6/:

$$
\begin{array}{c}
\text{DH} \;
\begin{array}{c}
X_7 \xrightarrow{\;k_7\;} X_1 \underset{\text{AA}}{\overset{\text{AA}}{\rightleftharpoons}} X_2 \\
\uparrow\downarrow \qquad\qquad\qquad \downarrow k_2 \\
X_6 \qquad\qquad\qquad X_3 \\
\;\;k_5 \searrow \quad k_4 \quad \nearrow O_2 \\
X_5 \xleftarrow{\quad} X_4 \\
O_2
\end{array}
\end{array}
\qquad (2)
$$

The first step of the process is
stoichiometrically predetermined absorption
of arachidonic acid on the enzyme active
site. At the second step arachidonic acid is
activated by acceptation of the hydrogen ion
from C-11. At the following two stages the
adding of oxygen and formation of intermediate
and unstable PGG_2 occur. The reduction of

the PGG_2 in the presence of reducers –
electron donors – terminates the catalytic
cycle.

Inactivation of PGH synthetase in the
course of the reaction.
Molecular mechanisms.

One of the most characteristic properties
of PGH synthetases is their inactivation
during the catalytic reaction. In the
experiments <u>in vitro</u> on PGH_2 synthesis
the enzymes completely lost the activity
for 2-4 min.
To struggle against this unfavourable
process very different "extinguishers" of
free radicals were tested, as well as very
different reducers – electron donors. The
effects of pH, ionic power, nature of the
matrix on which (in which) the enzyme is
immobilized, were being studied /5/. But
the velocity of PGH synthetase inactivation
did not decrease. The enzyme was inactivated
with a constant velocity and this inactivation
does not depend on whether the enzyme is
homogeneous and located in the solution,
or in a detergent micelle, or in the lipid
surrounding of microsomes, or in the
platelet. Therefore, we have come to the
conclusion that PGH synthetase inactivation
during the reaction is a specific and
invariant property of the enzyme. PGH
synthetase is a suicide enzyme.
The conclusion called for a detailed
kinetic study of the inactivation mechanism
and biological essence of the phenomenon.
A study on the kinetics of PGH synthetase
inactivation subject to the concentration of
the substrates allowed to conclude that the
reaction proceeds through intermediate
enzyme-substrate complexes /7/. Moreover, a
detailed studying of the observed dependence

of the rate constant of PGH synthetase
inactivation on the concentration of
arachidonic acid, oxygen and electron donor
shows that there are two intermediates X_4
and X_6 (see Scheme 2) in the catalytic
cycle, whose interaction with protein
results in the active site blocking and in
a complete irreversible loss of the
catalytic activity. Thus, PGH synthetase
accompleshes some thousands cycles; each
enzyme molecule synthesizes 10^3-10^4
prostaglandin molecules and then withdraws
from the synthetic process. That is the
mechanism of PGH synthetase operation.

Inactivation of PGH synthetase during
the reaction.
Regulatory role.

The discovered irreversible inactivation
of PGH synthetase in the course of the
reaction raises a number of questions.
Why does the organism need such an
unfavourable at first sight process? What
is its role in vivo? What are the regulari-
ties of enzymatic systems in which the
enzyme inactivation during the catalytic
reaction occurs?

It is necessary to analyse the kinetic
models of the processes in open systems
with the enzyme inactivation during the
reaction to answer all these questions /6-9/.

It is unexpected and principally important
conclusion, for in systems with enzymes
inactivated during the reaction the steady-
state concentration of product does not
depend on the concentration of the
substrate inflow.

The enzyme, inactivated in the course of
the reaction, plays the role of a valve
that is controlled by the substrate
concentration. An increase of the substrate

concentration results in the process acce-
leration, and simultaneously in a decrease
of the active enzyme concentration, while
the product concentration remains strictly
constant. Nowadays some types of conservative
mechanisms are known in the biochemical
kinetics that are able to struggle against
unfavourable changes in the substrate concentration and to maintain a constant
concentration of product. They are mechanisms
with a feed-back competitive or non-competitive inhibition by the reaction product.
These mechanisms were compared with the
mechanism that based on a process of the
enzyme inactivation during the reaction /8/.

These conservative mechanisms significantly
differ in the "regulation strictness". The
mechanism of competitive inhibition does not
cope with an increase of the substrate
concentration in the system. The mechanism
of non-competitive or allosteric inhibition
is considerably more efficient. A single
mechanism that is able to maintain steady-
state product concentration at a constant
level, not depending on changes in the
substrate concentration, is the mechanism
of enzyme inactivation in the course of the
reaction.

Thromboxane-prostacycline system

We set ourselves a task to study the
mechanism operation in the whole multienzyme
system of prostanoid synthesis. For this we
have "mathematically inserted" the enzyme
in the multienzyme system of thromboxane and
prostacycline synthese /9/. A kinetic scheme
for the multienzyme system of thromboxane
and prostacycline synthesis is presented:

317

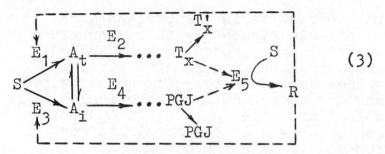

$$(3)$$

The multienzyme chains include phospholipases
(E_1, E_3), liberating unsaturated fatty acids
(A_t, A_i), PGH synthetase (E_2, E_4), producing
PGH_2 and PGH convertases, producing thromboxane
(Tx) and prostacycline (PGJ). We have taken
into account regulatory effects of thromboxane
and prostacycline on adenylate cyclase (E_5)
and a possible feed-back at the level of the
effect on phospholipases.

Summing up the findings of the analysis we
should state that systems with enzyme
inactivation in the course of the reaction
offer a number of very interesting regulation
properties, the most important of which is
their ability to maintain the product concentration at a constant level.

These experimental and theoretical studies
on the regulatory mechanisms of enzymatic
systems of prostaglandin and thromboxane
synthesis enable to solve a number of
questions on a purposeful specific control
of prostanoid concentration by various drugs.

Recently we have completed a kinetic analysis
of PGH synthetase inhibition by non-steroidal
anti-inflammatory drugs (aspirin, brufen,
indomethacin, voltaren, analgin and many
others /10,11/). The kinetic analysis has
revealed that ver efficient complex preparations can be found which can change
specifically the concentration ratio of various
prostanoids. The data are presented on two-
component inhibition of platelet aggregation

318

by nonylimidazole and brufen, induced by arachidonic acid. None of the above drugs at low concentrations influences by itself the rate of platelet aggregation, but their combined effect blocks completely platelet aggregation - the first stage of clotting.

In our opinion, it is the most promising trend of the research on the regulatory mechanisms of enzymatic systems of prostaglandin synthesis.

REFERENCES

1. Lands, W.S.M., Smith, W.L. (eds) (1982) Methods in Enzymology. Academic Press, v. 86.
2. Mevkh, A.T., Basevich, V.V., Varfolomeev, S.D..(1982) Study of endoperoxide prostaglandin synthetase from microsomal fraction of human platelet. Biochemistry (Russ.) 47, 1635-1640.
3. Mevkh, A.T., Basevih, V.V., Jarving, I., Varfolomeev, S.D. (1982) Inactivation of prostaglandin endoperoxide synthetase from the microsomal fraction of human platelets during the reaction. Biochemistry (Russ.) 47, 1852-1858.
4. Mevkh, A.T., Vrzhesch, P.V., Sviadas, V.Ju.K., Varfolomeev, S.D., Myagkova, G.I., Yakusheva, L.A. (1981) Prostaglandin synthetase. Inactivation of endoperoxide prostaglandin synthetase, a limiting enzyme in the synthesis of prostaglandins. Bioorg.Chem. (Russ.) 7, 695-702.
5. Mevkh, A.T., Vrzhesch, P.V., Basevich, V.V., Varfolomeev, S.D. (1983) Multienzyme system of prostaglandin synthesis.In: Chemical and Biochemical Kinetics, Emanuel N.M., Berezin I.V., Varfolomeev S.D. (eds) Moscow University Publishing house, pp. 224-292.

6. Varfolomeev, S.D., Mevkh, A.T. (1985) Prostaglandins-molecular bioregulators: Biokinetics, Biochemistry, Medicine. Moscow University Publishing House.
7. Varfolomeev, S.D. (1982) Enzyme inactivation in the course of the reaction. Kinetic description and discrimination of mechanisms. Biochemistry (Russ.) 47, 343-354.
8. Varfolomeev, S.D. (1984) Enzyme inactivation in the course of the reaction. Possible regulatory role. Biochemistry (Russ.) 49, 723-735.
9. Varfolomeev, S.D., Gachok, V.P., Mevkh, A.T. (1984) Kinetic model and mechanisms of regulation in a multienzyme system of thromboxane synthesis. The preprints of the Institute for Theoretical Physics, 1-35.
10. Muratov, V.K., Igumnova, N.D., Basevich, V.V., Churyukanov, V.V., Mevkh, A.T. (1983) Mechanisms of interaction of acetylsalicyl acid and indomethacin with endoperoxide prostaglandin synthetase. Pharmacol. and Toxicol. (Russ.) 5, 44-48.
11. Muratov, V.K., Varfolomeev, S.D., Igumnova, N.D., Mevkh, A.T., Churyukanov, V.V. (1984) On the mechanism of interaction of ibuprophen and naproxen with endoperoxid prostaglandin synthetase. Pharmacol. and Toxicol. (Russ.) 1, 71-74.

Symposium IV

BIOCHEMISTRY OF THE CELL CONTACT
INTERACTIONS

DYNAMIC ASPECTS OF MEMBRANE-MICROFILAMENT INTERACTION IN AREAS OF CELL CONTACT

BENJAMIN GEIGER, ZAFRIRA AVNUR, TOVA VOLBERG AND TALILA VOLK. Department of Chemical Immunology, The Weizmann Institute of Science, Rehovot 76100, Israel

Adherens junctions are a family of cell contacts which share a similar mode of interaction with the cytoskeleton; they all interact at their cytoplasmic aspects with actin-containing microfilaments through a plaque enriched with the protein vinculin (1,2). In the recent few years much information was collected on the topology of different junctional constituents and their interaction in vitro or within the living cell. Based on that information it was hypothesized that the formation of adherens junctions involves a cascade of nucleation events. It was proposed that local contacts formed between specific cell surface receptor(s) and extracellular components (on the substrate or on the membrane of neighbouring cells) develop into "adhesive patches" in which the respective receptors become clustered. This clustering or immobilization lead to a local changes at the cytoplasmic faces of the nascent junctional membrane. One of the apparent changes is the capacity to bind elements of the junctional plaque (such as vinculin). This membrane-bound layer serves as a nucleation site for the assembly of actin into bundles. This hypothesis implies, in fact, that adherens junctions contain four major subdomains whose assembly is unidirectionally interdependent.

Junctional subdomains and their experimental manipulation

The information concerning the molecular nature of the various junctional subdomains was largely derived from immunocytochemical localizations combined with limited and controlled disruption of the junction. This approach has recently been reviewed (3) and we will, therefore, only briefly symmarize the results.

The outermost components of the junction are probably the extracellular constituents to which the cells attach.

Proceedings of the 16th FEBS Congress
Part A, pp. 323–329
© 1985 VNU Science Press

These may include cellular or non-cellular materials and may display considerable heterogeneity. Next are the membrane receptors which bind to the extracellular domain and which are expected to be integral membrane proteins. At the interior of the cells, peripherally attached to the membrane are the junctional plaque proteins. Unlike the extracellular and membrane domains whose constituents are largely unknown, the plaque is somewhat better characterized in as much as it contains vinculin (1) and, in some cases, talin (4). The membrane-bound plaque provides the anchorage sites for the innermost cytoskeletal domain. The constituents of the latter are actin, myosin, tropomyosin, α-actinin, filamin and probably also other proteins which have not yet been characterized.

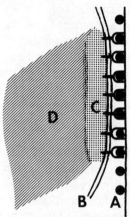

Fig. 1. A schematic representation of the different subdomains of adherens junctions. Subdomain A is the external surface (non-cellular or cellular) to which the cells bind; B is the membrane domain with specific contact receptors; C is the junctional plaque and D the bundle of actin microfilaments.

Beside the immunocytochemical localization of molecules within the last two compartments, we have recently dissected the junction and separated the domains from each other; We have shown that isolated ventral membranes or permeabilized cells, treated with fragmin, rapidly lose the focal contact-bound actin as well as the other cytoskeletal elements listed above. Vinculin and talin remained attached after this treatment (5,6). Another approach for the separation of junctional domains from each other was successfully performed with the intercellular junctions of cultured bovine kidney cells (MDBK). When treated with 2-4 mM EGTA the intercellular contact was rapidly disrupted and neighbouring cells separated from each other. Consequently, the junctional plaque detached from the membrane and, along with the cytoskeletal elements contracted towards the cell center. It thus appears that the anchorage of the latter two domains to the membrane depends strictly on the continuous maintenance of the contact at the exterior of the cell.

The extracellular domain of cell-substrate contacts: Active modulation by the cells

For several years we, as well as others, have tried to identify extracellular components uniquely associated with focal contacts. These attempts met difficulties since it was found that the junctional space is not accessible to antibodies (this observation was eventually used for the localization of focal contacts, as an alternative to interference-reflection optics (7)). After extensive permeabilization, the accessibility barrier was no longer a problem and the cell cultures could be directly immunolabeled with antibodies to extracellular matrix components. In such experiments we have found that fibronectin as well as chondroitin sulfate-containing proteoglycan (CSPG) were generally absent from stable focal contacts. Moreover, plating of fibroblasts on a uniform layer of fibronectin resulted in a progressive removal of the matrix protein from underneath focal contacts and its packing into cables (see Fig. 2a). Careful examination of this process indicated that cells readily form contacts with extracellular fibronectin which develop into vinculin-rich focal contacts. Nevertheless, during that stage the underlying fibronectin is displaced towards the cell center. Nevertheless, electron microscopic examination of saponimpurified focal contacts indicated that thin bridging fibers are detected between the membrane and the substrate (8). The nature of these fibers is still unknown. Is there a ubiquitous and defined linker molecule on the substrate, or between cells, which is specific for adherens junctions? The answer to that question is not clear yet.

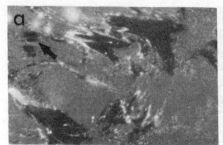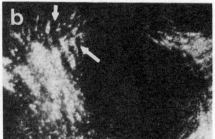

*Fig. 2. The absence of fibronectin (a) and chondroitin
sulfate proteoglycan (b). The arrows point to matrix-
free areas which coincide with cell-substrate focal
contacts.*

The contact "receptor(s)" of adherens junctions

Apparently key molecules in the establishment and maintenance of cellular contacts are the membrane receptors.
Considerable efforts directed in recent years towards the
identification of "cell adhesion molecules" have revealed
a family of functionally interesting surface molecules
though most (if not all) of them were not confined to
adherens junction areas.

We have recently identified a new surface molecule which
is specifically associated with intercellular adherens
junctions (for details see (9)). This molecule was

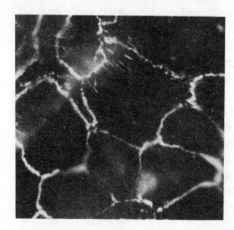

*Fig. 3. Immunofluores-
cent labeling of
cultured chick lens
cells for the 135 Kd
protein using ID-7.2.3
monoclonal antibodies.
The intensely labeled
lines coincide with the
subapical adherens
junctions of these
cells. Notice that
focal contacts are not
labeled.*

326

present in several cell-cell contacts including zonula
adhaerens and fascia adhaerens of intestinal epithelium
and cardiac muscle, respectively, in contacts between lens
cells and in a large variety of cultured cells. In all
these locations the new antigen coincided with vinculin.
In vinculin-containing adherens junctions formed with non
cellular substrates (focal contacts, dense plaques of
smooth muscle, etc.) the new antigen could not be detected. Not much is known, as yet, on the molecular properties of the new component but it has been shown to be a
surface polypeptide with an apparent molecular weight of
135,000 (somewhat bigger than vinculin). At present, we
direct much effort towards the characterization of this
protein and its interactions at the exterior, inside the
membrane and at the cytoplasmic faces of the junction.

The dynamics of junctional structures: Concluding remarks

In this last topic we would like to comment on the dynamic
properties of junctional molecules and discuss the possible modes of their assembly (for an elaborate discussion
of these aspects see (2).

As has been shown the formation of adherens junctions involves "immobilization" of the various junctional elements, yet the junction remains a dynamic structure. As
described above, extracellular matrices to which the membrane attaches may be actively mobilized from underneath
focal contacts. This suggests that force is generated in
that area, leading to the centripetal movement of fibronectin, probably along with its membrane receptors. Direct
analysis of lateral mobilities of lipids and proteins in
focal contacts using fluorescence photobleaching recovery
experiments has shown that focal contacts were not major
diffusion barriers. Thus a lipid probe showed complete
recovery after photobleaching with retardation of diffusion coefficients by only 50%. The same type of analysis
indicated that two quantitatively comparable populations
of membrane proteins exist, one being immobile and the
other free to move in or through the contact area.

A different approach was selected for studying the dynamic

properties of the plaque constituents (represented by vinculin) and components of the cytoskeletal domain (actin and α-actinin). Fluorescent derivatives of these proteins were prepared and injected into living cells. Within relatively short time each of the injected proteins became incorporated into the respective junctional domain and subjected to FPR analysis. While these experiments were described and discussed in detail elsewhere (10) the general conclusion was that all three proteins tested maintain a dynamic equilibrium between soluble cytoplasmic pools and immobile forms at the junction.

Based on these results as well as those described in previous sections we may summarize some of the molecular features of adherens junctions:
(1) Adherens junctions, defined by the presence of actin and vinculin are composed of 4 major domains - extracellular, membranal, plaque-bound and cytoskeletal.
(2) These junctions may show some molecular diversity as shown here by the presence of the 135 Kd protein in intercellular adherens junctions only.
(3) All the junctional elements appear to maintain a dynamic equilibrium with mobile extrajunctional pools. This suggests that changes in this equilibrium process play major role in the assembly and disassembly of the junction.

REFERENCES

1 Geiger, B. (1983). Membrane-cytoskeleton interaction. Biochim. Biophys. Acta 737, 305-341.
2 Geiger, B., Avnur, Z., Kreis, T.E. and Schlessinger, J. (1984). The dynamics of cytoskeletal organization in areas of cell contact. Cell and Muscle Motility 5, 195-234.
3 Geiger, B., Avnur, Z., Volberg, T. and Volk, T. Molecular domains of adherens junctions. Neuroscience (in press).
4 Burridge, K. and Connel, L. (1983). A new protein of adhesion plaques and ruffling membranes. J. Cell Biol. 97, 359-367.
5 Avnur, Z., Small, J.V. and Geiger, B. (1983). Actin-independent association of vinculin with the cytoplasmic aspect of the plasma membrane in cell-contact areas. J. Cell. Biol. 96, 1622-1630.

6 Geiger, B., Avnur, Z., Rinnerthaler, G., Hinssen, H. and Small, J.V. (1984). Microfilament-organizing centers in areas of cell contact:Cytoskeletal interactions during cell attachment and locomotion. J. Cell Biol. 99(1), 835-915.
7 Neyfakh, A. Jr., Tint, I.S., Svitkina, T.M., Bershadsky, A.D. and Gelfand, V.I. (1983). Exp. Cell. Res. 149, 387-396.
8 Neyfakh, A. Jr. and Svitkina, T.M. (1983). Isolation of focal contact membrane using saponin. Exp. Cell. Res. 149, 582-586.
9 Volk, T. and Geiger, S. (1984). EMBO J. 3, 2249-2260.
10 Kreis, T.E., Avnur, Z., Schlessinger, J. and Geiger, B. Dynamic properties of cytoskeletal proteins in focal contacts. Cold Spring Harbor Symp. (in press).

MEMBRANE-CYTOSKELETON INTERACTIONS DURING CELL SPREADING ON NON-CELLULAR SUBSTRATA.

J.M.VASILIEV and I.M.GELFAND
Moscow State University and USSR Cancer
Research Center, Moscow, USSR.

Focal contacts are the main structures
responsible for the attachment of cultured
cells to the surfaces of non-living substrata such as plastic, glass etc. Here we
will discuss dependence of focal contacts
on the state of cellular cytoskeleton. The
spread cultured fibroblast forming focal
contacts is a polarized cell with active
and non-active zones edges; pseudopods are
continuously formed and attached at these
edges /I/. As shown by examination of
electron-microscopic replicas /2/ and by
other methods, actin cytoskeleton of these
cells is also highly vectorized and differentiated.

How is formation of focal contacts
related to this dynamic organization? Our
early studies /I/ and recent interference-
reflection observations of Izzard and Lochner /3/ indicated that new focal contacts
appear under the advancing pseudopods. However, study of small focal contacts by
usual method of interference-reflection
alone meets many technical difficulties.

Useful addition to the methods of visualization of focal contacts is a new antibody exclusion technique /4/. This method permitted to distinguish two variants
of contacts: usual elongated dash-like
contacts and small dot-like contacts. Dots
are localized near the active edges, while
dash-like contacts are predominant at the

Proceedings of the 16th FEBS Congress
Part A, pp. 331–335
© 1985 VNU Science Press

more central parts of surface. Both dash
and dot contacts contain a characteristic
protein-vinculin. Dots, in contrast to
dashes, are not associated with the bundles
of actin microfilaments. However, they are,
probably, associated with the dense network
of microfilaments at the active edge /2/.

These data give reason to distinguish
two processes: initiation of focal contacts,
and their maturation, that is, growth,
elongation and association with actin
bundle. Initiation takes place at the active edge. Our observations indicate that
maturation of contacts depends on the tension exerted by actin cortex. When partial
retraction of the cell edge is caused by
trypsin, EDTA or by transfer of the cells
into the room temperature and the tension,
probably, increases, elongation of some
contacts located near this edge is regular-
ly observed. Spontaneous retraction of the
edge is also accompanied by the simultaneous elongation of many focal contacts.
Centripetal tension can orient microfilaments tangentially to the substratum so
that larger areas of the membrane will come closer to the substrate and to the bundle. We suggest that this physical nearness
can promote some chemical interactions
between the components of contact and thus
trigger its maturation. This new phenomenon clearly demonstrates the control of
membrane components by cytoskeleton in the
contacts and therefore deserves further
study.

Dynamic actin organization, in which
pseudopods and actin network can be formed
at the periphery and tension is developed
toward the center, can arise not only in
large cell but also in small anuclear

cells, like platelets. Antibody exclusion
method had shown that spreading platelets
form focal contacts under attached pseudopods /5/. Small fragment surgically detached from the fibroblast can form pseudopods and develop focal contacts at its periphery. Periphery and center are determined in this case de novo with regard to
the fragment and not to the cell from which
it was detached. It would be very important
to study mechanism of self-organization of
these mini-systems.

Besides actin cortex, large nucleated
cells have also another cytoskeletal component which can be essential for the determination of distribution of focal contacts. These components are microtubules;
their role is shown clearly in the experiments with colcemid which depolymerises
these structures. After addition of colcemid polarized fibroblast acquires non-
elongated polygonal shape /I/; focal contacts are enlarged and form the circle
around the periphery; actin bundles acquire arc-like or irregular circular pattern.
These results suggest that microtubules
are essential for the maintenance of elongated polarized shape, but non-polarized
shape with peripheral circular pattern of
contacts and bundles can be maintained
winhout microtubules. This suggestion is
supported by the experiments with epithe-
liocytes of liver-derived IAR-2 line. These cells spread to discoid non-polarized
shape on usual substrata. They have peripheral circular focal contacts associated
with circular actin bundle. When the same
cells apread on the narrow strips of glass,
they are forced to acquire the elongated
shape. Colcemid does not significantly al-

ter the shape of discoid cells, but causes retraction of elongated cells. We suggest that microtubules prevent the contraction of actin cortex. The cortex of elongated cell is highly stretched between the few contacts; microtubules are essential here to prevent contraction. In contrast, discoid cell has more numerous contacts at the edge and can be stable even without the microtubules. The role of actin cortex in the retraction induced by colcemid is confirmed by the experiments showing that cytochalasin prevents this retraction.

Morphologically transformed cells are badly spread and have deficient microfilament bundules /I/. Antibody exclusion method permitted to study in detail the state of focal contacts in the cells of I6-Q quail line, transformed by RSV. We have found that formation of the initial focal contacts at the edge takes place in these transformed cells but large central bundle-associated structures are not formed. This absence of maturation is possibly, associated with decreased tension exerted by transformed cell cortex on the initial contact. In other words, contact changes can be secondary to alterations of actin cytoskeleton. Thus, there are several types of control of focal contacts by cytoskeleton. Actin cortex determines the sites of formation of pseudopods, which initiate focal contacts. Tension of cortex determines maturation on of focal contact. Microtubules perform the higher level of control by stabilizing the state of actin cortex.

References

I. Vasiliev J.M. and Gelfand I.M. (I98I).

Neoplastic and Normal Cells in Culture
Cambridge University Press, Cambridge,
UK.
2. Svitkina T.M., Shevelev A.A., Bershadsky
A.D. and Gelfand V.I. (1984). Cytoskeleton of mouse embryo fibroblasts. Electron microscopy of platinum replicas.
Eur. J.Cell Biol. 34, 64-74.
3. Izzard C.S. and Lochner L.R. (1980).
Formation of cell-to-substrate contacts
during fibroblast motility; an interfe-
rence - reflection study. J.Cell Sci.,
42, 81-116.
4. Neyfakh A.A. Jr., Tint I.S., Svitkina
T.M., Bershadsky A.D. and Gelfand V.I.
(1983). Visualization of cellular focal
contacts using a monoclonal antibody to
80 kD serum protein adsorbed on the
substratum. Exp. Cell Res., 149, 387-396.
5. Alexandrova A.Y. and Vasiliev J.M.
(1984). Focal contacts of spreading platelets with the substratum, Exp. Cell
Res., 153, 254-258.

Symposium V

BIOCHEMISTRY OF VIRUSES

ON THE MOLECULAR BASIS OF BIOLOGICAL DIFFERENCES BETWEEN POLIOVIRUS STRAINS

VADIM I. AGOL
Institute of Poliomyelitis & Viral Encephalitides, Academy of Medical Sciences, and Moscow State University, Moscow, USSR

It is well known that some poliovirus strains bring about epidemics in non-immune human populations. Other strains can safely be used as live vaccines. The molecular basis of this difference is obscure. Here, I am going to show that the major determinants of poliovirus neurovirulence are located in the 5' half of the viral genome, perhaps, at least partly, in the untranslated nucleotide sequence. The capacity of the RNA of attenuated strains to initiate translation appears to be diminished.

For mapping determinants of neurovirulence we made use of genetic analysis. Recombinants with a centrally located crossover point were constructed by the following method /1/. A guanidine-sensitive (gs) strain of poliovirus type 3 was crossed with a guanidine-resistant (gr) strain of type 1. Then gr clones with the type 3 antigenicity were selected. The locus determining resistance to guanidine was known to be located in the central region of the genome. The nucleotide sequence coding for antigenic determinants should be located not very far away toward the 5' end. Therefore the recombinants obtained in this was should inherit a half of the genome from one parent, and the other half from the second parent. Indeed, the capsid proteins of such recombinants were identical to those of their type 3 parent, whereas the noncapsid polypeptides X, 2 and 4 of the recombinants were indistinguishable from the corresponding polypeptides of the

Proceedings of the 16th FEBS Congress
Part A, pp. 339–345
© 1985 VNU Science Press

type 1 parent /1,2/.

The approximate position of the crossover region could tentatively be deduced from the analysis of the RNase T1 oligonucleotide maps of the genome. When the maps of the recombinants were compared with those of the parental viruses, it could be seen that the recombinant genomes included RNA sequences originating from both parents /3/. The exact genomic position of many large type 1-derived oligonucleotides of the recombinant genomes were known from the published studies. We have sequenced one of the type 3-derived oligonucleotides of the recombinant RNA, and using the published primary structure of the polivirus type 3 RNA, we have located this oligonucleotide (1*) on the viral genome. Fig. 1 presents the deduced genome structure of two recombinants. For one of them (a3/a1-2) the crossover region could be defined with a relatively great precision, namely between oligonucleotides 1* and 7, that is within a sequence 202 nucleotides-long. In both cases, the crossover point lies in the central region of the genome, as expected.

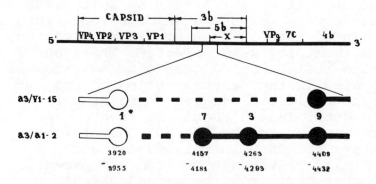

Fig. 1. Tentative structure of the genomes of two recombinants. The type 3- and type 1-derived oligonucleotides are represented by open and closed circles, respectively.

After being convinced that we knew how to
manipulate with the genome halves, we have
constructed intertypic (type3/type1) recombinants
between attenuated and virulent polio strains/3/.
Four such recombinants had all the possible
arrangements of "attenuated" and "virulent"
genome halves: attenuated/virulent, attenuated/
/attenuated, virulent/virulent and virulent/at-
tenuated. The virulence of these recombinants
was assayed by intracerebral inoculation of
monkeys. The recombinants that inherited the 5'
half of the genome from the virulent parent
proved to be virulent, irrespective of the
origin of the 3' half and despite the fact that
one of them exhibited the ts RNA⁻ phenotype;
the recombinants that inherited the 5' half
from the attenuated parent exhibited the
attenuated phenotype (Fig. 2). This demonstrates
that the major determinants of poliovirus
attenuation are located in the 5' half of the
genome.

A similar conclusion emerged also from the
experiments with homotypic (type 1) recombinants
between attenuated and virulent polio strains
that were constructed by means of a specially
developed procedure /4/. Again, it was the
5' half of the genome that primarily determined
whether a particular strain expressed attenuated
or virulent phenotype.

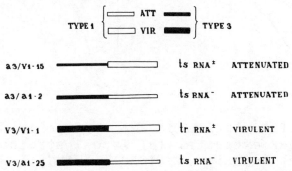

Fig. 2. Neurovilence of polio recombinants.

The 5' half codes for the capsid proteins. It is conceivable that properties of these proteins may affect the virulence. The 5' half, however, encompasses also an untranslated region, which may well contain diverse signals involved in the control of replication and translation of the viral RNA. In an attempt to learn whether some of these signals function differently in virulent and attenuated polio strains, we compared efficiencies of translation of the respective genomes in extracts from Krebs-2 cells (Y. Svitkin, S. Maslova and V. Agol, in preparation).

Fig. 3 shows that the RNA of type 1 attenuated Sabin strain was translated with a markedly lower efficiency, as compared to the RNA of its virulent relative, strain Mahoney. Among several type 3 strains studied, the lowest activity was again exhibited by the vaccine strain RNA. Moreover, the reversion of the latter to neurovirulence appears to be accompanied by restoration of the wild-type level of template activity of its genome (Fig. 3).

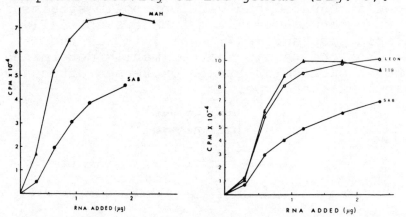

Fig. 3. Translation of RNA's of polio strains in Krebs-2 extracts. (a) Type 1 strains Mahoney (MAH) and LSc 2ab (SAB). (b) Type 3 strains Leon, Leon 12a$_1$b (SAB) and a neurovirulent revertant of the latter (119).

342

Thus, there exists a striking correlation between the attenuated phenotype of a strain and the diminished ability of its RNA to promote translation in an in vitro system. We propose that the diminished translation efficiency is a factor contributing to the attenuated phenotype of the relevant virus. How great this contribution is remains, however, an open question.

Not less than in the nature of neurovirulence, we are interested in the control of translation in eukaryotic cells. The observed difference in the template efficiencies of closely related genomes gives us a promising tool for elucidating some of these control mechanisms. This study has begun only quite recently, and I shall briefly summarize our initial observations.

We found that the genomes of attenuated and virulent polio strains, exhibiting as already demonstrated different template activities in the Krebs extracts, were translated with a nearly equal efficiency in reticulocyte lysates. Thus, we have to explain not only the reasons for the template-to-template variation but also why this variation was not revealed in certain cell-free systems. A tentative explanation is as follows. The genomes of attenuated strains are deficient in promoting initiation of translation at the proper site, which corresponds to the N-terminus of the polyprotein. Such a deficiency will obviously result in a decrease of template activity, but only under condition that translation is initiated predominantly at the correct site. The Krebs extract is just such a correctly-initiating cell-free system. By contrast, the reticulocyte lysates translate polio RNA largely from incorrect, internally located sites /5/. Since the RNA's of virulent and attenuated strains are equally active in this incorrect initiation, they exhibit a comparable level of the overall template activity in reticulocyte lysates.

This hypothesis was supported by electrophoretic analyses of the in vitro products. The efficiency of correct initiation could be judged by the accumulation of polypeptide 1a, the precursor of capsid proteins. We found that in Krebs extracts the RNA's of virulent strains directed the synthesis of considerably greater amounts of 1a than did the RNA's of attenuated strains. Irrespective of the strain, polio RNA's induced predominantly the synthesis of comparable amounts of abnormal polypeptides in reticulocyte lysates.

There is some evidence suggesting that the difference in the translation efficiencies of the respective templates are due to a mutation in the central region of the 5'-untranslated part of the viral genome. As a result of this mutation, the RNA of attenuated strains requires a greater concentration of certain initiation factors to promote correct initiation of translation.

REFERENCES

1. Tolskaya, E.A., Romanova, L.I., Kolesnikova, M.S. and Agol, V.I. (1983) Intertypic recombination in poliovirus. Virology 124, 121-132.
2. Romanova, L.I., Tolskaya, E.A., Kolesnikova, M.S. and Agol, V.I. (1980) Biochemical evidence for intertypic genetic recombination of polioviruses. FEBS Letters 118, 109-112.
3. Agol, V.I., Grachev, V.P., Drozdov, S.G. Kolesnikova, M.S., Kozlov, V.G., Ralph, N.M., Romanova, L.I., Tolskaya, E.A., Tyufanov, A.V., and Viktorova, E.G. (1984) Construction and properties of intertypic poliovirus recombinants: First approximation mapping of the major determinants of neuro-virulence. Virology 136, 41-55.

4. Tolskaya, E.A., Kolesnikova, M.S.,
   Romanova, L.I., Viktorova, E.G. and
   Agol, V.I. (1984) Construction of recombinants between attenuated and virulent
   poliovirus type 1 strains with a crossover
   point in the central region of the genome.
   Mol. genetika, mikrobiol. i virusol. No.9,
   22-28.
5. Dorner, A.J., Semler, B.L., Jackson, R.J.,
   Hanecak, R., Duprey, E. and Wimmer, E.
   (1984) In vitro translation of poliovirus
   RNA: Utilization of internal initiation
   sites in the reticulocyte lysate. J. Virol.
   50, 507-514.

ALFALFA MOSAIC VIRUS NON-STRUCTURAL PROTEINS INVOLVED IN VIRAL RNA AND PROTEIN SYNTHESIS

JOHN F. BOL, MARIANNE J. HUISMAN, FIEKE ALBLAS AND
LOUS VAN VLOTEN-DOTING

Department of Biochemistry, State University,
P.O. Box 9605, 2300 RA Leiden, The Netherlands.

INTRODUCTION

Our research is focussing on the structure and function of the tripartite RNA-genome of alfalfa mosaic virus (AlMV). Recently, the complete nucleotide sequence of this genome has been deduced (1,2,3). The sequence data indicate that the AlMV-genome encodes four primary gene products: a 126K protein encoded by RNA 1, a 90K protein encoded by RNA 2 and a 32K protein and the coat protein encoded by RNA 3. The coat protein is not translated from RNA 3 but from a subgenomic messenger, RNA 4. We are investigating the function of these four proteins in AlMV replication. The observation that a mixture of RNAs 1 and 2 is able to replicate in cowpea protoplasts in the absence of RNA 3 indicates that the 126K and 90K proteins are involved in viral RNA synthesis (4). This work also permitted the conclusion that an RNA 3 encoded protein regulates the balance between viral plus- and minus-strand RNA synthesis. In addition to its structural role, the coat protein is required to initiate infection: a few coat protein subunits have to be bound to the 3'-end of each genome segment to start the replication cycle (5).

To learn more about the function of the four AlMV proteins we are studying the replication of temperature-sensitive mutants in cowpea protoplasts. Here, we present the results obtained with two RNA 1 mutants (Bts 04 and Bts 03) and two RNA 2 mutants (Mts 04 and Mts 03).

RESULTS AND DISCUSSION

Table 1 shows the production of infectious virus by these mutants at the restrictive temperature (30°) compared to virus production at the permissive temperature (25°).

Proceedings of the 16th FEBS Congress
Part A, pp. 347–351

Table 1

Relative virus production in cowpea protoplasts at the restrictive temperature [a)]

Mutation in RNA	Mutant	Production of Infectious Virus $\dfrac{\text{at } 30^{\circ}}{\text{at } 25^{\circ}}$ x 100%
-	Wild Type	71
1	Bts 04	84
1	Bts 03	2
2	Mts 04	5
2	Mts 03	6

[a)] Virus production in protoplasts was measured by local lesion assay.

The wild type replicates well at 30° but virus production by Bts 03, Mts 04 and Mts 03 is greatly reduced at this temperature. Bts 04 shows a normal virus production at 30° but as we will see it is a useful mutant.

To localize the temperature sensitive-defects in the replication cycle of these mutants more precisely, we have analyzed the synthesis of viral minus-strand and plus-strand RNA and coat protein at 25° and 30°. ^{32}P-labeled virion RNA and ^{32}P-labeled viral cDNA were used as probes to detect viral minus-strand and plus-strand RNA, respectively, on Northern blots; incorporation of ^{35}S-Methionine and PAGE were used to analyse the coat protein in extracts from infected protoplasts. The results are summarized in Table 2. The synthesis of viral minus-strand RNA by both the RNA 1 and RNA 2 mutants is reduced by 70 to 90%. However this reduced amount of minus-strand RNA acts as the template for a normal production of plus-strand RNA for all four mutants. In Bts 04 infected protoplasts the plus-strand RNA 4 is translated into coat protein at 30° and the genome is encapsidated to give infectious virus. In Bts 03 and Mts 04 infected

Table 2

Production of viral material at the restrictive temperature [a)]

Mutation in RNA	Mutant	Production at 30° of			
		⊖ RNA	⊕ RNA	coat protein	infectious virus
1	Bts 04	−	+	+	+
1	Bts 03	−	+	−	−
2	Mts 04	−	+	−	−
2	Mts 03	−	+	N.D.	−

a)
    A plus sign means that synthesis is comparable to
    that of the wild type; a minus sign means that
    synthesis is considerably reduced.

protoplasts the RNA 4 produced at 30° is not translated into coat protein and consequently there is no
assembly of infectious virus. The batch of Mts 03
was exhausted before coat protein production could
be assayed; upon isolation of a second batch of Mts
03 the mutant character appeared to be lost.
    From the results in Table 2 we conclude that the
126K and 90K proteins encoded by RNAs 1 and 2 are
both involved in the synthesis of viral minus-strand
RNA and the translation of RNA 4. The first function
may suggest that they are both subunits of a viral
replicase; the second function is more difficult to
explain. As replicase subunits, the RNAs 1 and 2
encoded proteins may be involved in capping of the
viral RNAs. If the mutants produce uncapped viral
mRNAs at 30° these may be translated less efficiently.
Another possibility is that the 126K and 90K proteins

constitute a factor that enhances RNA 4 translation in wild type infected cells. If this function is defective with the mutants, RNA 4 translation may fall back to the same low level at which translation of the genomic RNAs does occur.

The results with the RNA 1 mutants show that the two functions of the 126K protein can be mutated separately. Moreover, they show that a reduction in minus-strand RNA-synthesis does not necessarily affect the production of infectious virus. It is the defect in coat protein production that is responsible for the lack of virus production by Bts 03 and Mts 04.

To see whether the mutations in Bts 03 and Mts 04 affect early or late functions in virus replication, the following experiment was performed. Samples of infected protoplasts were incubated at 25°; at different times after inoculation the temperature was shifted up to 30° and the protoplasts were incubated for an additional time at 30°. The total time of the first incubation at 25° and the second incubation at 30° was 24 hours for each sample. After that period the samples were assayed for the production of infectious virus, minus-strand RNA, plus-strand RNA or coat protein. Similar amounts of virus were produced in wild-type infected protoplast⸱ incubated for 24 hr at 25° or 24 hr at 30°. However, if the first half of this incubation is done at 25° and the second half is at 30° there is a twofold stimulation in virus production. Possibly, early steps in the replication cycle are functioning better at 25° whereas late steps are more efficient at 30°. Mutants Bts 03 and Mts 04 produce hardly any virus, minus-strand RNA or coat protein when the protoplasts are incubated for 24 hr at 30°. However, when the protoplasts are incubated for 6 hours at 25° the two mutants produce a normal amount of virus, minus-strand RNA and coat protein during the subsequent incubation at 30°. This suggests that the temperature-sensitive functions of the RNA 1 and RNA 2 mutants are confined to early steps in the replication cycle. To explain this, we propose that after their translation from RNAs 1 and 2, the 126K and 90K polypeptides assume a functional conformation and are subsequently incorporated in a multi-subunit complex. This complex could be the replicase or a factor controlling RNA 4 translation. Our hypothesis is that when the temperature is raised to 30° during translation of RNAs 1 and 2 the polypeptides becomes denatured and are not incorporated in the putative complex. However, once this complex is assembled at the permissive temperature it may be protected from denaturation at 30° by protein-protein interactions. When the 126K and 90K proteins are synthesized in sufficient quantities during the first 6 hr at 25°, they may be functional when the temperature is raised to 30° later on.

At present we are screening other mutants from our collection of over 40 ts-mutants, hoping that they will permit us to unravel other functions of the AlMV proteins.

REFERENCES

1. Cornelissen, B.J.C., Brederode, F.Th., Moorman, R.J.M., and Bol, J.F. (1983). Complete nucleotide sequence of alfalfa mosaic virus RNA 1. Nucl. Acids Res. 11, 1253-1265.
2. Cornelissen, B.J.C., Brederode, F.Th., Veeneman, G.H., Van Boom, J.H., and Bol, J.F. (1983). Complete nucleotide sequence of alfalfa mosaic virus RNA 2. Nucl. Acids Res. 11, 3019-3025.
3. Barker, R.F., Jarvis, N.P., Thompson, D.V., Loesch--Fries, L.S., and Hall, T.C. (1983). Complete nucleotide sequence of alfalfa mosaic virus RNA 3. Nucl. Acids Res. 11, 2881-2891.
4. Nassuth, A., and Bol, J.F. (1983). Altered balance of the synthesis of plus- and minus-strand RNAs induced by RNAs 1 and 2 of alfalfa mosaic virus in the absence of RNA 3. Virology 124, 75-85.
5. Smit, C.H., Roosien, J., Van Vloten-Doting, L., and Jaspars, E.M.J. (1981). Evidence that alfalfa mosaic virus infection starts with three RNA--protein complexes. Virology 112, 169-173.

tRNA-RELATED CONFIGURATIONS IN NUCLEIC ACIDS

A.L. HAENNI, S. JOSHI and R.L. JOSHI

Département de Biologie du Développement, Institut
Jacques Monod, CNRS and Université Paris VII, 2 Place
Jussieu, 75251 Paris Cedex 05, France.

INTRODUCTION

In recent years, the study of RNAs has led to the observation that certain viral RNAs resemble tRNAs in so far
as they can be aminoacylated in vitro by a specific
amino acid and are capable of interacting with several
enzymes thought to be specific of tRNAs; such RNAs are
said to possess a 'tRNA-like' region. In addition, based
on sequence analogies with tRNAs and similar secondary
folding, various other RNAs have been reported to possess
elements in common with tRNAs; these are designated here
'pseudo tRNAs'.
  This paper reviews the recent developments in the area
of tRNA-related RNAs and considers how these molecules
might have evolved to acquire features of tRNAs.

tRNA-LIKE REGIONS IN PLANT VIRAL RNAs

Since the first reports in 1970 that turnip yellow
mosaic virus (TYMV) RNA could be aminoacylated in vitro
with valine (1,2), several groups have demonstrated that
various other viral RNAs can similarly be esterified by
an amino acid (for reviews see ref. 3,4). The list of
viruses whose RNAs can be esterified in vitro, the group
to which they belong and the amino acid their RNAs can
accept are presented in Table 1. Most of these are plant
viruses and the amino acid is bound to the 3' end of the

Proceedings of the 16th FEBS Congress
Part A, pp. 353–362
© 1985 VNU Science Press

Table 1. In vitro amino acid acceptor activity of viral RNA genomes (adapted from ref. 3,4 and from unpublished results of the authors).

Virus group	Source of viral RNA	Amino acid bound
Plant viruses		
Tymovirus	Turnip yellow mosaic virus (TYMV)	Valine
	Cacao yellow mosaic virus (CYMV)	Valine
	Eggplant mosaic virus (EMV)	Valine
	Okra mosaic virus (OMV)	Valine
	Wild cucumber mosaic virus (WCMV)	Valine
Tobamovirus	Tobacco mosaic virus (TMV)	Histidine
	Cowpea strain of TMV (C$_C$TMV)*	Valine
	Cucumber green mottle mosaic virus (CGMMV)	Histidine
Bromovirus	Brome mosaic virus (BMV)	Tyrosine
	Broad bean mottle virus (BBMV)	Tyrosine
	Cowpea chlorotic mottle virus (CCMV)	Tyrosine
Cucumovirus	Cucumber mosaic virus (CMV)	Tyrosine
Hordeivirus	Barley stripe mosaic virus (BSMV)	Tyrosine
Animal viruses		
Picornavirus	Mengovirus	Histidine
	Encephalomyocarditis virus (EMCV)	Serine

*Identical to Sun hemp mosaic virus (SHMV).

354

non-coding region of the RNAs; furthermore, apart from one exception among the tobamoviruses, the RNAs of the viruses of a given taxonomic group accept the same amino acid. The bromo-, cucumo- and hordeiviruses usually contain a tripartite genome; the 3' end of each RNA can be tyrosylated in vitro. In the case of the two animal viruses, it is still unclear whether aminoacylation occurs at the 3' end of the genomic RNA or at an internal position after prior fragmentation.

The tRNA-specific enzymes capable of interacting in vitro with the 3' region of the plant viral RNAs listed in Table 1 include, in addition to the aminoacyl-tRNA synthetases, the tRNA nucleotidyltransferase, the peptidyl-tRNA hydrolase, the protein elongation factors EF-Tu or EF-1, 'RNase P' and a tRNA-specific cytosine methylase (for a review see ref. 3). TYMV RNA is valylated in vivo either when microinjected into Xenopus laevis oocytes (5), or in TYMV-infected Chinese cabbage leaves (6). Likewise, BMV RNA and BSMV RNA are tyrosylated in vivo in barley protoplasts (7).

In spite of the fact that certain viral RNAs and tRNAs share common properties, sequencing of the 3' region of the viral RNAs has revealed remarkably little similarity with tRNAs. The tRNA-like regions are devoid of modified nucleosides, they contain only few sequences in common with tRNAs acceptor of the same amino acid, and they do not fold into the classical clover-leaf pattern of tRNAs.

Within the last few years, several groups have examined the folding that confers tRNA-like properties to the 3' region of viral RNAs (8-14). These studies have comprised the following approaches: 1. the determination of the length of the shortest RNA fragment from the 3' end of the viral RNA capable of being aminoacylated: this delineates the tRNA-like region. Similarly, the length of the shortest RNA fragment from the 3' end required for adenylation has been established; 2. the determination of possible base-pairings within the tRNA-like region using chemical reagents or specific RNases under various experimental conditions; 3. computation; 4. oligonucleotide band compressions in sequencing gels.

As detailed below, folding of the 3' part of the tRNA-like regions appears to fall into two classes, that of

the tymoviruses (possibly also of the tomaboviruses) and
that of the bromo-, cucumo- and hordeiviruses. Both types
of folding are greatly different from that of tRNAs (for
a review see ref. 4).

Tymoviruses

The minimum length of TYMV RNA required for valylation is
∿86 nucleotides. The model proposed for the tRNA-like
region of this viral RNA is presented in Fig. 1; in its
'L'-shaped conformation it is schematized in Fig. 2. In
this model, the acceptor stem results from a very unexpected folding: it is composed exclusively of nucleotides
from the 3' part of the tRNA-like region without participation of nucleotides from the 5' part. Furthermore, two
short bridges link the two sides of the stem.

Bromo-, cucumo- and hordeiviruses

The last ∿160 nucleotides from the 3' end of the RNAs that
constitute the genome of the bromoviruses and of CMV are
remarkably conserved even though the coding sequences
which precede them are totally different. In addition to
this strong intraviral sequence conservation, there also
exists considerable interviral sequence similarity between these tRNA-like regions (9).

The minimum length of BMV RNA required for tyrosylation
is ∿134 nucleotides. The biochemical and biophysical data
available for the tRNA-like region of this RNA are compatible with the model presented in Fig. 1, and schematized
in Fig. 2. This model can be extrapolated to the tRNA-
like regions of the other bromo- and cucumoviruses in
view of the great sequence similarity that exists between
these regions. The 3' region of BSMV RNA also appears to
fold according to this model (15), even though it does
not contain significant sequence homology with the corresponding region of the bromo- and cucumovirus RNAs.

It is noteworthy that the folding of these regions
adopts an 'L'-shaped rather than a clover-leaf configuration. Here again the 'aminoacyl arm' (corresponding to
the continuous stacking of the acceptor stem and the T
stem and loop of tRNAs) is formed in an unexpected manner

356

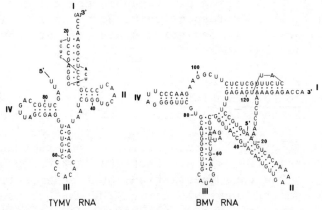

Fig. 1. The secondary structure of the tRNA-like region of TYMV RNA and of BMV RNA. I to IV correspond to stems and loops. Every 20th nucleotide is numbered.

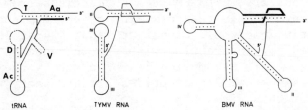

Fig. 2. Schematic representation of the 'L'-shaped configuration of tRNAs and of viral tRNA-like regions. The thick lines correspond to the contribution of the 5' region to the formation of the 'aminoacyl arm'. Aa = acceptor stem; T = T stem and loop; V = variable stem and loop; Ac = anticodon stem and loop; D = D stem and loop. I to IV are as in Fig. 1. (adapted from ref. 14).

(Fig. 2): one half of this arm involves the participation of nucleotides from the 3' and 5' part of the molecule as it does in tRNAs. The other half, however, is composed of nucleotides exclusively from the 5' part of the tRNA-like region, whereas in tRNAs the other half of this arm is made up of nucleotides from only the 3' part of the molecule. Furthermore, in the tRNA-like structure a short bridge links both sides of the 'aminoacyl arm'. Stems and loops II and III are reminiscent of the variable stem and loop and of the 'anticodon arm' (corresponding in tRNAs to

357

the continuous stacking of the anticodon and the D stems
and loops) of tRNAs respectively. Stem and loop IV are
not mandatory for tyrosylation since they are absent from
the BBMV and BSMV RNAs.

Requirements for adenylation

In TYMV RNA the last ∿50 nucleotides are required for adenylation. This has led us to propose that the 'aminoacyl
arm' is sufficient for recognition by the tRNA nucleotidyltransferase (11,14), and that the 'anticodon arm' is
not involved in this interaction. Such a demonstration
has been rendered possible using TYMV RNA because the
'aminoacyl arm' of this viral RNA only contains nucleotides from the 3' part of the molecule and thus constitutes an independent 'domain'.

On the contrary, with BMV RNA nucleotides from the 5'
part are involved in the formation of the 'aminoacyl arm'.
Consequently, one would expect at least 124 nucleotides to
be required for interaction with the tRNA nucleotidyltransferase. This assumption is borne out by the results
obtained, since ∿132 nucleotides are necessary for adenylation of this viral RNA.

ELEMENTS OF tRNAs IN OTHER VIRAL AND CELLULAR RNAs: 'PSEUDO tRNAs'

In recent years a few reports have appeared of examples
of regions in RNAs that in view of sequence homologies
and possible secondary folding are reminiscent of tRNAs.
These are reviewed here.

One such example is observed upon infection of Escherichia coli by certain DNA bacteriophages such as T2, T4 or
T6; this leads to the appearance of a stable RNA species
(species I) of 140 nucleotides whose 3' end terminates by
the sequence -CCA. Two parts of this RNA, nucleotides 46
to 67 and 87 to 140, both of which resemble about one
half of a tRNA molecule, can be folded into a clover-leaf
structure; the function of this RNA is still unknown (16).

It is well established that in the bacterial operons

for the biosynthetic pathways of certain amino acids, one
of the controls at the transcription level is by attenuation, i.e. by translational control of transcription termination. In the his operon of Salmonella typhymurium,
the region upstream of the corresponding messenger RNA
can adopt two mutually exclusive configurations. One of
them is reminiscent of the clover-leaf structure of tRNAs
with base-pairings analogous to those found in tRNAHis. It
has been suggested that enzymes specific of tRNAHis might
interact with this 'pseudo tRNA' and modulate the stability of this configuration to either favor or hinder early
transcription termination (17). Likewise, the leader
sequence of the E. coli mRNA coding for the threonyl-tRNA
synthetase can be folded into a clover-leaf configuration;
it has been postulated that the threonyl-tRNA synthetase
could bind to this 'pseudo tRNA' and thereby inhibit
translation (18). Finally, it is noteworthy that in the
E. coli glycyl-tRNA synthetase gene there exists a 12
nucleotide-long sequence similar to that found in the
anticodon region of tRNAGly (19).

Serial high multiplicity passage of DNA or RNA viruses
in animal cell culture leads to the appearance of viral
preparations enriched in particles known as defective
interfering (DI) particles. The nucleic acid contained in
the DI particles is smaller than the one contained in the
standard virus. It has been demonstrated (20) that the RNA
extracted from certain DI particles of Sindbis virus
contains at its 5' end a region which is remarkably similar to cellular tRNAAsp. Although this region lacks the
nine 5' terminal nucleotides of the acceptor stem of
tRNAAsp, it differs by only two bases from this tRNA. The
3' -CCA is not free, but is covalently bound to the re-
mainder of the RNA of the DI particle, and consequently
cannot be aminoacylated. One does not understand the role
that such a sequence — present in the RNA of DI particles
but absent from the RNA of standard virus — plays in
virus propagation.

Sequencing of satellite tobacco necrosis virus (STNV)
RNA has revealed that its 3' region can be folded into a
clover-leaf structure with an anticodon for AUG in an
appropriate position (21). However, it is not known whether STNV RNA can be charged with methionine or with any

other amino acid.

In addition to these examples of RNA regions containing features of tRNAs, another example has been provided by sequence analyses of Polyoma virus DNA: two regions of the DNA (between positions 715-799 and between positions 5160-5231) can be made to fold each into a clover-leaf-like manner (22,23).

CONCLUDING REMARKS

In the examples of the 'pseudo tRNAs' presented above, one must bear in mind that a similarity between a given region in an RNA (or DNA) and tRNA has so far been based solely on sequence homology and folding of the RNA molecule. As yet, no direct evidence has been provided that these RNA regions can indeed interact with tRNA-specific enzymes. This contrasts with the viral tRNA-like regions described in the first part of this paper, whose presence was detected primarily because of the biochemical reactions that these RNAs could undergo in the presence of tRNA-specific enzymes.

tRNAs, whose only function was for many years thought to be to provide amino acids in mRNA-dependent protein synthesis, have in recent years been shown to possess various other functions in the cell. In addition, tRNA-like regions and 'pseudo tRNAs' have been detected in cellular and viral RNAs, but their function remains a matter of speculation. One can postulate that 'pseudo tRNAs' and tRNAs might have originated from common ancestors and then diverged. As a result, certain 'pseudo tRNAs' might now correspond to 'silent' tRNA genes whose maintenance within an RNA sequence would be required as regulatory signals. On the other hand, the tRNA-like regions of plant viral RNAs and tRNAs can hardly be thought as originating from common ancestors. Rather, one is led to suppose that the viral RNAs have been forced to adopt a configuration which although distantly related to that of tRNAs, nevertheless enables them to interact with tRNA-specific enzymes. The reason for this convergence is unknown. The recent results obtained on the folding of the tRNA-like regions has revived interest in the search of a possible role of these 3' regions in the life-cycle of the virus.

ACKNOWLEDGEMENTS

We are grateful to François Chapeville for his constant interest in this work and for stimulating discussions. R.L.J. is recipient of a Fellowship of the 'Ministère de l'Industrie et de la Recherche'. This work was supported in part by a grant from the 'ATP : Interactions entre plantes et microorganismes', Centre National de la Recherche Scientifique.

REFERENCES

1. Pinck, M., Yot, P., Chapeville, F. and Duranton, H. (1970). Nature 226, 954-956.
2. Yot, P., Pinck, M., Haenni, A.L., Duranton, H.M. and Chapeville, F. (1970). Proc. Natl. Acad. Sci. USA 67, 1345-1352.
3. Haenni, A.L., Joshi, S. and Chapeville, F. (1982). Prog. Nucl. Acid Res. Mol. Biol. 27, 85-104.
4. Joshi, S., Joshi, R.L., Haenni, A.L. and Chapeville, F. (1983). Trends Biochem. Sci. 8, 402-404.
5. Joshi, S., Haenni, A.L., Hubert, E., Huez, G. and Marbaix, G. (1978). Nature 275, 339-341.
6. Joshi, S., Chapeville, F. and Haenni, A.L. (1982). EMBO J. 1, 935-938.
7. Loesch-Fries, L.S. and Hall, T.C. (1982). Nature 298, 771-773.
8. Symons, R.H. (1979). Nucl. Acids Res. 7, 825-837.
9. Ahlquist, P., Dasgupta, R. and Kaesberg, P. (1981). Cell 23, 183-189.
10. Rietveld, K., Van Poelgeest, R., Pleij, C.W.A., Van Boom, J.H. and Bosch, L. (1982). Nucl. Acids Res. 10, 1929-1946.
11. Joshi, S., Chapeville, F. and Haenni, A.L. (1982).

Nucl. Acids Res. 10, 1947-1962.

12. Florentz, C., Briand, J.P., Romby, P., Hirth, L., Ebel J.P. and Giégé, R. (1982). EMBO J. 1, 269-276.

13. Rietveld, K., Pleij, C.W.A. and Bosch, L. (1983). EMBO J. 2, 1079-1085.

14. Joshi, R.L., Joshi, S., Chapeville, F. and Haenni, A.L. (1983). EMBO J. 2, 1123-1127.

15. Kozlov, Yu.V., Rupasov, V.V., Adyshev, D.M., Belgel-askaya, S.N., Agranovsky, A.A., Mankin, A.S., Morozov, S.Yu., Dolja, V.V. and Atabekov, J.G. (1984). Nucl. Acids Res. 12, 4001-4009.

16. Paddock, G. and Abelson, J. (1973). Nature New Biol. 246, 2-6.

17. Ames, B.N., Tsang, T.H., Buck, M. and Christman, M.F. (1983). Proc. Natl. Acad. Sci. USA 80, 5240-5242.

18. Lestienne, P., Plombridge, J.A., Grunberg-Manago, M. and Blanquet, S. (1984). J. Biol. Chem. 259, 5232-5237.

19. Keng, T., Webster, T.A., Sauer, R.T. and Schimmel, P. (1982). J. Biol. Chem. 257, 12503-12508.

20. Monroy, S.S. and Schlesinger, S. (1983). Proc. Natl. Acad. Sci. USA 80, 3279-3283.

21. Ysebaert, M., Van Emmelo, J. and Fiers, W. (1980). J. Mol. Biol. 143, 273-287.

22. Soeda, E., Arrand, J.R., Smolar, N., Walsh J.E. and Griffin, B.E. (1980). Nature 283, 445-453.

23. Katinka, M., Vasseur, M., Montreau, N., Yaniv, M. and Blangy, D. (1981). Nature 290, 720-722.

PRELIMINARY ATOMIC MODEL FOR TOBACCO MOSAIC VIRUS

ALFONSO MONDRAGON and ANNE C. BLOOMER
Medical Research Council Laboratory of Molecular Biology
Hills Road, Cambridge CB2 2QH, U.K.

WERNER GEBHARD and KENNETH C. HOLMES
Max-Planck-Institut für Medizinische Forschung
Jahnstr. 29, 6900 Heidelberg, FRG

INTRODUCTION

TMV particles are rod-like, 300 nm long and 18 nm in
diameter with a central hole of diameter 4.0 nm (1). The
particles consist of 94% protein and 6% nucleic acid. A
particle contains 2140 identical protein subunits, each
of molecular weight 17,420 Daltons (158 residues) (2),
arranged on a helix of pitch 2.3 nm with 16 1/3 subunits
per turn. Winding through this helix is a single strand
of RNA 6400 nucleotides long with three bases bound to
each protein subunit.

The isolated nucleoprotein particle can readily be
taken apart (3) and re-assembled (4). The re-assembly
of the coat protein in vitro without RNA leads
primarily to the production of double layer disks
containing two rings each comprised of 17 protein subunits. The two rings have the same orientation but are
not equivalent. Butler and Klug (5) were able to show
that the disk is the major precursor for the initiation
and growth of the virus. The disk crystallises and has
been analysed by X-ray diffraction to a resolution of
0.28 nm (Bloomer et al) (6). This shows the structure
of the subunit in the two rings of a disk to be
essentially identical, although their inclinations
with respect to the 17-fold axis differ by 10°.

Proceedings of the 16th FEBS Congress
Part A, pp. 363–373
© 1985 VNU Science Press

STRUCTURE OF THE TWO-LAYER DISK

The general appearance of the subunit, as deduced from the high resolution studies of Bloomer *et al.* is shown in Fig. 1.

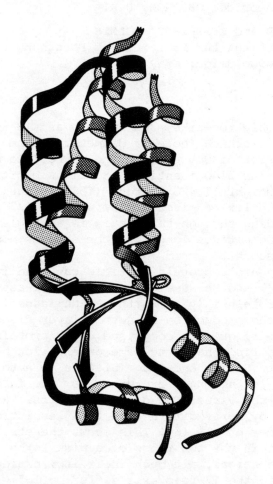

Schematic view of the protein subunit in the disk - by courtesy of Jane Richardson. Note the LS and RS helices (black) overlying the truncated RR and LR helices (grey).

Both the N and C termini are located distally. Starting from the N-terminus the chain builds a short helical structure followed by a strand of the distal beta-pleated sheet. Then follows (20-30) the LS (left slewed) helix and after a tight turn (31-37) the chain proceeds distally along the RS (right slewed) helix (38-51) which is roughly parallel to the LS helix. The chain now builds two strands of the beta-sheet before starting the RR (right radial) helix (76-89) which proceeds proximally to a radius of about 4.5 nm before the electron density fades out. Then follows a flexible loop (90-113) which has been shown by proton NMR to be highly mobile in the disk but not in the virus (7). The map shows clearly two turns of helical structure at one end of the mobile loop, adjacent to the well-ordered helix from residue 114 in the LR (left radial) helix. This helix runs roughly horizontally from 4.0 nm to 7.0 nm radius (134), terminating next to the final strands of the beta-sheet. The chain then continues to high radius with a short section of helix before the C-terminus. Thus the major part of the subunit comprises four alpha-helices. These are abutted on their distal ends by a beta sheet outside of which is a girdle of hydrophobic interactions extending around the disk both within and between subunits.

Interactions between the subunits within one ring of the disk are extensive and occur in alternating patches of polar and hydrophobic contacts. These lateral interactions are similar to those found in the virus, whereas the axial interactions between the two rings of a disk are quite different from the intimate contacts found in the virus. The two rings of a disk are widely separated towards the central hole of the disk, allowing access of the RNA which is entrapped between the two rings during the assembly process (Butler et al.) (8). At high radius the most extensive interaction between the upper and lower rings of the disk is mediated by salt bridges.

Concentrated solutions of TMV form spontaneously
birefringent tactoids which may be easily persuaded to
fuse to form a highly orientated gel (9). From such gels
it is possible to obtain X-ray fibre diagrams of
unsurpassed quality (10). Stubbs et al.(11) were able
to calculate an electron density map of the virus by a
Fourier-Bessel synthesis using all data to 0.4 nm.
Analysis of the fibre diffraction pattern of the gels
made use of the method of isomorphous replacement both
to phase the diffraction pattern and to separate the
overlapping Bessel function terms. The low radius region
of the map appeared to be well resolved, showing several
details within the protein density. Furthermore, the
nucleic acid and its environment could be clearly
identified.

Three nucleotides are associated with each protein
subunit. Studies by Mandelkow et al. (12) on the
re-polymerised helical form of the coat protein without
RNA allowed the allocation of certain electron density
to RNA. A least-squares refinement into this density
was made by Stubbs and Stauffacher (13). The phosphates
are clustered around a radius of 4.0 nm and the bases
cluster round the LR helix with two at about the same
radius as the phosphates and one at higher radius. The
RNA binding site lies between the rings of a disk, in
agreement with the model for TMV assembly proposed by
Butler et al. (8).

The identification of the helices LS, RS, RR and LR in
the 0.4 nm virus electron density map was clear. Outside
6.0 nm radius the use of only three Bessel functions
in the Fourier-Bessel synthesis resulted in a loss of
resolving power so that an unambiguous interpretation
of the electron density was no longer possible, although
a general similarity to the electron density of the disk
was apparent. In the virus map it was apparent that
proximally from 4.0 nm radius (where the density in
the disk fades out), the LR and RR helices continue
to low radius (2.5 nm) where they are joined together
by a vertical column of density (the V-column).

BUILDING THE ATOMIC MODEL OF THE DISK INTO THE VIRUS MAP

It is clearly desirable to combine the resulting detailed
model of the subunit in the disk with the virsu map.
Bloomer et al.(14) analysed the relationship between
the A-ring , the B-ring, and the virus and have shown
that, in addition to a small radial movement, the
subunits must be rotated by 10° (A-disk) or 20° (B-disk)
about an axis perpendicular to the disk or helix axis
in order to bring them into the same orientation as
the virus.

In the present study, a least-squares procedure has
been used to obtain the best match of the intensities
calculated from the transformed disk atomic model
(fitted initially as a rigid body) to the diffracted
intensities from the virus. To a first approximation,
the disk and helix structures may be related by a rigid-
body transformation which is most easily visualised as
a translation of 0.3 nm radially inwards and three
rotations corresponding to changes of about 15° in the
pitch of the subunit followed by 5-10° in the slew of
the molecule with respect to the radius vector and less
than 5° in the roll about this vector.

Having positioned the disk subunit in the virus map,
the residues missing from the disk model have now been
built into the model using the electron density of the
4.0 nm virus map as a guide.

Further refinement is in progress with the protein
molecule divided into several separate rigid pieces, to
allow for local deformations and reveal the nature of
any departures from a strict rigid-body transformation.
With the present model the crystalllographic R-factor
is 32% between the intensities observed in the diffraction
pattern (from 1.0 to 0.5 nm) and those calculated from
the coordinates.

Figure 2 shows an example of the agreement between
this model and the 0.4 nm virus map of Stubbs et al.(11).

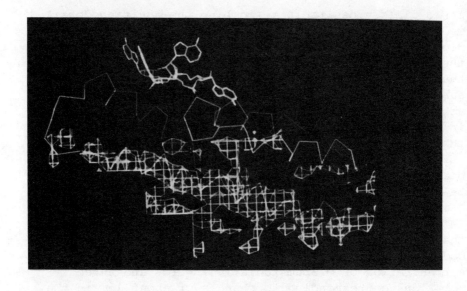

Fig. 2.
To illustrate the measure of agreement between the
extended LR helix of the present model and the 4.0 nm
virus map of Stubbs et al. (11).

As proposed by Stubbs et al.(11), both the LR and
RR helices are longer in the virus than the disk and
extend inwards to 2.5 nm radius. The vertical column
appears to be a nearly extended chain of 5 residues
joining the two helices. The resolving power of a 4.0 nm
electron density map does not generally allow one to
locate side chains other than by model-building so that
most side chain positions in the virus remain to be
determined. The configuration of the RNA has been taken
from the coordinates of Stubbs and Stauffacher (13).
The RNA coordinates are combined with those of the
protein subunit to give an atomic model of the virus
(Fig. 3).

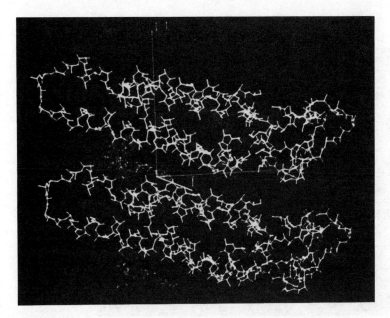

Fig. 3
Side view of the main chain of two protein subunits
and the RNA entrapped between the two turns of the
viral helix (axis of virus is vertical). Note the
lengthened RR and LR helices which now extend from
76-100 and from 108-134. One base (at high radius)
makes contact with the band region between the RS and LS
helices and with the LR helix. The phosphates lie between
the LR helix of one subunit and the RR helix of the
adjacent subunit one turn down.

   The protein subunits are closely associated across
the lateral interface with the neighbouring molecule
in the helix (Fig. 4). The increase in the slew angle
of a protein subunit in the virus compared with that
in the disk results in the virus lateral contacts being
even more intimate and extensive than those in the disk.
The axial bonding between turns of the helix is also
more extended in the virus and is mediated by salt
bridges. The network of salt bridges, covering much of
the interface at higher radius than the RNA, involves
residues on the lower surface of one subunit with those

on the upper surface of <u>two</u> adjacent molecules in the
neighbouring turn of the viral helix.

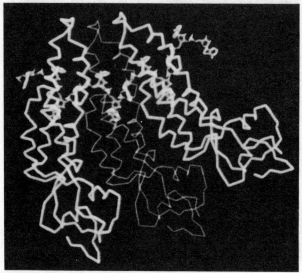

Fig. 4a The adjacent protein subunits with the RNA
below (looking along the helix axis).

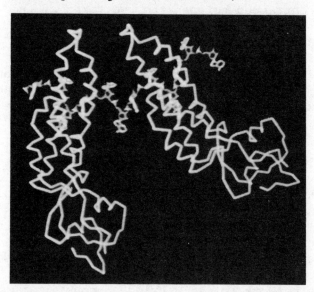

Fig. 4b As in 4a but with centre unit removed for
clarity.

PROTEIN-RNA INTERACTIONS

Some aspects of the protein-RNA interaction become clear from the present model. The RNA fits snugly into the "jaws" formed between two adjacent turns of the helix. The high radius base of the RNA can be seen to be inserted into the gap between the LS and RS helices of the lower subunit and the LR helix from a molecule in the turn above. There are several possible hydrogen bonds which can be made by a purine or pyrimidine base in this position. The phosphate group of this nucleotide probably bonds to ARG 41 where the side chain may swing up from the half-buried position within the disk. The other two bases lie close to the LR helix, as proposed by Stubbs et al. (11). The remaining phosphate groups form salt bridges with residues ARG 90 and 92 from the subunit below.

The vertical column at small radius (2.5 nm) consists of five residues which run at an oblique angle (Fig. 5) so that the chains from neighbouring subunits are only 0.7 nm apart forming a pallisade on the lumen-side of the RNA.

ACKNOWLEDGEMENTS

We gratefully acknowledge the expert photographic assistance of Ken Harvey and Gabriele Eulefeld. We thank Jane Richardson for permission to reproduce Fig. 1. We thank Arthur Lesk for his help with the computer graphics. A. Mondragon thanks the National University of Mexico and ORS for support.

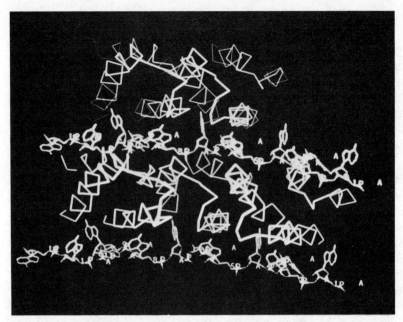

Fig. 5 View from the centre looking outwards; 5
subunits and two turns of RNA. Note the five residues
running diagonally which join the RR and LR helices.
Although these chains come from different subunits
they are in close contact (approx. 0.7 nm) and form
a wall protecting the RNA from the lumen of the virus.

REFERENCES

1. Klug, A., Caspar, D.L.D. (1960). Adv. Virus Res. 7,
   225-325.
2. Anderer, F.A. (1963). Adv. Protein Chem. 18, 1-35.
3. Schramm, G. (1947). Z. Naturforsch. 2b, 112-118
   and 249-257.
4. Fraenkel-Conrat, H., Williams, R.C. (1955). Proc.
   Natl. Acad. Sci. USA 41, 690-704.
5. Butler, P.J.G., Klug, A. (1971). Nature New Biol.
   229, 47-50.
6. Bloomer, A.C., Champness, J.N., Bricogne, G.,
   Staden, R., Klug, A. (1978). Nature (London) 276,
   362-368.

7. Jardetzsky, O., Akasaka, K., Vogel, D., Morris, S., Holmes, K.C. (1978) Nature (London) 273, 564-566.

8. Butler, P.J.G., Bloomer, A.C., Bricogne, G., Champness, J.N., Graham, J., Guilley, H., Klug, A., Zimmern, D. (1976). In: Structure -Function Relationships in Proteins, Markham, R. and Horne, R. (Eds). 3rd John Innes Symposium, North Holland, Amsterdam, pp 101-110.

9. Gregory, J., Holmes, K.C. (1965). J. Mol. Biol. 13, 796-801.

10. Franklin, R.E.F. (1955). Nature (London) 175, 379-384.

11. Stubbs, G., Warren, S., Holmes, K.C. (1977). Nature (London) 267, 216-221.

12. Mandelkow, E., Stubbs, G., Warren, S. (1981). J. Mol. Biol. 152, 375-386.

13. Stubbs, G., Stauffacher, C.V. (1981) j. Mol. Biol. 152, 387-396.

14. Bloomer, A.C., Graham, J., Hovmoeller, S., Butler, P.J.G., Klug, A. (1981). In: Structural aspects of recognition in biological macromolecules. Balaban, M., Sussman, J., Traub, W., Yonath, A. (Eds). Balaban ISS, Rehovoth, pp. 851-864.

TRANSPORT OF VIRUS GLYCOPROTEINS IN EUKARYOTIC CELLS

L. KÄÄRIÄINEN,[1] E. KUISMANEN[1], R. PETTERSSON[1], M. PESONEN[1], N. GAHMBERG[1], AND J. SARASTE[2]

[1] Recombinant DNA Laboratory, University of Helsinki, Valimotie 7, SF-00380 Helsinki, Finland

[2] Department of Virology, University of Helsinki, Haartmaninkatu 3, SF-00290 Helsinki, Finland

INTRODUCTION

The integral membrane glycoproteins of enveloped viruses have been used as models to study the translation, glycosylation and transport of cellular membrane proteins in eukaryotic cells (for reviews see 1, 2). As compared to cellular glycoproteins the viruses have many advantages i) The glycoproteins are produced in large amounts and can be purified easily with the released virus particles, ii) Virus-specific mRNAs are easy to obtain to allow *in vitro* translation studies and even determination of the primary structure of the proteins by sequencing of the cloned cDNA, iii) Use of temperature-sensitive virus mutants with defects in the transport of glycoproteins has enabled studies of the different steps involved in the transport by simple temperature shifts.

We have used Semliki Forest (SFV) and Uukuniemi virus (UUK) as models to study the biogenesis of plasma and Golgi membranes, respectively. SFV consists of a nucleocapsid and a lipoprotein envelope with 210 glycoprotein trimers consisting of E1, E2 and E3 (3, 4). E1 and E3 carry one complex glycan, whereas E2 has two high mannose glycans (5). The virus matures at the host cell plasma membrane where the nucleocapsid recognizes the cytoplasmic extension of E2 resulting into budding of the

Proceedings of the 16th FEBS Congress
Part A, pp. 375–381
© 1985 VNU Science Press

virions into the extracellular space (for reviews see 3, 6,7).

We have isolated temperature-sensitive mutants of SFV (8), one of which, ts-1, turned out to have a temperature-dependent transport defect. At the restrictive temperature 39°C the virus glycoproteins are arrested in rough ER. Once the infected cultures are transferred to 28°C (permissive temperature) the glycoproteins are transported to the plasma membrane (9, 10, 11).

Some of our recent experiments describing the transport of SFV envelope proteins to the host cell plasma membrane are demonstrated as an example of the pathway of plasma-membrane-specific membrane glycoproteins.

Uukuniemi virus is a member of a large Bunyaviridae family, which mature at the Golgi complex (12). The UUK virus has two glycoproteins, G1 and G2, 75,000 and 65,000 daltons, respectively. G1 has complex, endo-glycosidase H resistant, oligosaccharide chains, whereas G2 has both high mannose and complex glycans (13, 14). Here we show that the kinetics of transport of UUK glycoproteins from ER to Golgi complex is considerably slower than that of SFV glycoproteins. The UUK glyco-proteins are arrested in the Golgi complex where they associate with virus nucleocapsid in normal infection. Part of the proteins are, however, transported to the plasma membrane.

RESULTS AND DISCUSSION

When SFV ts-1 mutant is grown in chick embryo or BHK21 cells at 39°C, no infectious virus is released into the medium. The viral structural proteins are synthesized in almost normal amounts (15). Typically, capsid protein, E1 glycoproteins and the precursor of E2 and E3, p62, are seen in polyacrylamide gels with or without immuno-precipitation. Both E1 and p62 are sensitive to endo-glycosidase H, indicating the absence of complex glycans. Glycan analysis has shown that only high mannose oligo-saccharides are present in both proteins (5). Interestingly the glycans were partly resistant to digestion to mannosidases suggesting that all of terminal glucose residues had not been removed. Immunoelectron microscopy using immunoperoxidase labeling has shown that in fact the glycoproteins are arrested in RER (11).

If the ts-1 infected cells are transferred to 28°C the glycoproteins are transported to the cell surface within 60 to 90 minutes as evidenced by immunofluorescence and more quantitatively by radioimmuno assay (9, 10) or by immunoelectron microscopy (11). At the same time part of the high mannose glycans are converted into complex ones (5).

Saraste and Kuismanen (16) have recently shown that if the ts-1 infected cultures are shifted from 39°C to 15°C the virus glycoproteins leave the ER but remain endo H sensitive. Immunoelectron microscopy revealed that the proteins accumulated in pre-Golgi vacuolar elements. If the temperature was again shifted to 28°C or 20°C a synchronous passage of viral glycoproteins could be followed. As a first step was the entrance of glyco-proteins via tubular extensions, which seemingly generated the first Golgi cisterna. The suggested cisternal progression was rapid (less than 5 min) followed by exit of proteins in vacuolar elements, which apparently fused with the plasma membrane within 5 to 10 min.

The appearance of ts-1 glycoproteins on the cell surface is effectively inhibited by 1 to 10 µM monensin. If the drug is administered just prior to shift down to 28°C of ts-1 infected cultures, the glycoproteins migrate from the RER to the Golgi complex but not to the plasma membrane (10, 17).

Typical features of the transport of SFV and ts-1 glycoproteins are a fairly rapid transfer from RER to Golgi in about 100 nm vesicles followed by entry via tubular extension of pre-Golgi vacuolar elements. Rapid passage of proteins through the Golgi cisternae by cisternal maturation and finally exit from Golgi via post-Golgi vacuoles in about 200 nm vesicles. The last step is evidently prevented by monensin, a drug known to inhibit the transport of many glycoproteins from Golgi to plasma membrane (18).

Uukuniemi virus was shown to mature through intracellular smooth membranes which morphologically were identified

as Golgi complex (19). Recent studies have shown that
the two Uukuniemi virus glycoproteins, G1 and G2, are
specifically concentrated in the Golgi membranes together
with nucleocapsid (N) protein (20). This is true even
after 6 h cycloheximide treatment. The SFV glycoproteins
disappear from the Golgi region already after 30 min
incubation with cycloheximide.

The "Golgi-specificity" of UUK glycoproteins is not
due to the association with N-protein. Nina Gahmberg
has isolated temperature-sensitive mutants (e.g. Uts-12),
which direct the synthesis of glycoproteins accumulating
into the Golgi complex, without associating with the
N-protein (21).

A typical feature for Uukuniemi virus infection is the
vacuolization of the Golgi complex in the middle of virus
growth cycle (10-12 h p.i.) (14). Again, this vacuolization is obtained also in Uts-12 -infected cells at
the restrictive temperature (39°C) in the absence of
virus maturation and binding of N protein (21). This
would mean that the UUK glycoproteins are alone responsible for the vacuolization of the Golgi membranes.

The transport of UUK glycoproteins has also been
followed by pulse-chase experiments using endo H as a
criterion of glycan processing (22). For the G1 protein,
which in mature virions contains only endo H resistant
glycans, it takes about 45 min for half of the glycoproteins to become resistant to the digestion by this
enzyme. This would suggest that the transport time for
UUK glycoproteins from the RER to the Golgi complex
is 2 to 3 times longer than that for SFV glycoproteins.

At present we do not know whether the transport of
UUK glycoproteins is retarded between the ER and the
proximal Golgi (cis-side) since endo H resistance is
attained at the trans-side of the complex (2). It is
also possible that the vacuolization of the Golgi
cisternae affect the transport kinetics in the Golgi
complex.

Part of the UUK glycoproteins are transported to the
cell surface as can be demonstrated by immunofluorescence
and radioimmune assays. This equally true for the wild
type virus and the Uts-12 mutant, indicating that transport

from Golgi to plasma membrane takes place without
virus maturation. In striking contrast to SFV glycoproteins, the transport of UUK glycoproteins was not
affected by 1 or 10 μM monensin.

The comparison of the events during the transport
of the glycoproteins of two different viruses has
revealed fundamental differences which are not spec-
ified by the host since both viruses have been grown in
the same cells (BHK21 and CEF). The SFV glycoproteins
can be regarded as plasma membrane proteins, whereas
UUK glycoproteins are "Golgi-specific" proteins. It
is tempting to assume that these virus proteins have
been derived from cellular anchestors during evolution.

REFERENCES

1. Kääriäinen, L. and Renkonen, O. (1977). Envelopes of
    lipid containing viruses as models of membrane
    assembly. In: The synthesis, assembly and turnover
    of cell surface components. Cell surface reviews.
    Vol. 4. G. Poste and G.L. Nicolson (eds). Elsevier
    North-Holland Biomedical Press, pp. 741-801.
2. Kääriäinen, L. and Pesonen, M. (1982). Virus glyco-
    proteins and glycolipids. Structure, biosynthesis,
    biological function and interaction with host. In:
    The glycoconjugates. M.I. Horowitz (ed). Academic
    Press, In. New York and London, PP. 191-242.
3. Kääriäinen, L. and Söderlund, H. (1978) Structure
    and replication of alphaviruses. Curr. Top.
    Microbiol. Immunol. 82:15-69.
4. Jacrot, B., Cuillel, M., and Söderlund, H. (1984)
    Molecular weight and structure of Semliki Forest
    virus. J. Mol. Biol. (in press).
5. Pesonen, M., Saraste, J., Hashimoto, K. and
    Kääriäinen, L. (1981) Reversible defect in the
    glycosylation of the membrane proteins of Semliki
    Forest virus ts-1 mutant. Virology 109:165-173.
6. Garoff, H., Kondor-Koch, C., and Riedel, H. (1982)
    Structure and assembly of alphaviruses. Curr. Top.
    Microbiol. Immunol. 92:1-49.
7. Strauss, E.G. and Strauss, J.H. (1983). Replication

strategies of single stranded RNA viruses of
eukaryotes. Curr. Top.Microbiol.Immunol. 105:1-98.
8. Keränen, S. and Kääriäinen, L. (1974). Isolation and
basic characterization of temperature-sensitive
mutants from Semliki Forest virus. Acta path.
microbiol. Scand. sect. B 82:810-820.
9. Saraste, J., von Bondsdorff, C.-H., Hashimoto, K.
Kääriäinen, L. and Keränen, S. (1980). Semliki
Forest virus mutants with temperature-sensitive
transport defect of envelope proteins. Virology
100:229-245.
10. Kääriäinen, L., Hashimoto, K., Saraste, J., Virtanen,
I. and Penttinen, K. (1980). Monensin and FCCP
inhibit the intracellular transport of alphavirus
membrane glycoproteins. J. Cell Biol. 87:783-791.
11. Saraste, J. and Hedman, K. (1983). Intracellular
vesicles involved in the transport of Semliki Forest
virus membrane proteins to the cell surface. EMBO
J. 2:2001-2006.
12. Bishop, D.H.L. and Shope, R.E. (1979). Bunyaviridae.
In: Comprehensive virology, vol. 14. H. Fraenkel-
Conrat and R.R. Wagner (eds). Plenum Publishing
Corp. New York, pp. 1-156.
13. Pesonen, M., Kuismanen, E., and Pettersson R.F. (1982)
Monosaccharide sequence of protein-bound glycans of
Uukuniemi virus. J. Virol. 41:390-400.
14. Kuismanen, E., Bång, B., Hurme, M., and Pettersson, R.
(1984). Uukuniemi virus maturation: an immunofluorescence microscopy study using monoclonal
glycoprotein-specific antibodies. J.Virol.(in press)
15. Keränen, S. and Kääriäinen, L. (1975) Proteins
synthesized by Semliki Forest virus and its 16
temperature-sensitive mutants. J. Virol. 16:388-396.
16. Saraste, J. and Kuismanen, E. (1984). Pre- and post-
Golgi vacuoles opearate in the transport of Semliki
Forest virus membrane glycoproteins to the cell
surface. Cell 38: (in press).
17. Kääriäinen, L., Virtanen, I., Saraste,J. and Keränen,
S. (1983). Transport of virus membrane glycoproteins
Use of ts-mutants and organelle-specific lectins.
In: Methods in enzymology, Vol. 96. S.Fleischer and
B. Fleischer (eds). Academic Press, New York,

pp. 453-465.
18. Pesonen, M. and Kääriäinen, L. (1982) Incomplete
complex oligosaccharides in Semliki Forest virus
envelope proteins arrested within the cell in the
presence of monensin. J. Mol. Biol. 158:213-230.
19. von Bonsdorff, C.-H., Saikku, P. and Oker-Blom, N.
(1970). Electron microscope study on the development of Uukuniemi virus. Acta Virol. 14:109-114.
20. Kuismanen, E., Hedman, K., Saraste, J. and Pettersson,
R.F. (1982). Uukuniemi virus maturation: accumulation of virus particles and viral antigens in the
Golgi complex. Mol. Cell Biol. 11:1444-1458.
21. Gahmberg, N. (1984). Characterization of two
recombination complementation groups of Uukuniemi
virus temperature-sensitive mutants. J. gen. Virol.
65:1079-1090.
22. Kuismanen, E. (1984). Post translational processing
of Uukuniemi virus glycoproteins G1 and G2.
J. Virol. (in press).

Symposium VI

BIOCHEMISTRY OF NITROGEN FIXATION AND NITROGEN ASSIMILATION IN PLANTS

RELATIONSHIP BETWEEN HYDROGENASE AND NITROGENASE IN NITROGEN-FIXING PHOTOTROPHS

I.N.GOGOTOV
Institute of Soil Science and Photosynthesis
Academy of Sciences of the USSR, Pushchino,
Moscow region, 142292 (USSR)

The majority of nitrogen-fixing microorganisms besides nitrogenase synthesize hydrogenase. However, the interrelation between these enzymes started coming to light only after the possibility of nitrogenase-mediated hydrogen evolution had been established.

According to some data (1-4) there exists for the purple bacteria and cyanobacteria that are able to assimilate N_2 a direct correlation between the light-induced H_2 production and nitrogen fixation. Both processes are inhibited by high concentrations of NH_4^+ and some other nitrogen compounds. Repression of nitrogenase synthesis or mutation leading to a loss of the enzyme in purple bacteria and cyanobacteria results in a loss of capacity for light-induced H_2 evolution. The green thermophilic bacterium Chloroflexus aurantiacus growing at temperatures of $60-70^\circ$C, which is incapable of nitrogen fixation, lacks the ability of light-induced H_2 evolution as well. CO, which inhibits hydrogenase activity, has only a slight effect on the light-induced hydrogen evolution by purple bacteria and cyanobacteria. Like nitrogen fixation, however, this process is suppressed in the presence of uncouplers and certain inhibitors of the electron transport chain (5). All this supports the view that the energy-dependent H_2 production in purple bacteria and cyanobacteria demands the participation of nitrogenase. Hydrogenases synthesized by the majority of these microorganisms take part in

Proceedings of the 16th FEBS Congress
Part A, pp. 385–390

H_2 production in the process of dark fermentation of some substrates, and in hydrogen consumption.

Nitrogenase-mediated H_2 production by the purple non-sulfur bacterium Rhodopseudomonas capsulata B10 depends on the nitrogen supply of the cells. Under N_2 - limiting conditions of growth, up to 55% of electrons are spent via nitrogenase on H_2 production (6). In many nitrogen-fixing microorganisms hydrogen evolved through nitrogenase may be rapidly utilized by the same organisms due to hydrogenase activity, i.e. the so-called process of H_2 recyclization takes place (5,7). This appears to be the reason why in some cases H_2 evolution by nitrogen-fixing organisms can be detected or is markedly increased with suppression of activity of hydrogenases functioning in the pathway of H_2 consumption, e.g. by adding CO or CO and C_2H_2 to the cells suspension (8). The H_2 recycling process is typical for nodule and purple bacteria, as well as for Azotobacter, Azospirillaceae, and a number of cyanobacteria (8). Thus, the ability for recycling hydrogen is characteristic of various nitrogen-fixing organisms, with the exception of bacterial strains that for some reason possess an underdeveloped system of H_2 consumption.

Investigations of the components of electron transport chain participating in nitrogen fixation and the recycling of H_2, evolved via nitrogenase in the nitrogen-fixing purple bacteria R.capsulata B10 and Thiocapsa roseopersicina BBS revealed that the enzymes and electron-transfer proteins are essentially different in these bacteria (5,8). Isolated hydrogenases differ not only in molecular weight and subunit composition but also in the ability to preferentially catalyze evolution or consumption of H_2 (Table 1). This is apparently related to the regulatory effect of the E_h of the medium that influences the FeS cluster in the active center, thus converting the enzyme into the active or inactive state. The natural electron

carriers that interact in vitro with hydrogenases of
the above mentioned purple bacteria are type "c"
and type "b" cytochromes (Table 1), but not ferredoxin (10), the latter being typical for clostridia
and some other organisms (8).

NAD(P)-reductases of T.roseopersicina catalyze
the ferredoxin-dependent reduction of NAD(P).
The ability to catalyze this reaction was not
observed for the NAD(P)-reductases of R.capsu-
lata. Unlike the reductases of T.roseopersicina,
this enzyme in R.capsulata interacts with electron
carriers having more positive redox potentials than
that of ferredoxin (Table 2).

On the basis of the studies of properties of
enzymes and electron carriers, as well as by
inhibitory analysis, one can put forward the following electron-transport pathways of H_2 metabolism
and nitrogen fixation in purple bacteria.

T.roseopersicina is characterized by high contents
of cytochrome c_{552}, flavodoxin and high-potential
Fe-S protein(8), whereas the amount of ferredoxin,
type "b" cytochromes and ubiquinones is low.
The latter compounds are present in the cells of
R.capsulata in considerable quantities (5). Cytochrome c', one of the natural electron acceptors
of hydrogenase in R.capsulata, was not detected
in T.roseopersicina. The R.capsulata hydrogenase
in vitro shows a higher rate of catalysis of H_2
consumption. Its natural acceptors possess higher
redox potentials than that of T.roseopersicina,
the hydrogenase of the latter catalyzing reactions
of H_2 oxidation and H_2 evolution at about the
same rate.

The initial electron donors of the nitrogen fixation chain in T.roseopersicina are H_2, thiosulfate
or organic compounds, which in all probability
reduce the immediate electron donors of nitrogenase, that is ferredoxins or flavodoxin.
Parallel with exogeneous H_2, the purple bacteria

Table 1 Properties of homogeneous preparations
of hydrogenases from purple bacteria

Properties of hydrogenases	T.roseopersicina	R.capsulata
Localization	membranes, cytoplasm	membranes
$\mathcal{E}$, $mM^{-1} \cdot cm^{-1}$	$\mathcal{E}_{280} = 115$ $\mathcal{E}_{400} = 29$	n.d. n.d.
M_r	68000	100000
Subunits	1x47000;1x25000	1x90000
Ni^{2+} per mol	1	1
Fe^{2+} per mol	4	4
S^{2-} per mol	4	4
SH per mol	10	n.d.
pI	1.15 and 4.2	4.25
EPR properties:		
ox.state	Hipip type, g=1.98; 2.03	Hipip type, g=2.019
red.state	EPR-silent	EPR-silent
Type of Fe-S cluster	4Fe-4S	4Fe-4S
E_o (pH 7.0), mV	$-200 \div -280$	-340
Natural electron donor/acceptor	cytochrome c'_3/ cytochromes c_3, c_3', c_{552} and Hipip-protein	n.d./cytochromes c', b_{560}
$T_{1/2}$, air, $+20^{o}C$	60 days	20 hours
Activity, μM produced /consumed $H_2 \cdot min^{-1} \cdot mg^{-1}$ protein	$30^{o}C$-100/21 $70^{o}C$-612/260	$30^{o}C$-1.3/30 $70^{o}C$-13/100

Table 2 Properties of NAD(P)-reductases of purple bacteria

Properties	T.roseopersicina		R.capsulata
	NADP-reductase	NAD-reductase	NAD(P)-reductase
Localization	cytoplasm	periplasm	cytoplasm
M_r	47000	44000	67000
Subunits	2x21000	2x22000	4x18000
Flavin	+	+	FMN
pI	n.d.	3.9	4.6
Temperature optimum, ^{o}C:	50	40	45
Thermostability, ^{o}C:	65	55	45
Half-inactivation time, h:			
Ar + glycerol ($-20^{o}C$)	n.d.	1440	n.d.
Ar ($-4^{o}C$)	240	24	n.d.
Ar + 5% O_2 ($-4^{o}C$)	120	12	n.d.
Activity:			
NAD(P)H + benzyl-viologen	+	+	+
+ ubiquinone R.capsulata	n.d.	n.d.	+
+ c' R.capsulata	n.d.	n.d.	+
+ c_3 T.roseopersicina	+	+	n.d.
+ c_3 -"-	+*)	+	n.d.
+ c_{552} -"-	+	+	+**)
+ ferredoxin -"-	+	+	-
+ Hipip-protein -"-	+	+	n.d.

*) Benzylviologen or ferredoxin added. **) FMN or menadione added.

388

are able to recycle the nitrogenase-produced hydrogen. This results in hydrogenase – mediated reduction of cytochromes c'_3, c_{552} and of the high-potential Fe-S protein. Subsequent electron transfer from the reduced cytochromes and Fe-S protein or NAD(P)H to ferredoxin (flavodoxin) in this bacterium is supposedly governed by NAD(P)- reductases (Table 2). Reduction of ferredoxin and flavodoxin in the case of T.roseopersicina is feasible with different electron carriers and enzymes, their composition depending on the nature of the initial electron donor, utilized by the cells in the process of nitrogen fixation. (Fig.1).

The electron transport chain composition fuctioning in H_2 metabolism of R.capsulata differs from that of T.roseopersicina. Hydrogenase mediates reduction of cytochromes c' or b_{560} by H_2, produced by nitrogenase with the assistance of ubiquinones and NAD(P)-reductases. The electrons may then be transferred to NAD(P). The formation of reduced NAD(P)H in R.capsulata apparently occurs in a reaction of a so-called reverse energy-dependent electron flow from the initial electron donors. As a result of a forward or reverse energy-dependent electron flow from H_2 the reduction of ferredoxins may take place as well, the latter being the immediate electron donors of nitrogenase in this bacterium (10). Thus, there exists a straightforward correlation between the abilities of purple bacteria for energy-dependent H_2 production and for nitrogen fixation. From the data presented here it follows also that the co- ordinated functioning of hydrogenase and nitro- genase is physiologically important and increases the nitrogen-fixation activity of microorganisms.

References

1. Gogotov, I.N. (1973). Hydrogen metabolism and nitrogen fixation in phototrophic bacteria. In: Abstracts of Symposium on Procaryotic Photosynthetic Organisms, G.Drews (ed.). Freiburg, pp.118-131
2. Gogotov, I.N. (1978). Relationships in hydrogen metabolism between hydrogenase and nitrogenase in phototrophic bacteria. Biochimie 60, 267-275
3. Wall, J.D., Weaver, P.F., Gest, H. (1975). Genetic transfer of nitrogenase - hydrogenase activity in Rhodopseudomonas capsulata. Nature 258, 630-631
4. Kelley, B.B., Meyer, C.M., Candy, C., Vignais, P.M. (1977). Hydrogen recycling by Rhodopseudomonas capsulata. FEBS Lett. 81, 281-284
5. Kondratieva, E.N., Gogotov, I.N. (1981). Molecular hydrogen in microbia metabolism. Moscow: Nauka, p.340.
6. Tsygankov, A.A., Gogotov, I.N. (1982). Effect of temperature and pH medium on nitrogenase activity in Rhodopseudomonas capsulata by nitrogen fixation. Microbiologija 51, 396-401
7. Dixon, R.O.D.(1978). Nitrogrnase-hydrogenase interrelationships in Rhizobia. Biochimie 60, 233-236
8. Kondratieva, E.N., Gogotov, I.N. (1983). Production of molecular hydrogen in microorganisms. In: Adv.Biochem.Eng., A.Fiechter (ed.), B.-H.-N.Y.-T.: Springer Verlag, 28, pp.139-191
9. Adams, M.W.W., Mortenson, L.E., Chen, J.S. (1980). Hydrogenase. Biochem.Biophis.Acta 594, 105-176
10. Yakunin, A.F., Gogotov, I.N. (1983). Properties and regulation of synthesis of two ferredoxins from Rhodopseudomonas capsulata. Biochem. Biophys.Acta 725, 298-308

ACTIVITY OF NITROGEN METABOLISM ENZYMES IN THE PROCESS OF KERNEL DEVELOPMENT IN DIFFERENT MAIZE GENOTYPES

VESNA HADŽI-TAŠKOVIĆ ŠUKALOVIĆ
Maize Research Institute, Zemun Polje
P.Box 89, 11081 Zemun, Yugoslavia

Since the discovery of high lysine mutants, which have a high nutritional value, there has been increasing interest in studying biochemical changes leading to increased lysine content and an altered proportion of amino acids in the endosperm.

High lysine maize endosperm has altered protein composition and increased lysine content (1). Besides prolamine synthesis in the endosperm being decreased, major differences exist in the metabolism in normal and high lysine varieties; it has been shown that high lysine varieties of barley as well as corn have an altered amino acid metabolism(2-4). The mechanism leading to such an altered proportion of amino acids is not known.

Since in plants all amino acids originate from either glutamine or asparagine and since glutamate, aspartate and alanine play the key role in amino acid metabolism, it was of interest to determine glutamine synthetase (GS), glutamate dehydrogenase(GDH),aspartate aminotransferase(GOT) and alanine aminotransferase (GPT) activity in the developing normal and mutant maize endosperm.

High lysine content in mutant maize endosperm is due to a lower rate of lysine catabolism to proline and glutamate(2,5). According to authors in(6),lysine-ketoglutarate reductase is involved in lysine catabolism in maize endosperm. This paper reports the activities of this enzyme during the development of normal and mutant maize endosperm.

Proceedings of the 16th FEBS Congress
Part A, pp. 391–396
© 1985 VNU Science Press

MATERIALS AND METHODS

For the determination of enzyme activity,crude enzyme preparations from endosperm of Oh 43 normal,Oh 43 opaque-2, Oh 43 sugary-2 and Oh 43 opaque-2 sugary-2 inbred lines taken at regular intervals from 15 to 45 days after pollination were used.

The activities of the investigated enzymes were determinated as described previously(6,7). The final activity of each enzyme was calculated on the basis of the amount of product produced or substrate utilized/endosperm per h.

RESULTS AND DISCUSSION

All the enzymes investigated were present in the immature endosperm in each variety(fig.1A-D,2). There is a general increase in the activity in the period of intensive storage-protein synthesis and accumulation of total nitrogen.

GS activity was higher in the opaque-2 mutant than in the normal endosperm throughout the experimental period,but that was not the case with the opaque-2 sugary-2 mutant and its sugary-2 conterpart(fig.1A). These results, and our previous results for opaque-2 maize hybrids(7) and synthetics(8) and those of authors in(9) suggest that the presence of different mutants in the same genetic background does not show any regular changes in GS activity.

Our results show that the level and pattern of development of GDH,GOT and GPT differ significantly in opaque-2 mutants from the normal variety, but only slightly in the opaque-2 sugary-2 mutant compared with the sugary-2 variety(fig.1B-D).

GDH activity in the endosperm of the opaque-2 mutant is much higher than in the normal during the period of intensive synthesis of storage proteins(fig.1B).

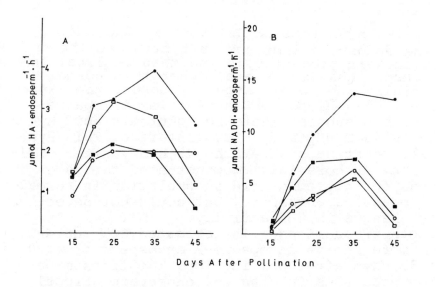

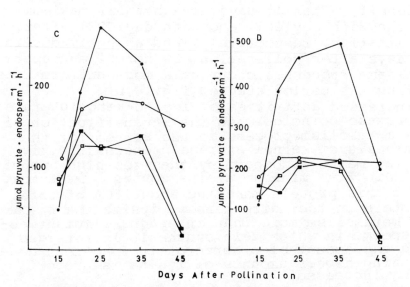

Fig.1. Changes in level of enzymes of nitrogen metabolism. GS (A), GDH (B), GOT (C), GPT (D) in developing endosperm of normal (o), opaque-2 (•), sugary-2 (□) and opaque-2 sugary-2 (■) maize.

It is known that NH_4^+ levels in the normal maize endosperm increase just prior to the onset of zein biosynthesis and then decline. In opaque-2, NH_4^+ levels are higher than normal initially and remain high throughout the experiment (9). Higher GDH activities in opaque-2 endosperm suggest increased glutamic acid synthesis from NH_4^+ and 2-ketoglutarate. This synthesis continues after the 45th day after pollination. Authors in(9) demonstrated the same trend for glutamic acid accumulation in normal and opaque-2 endosperm, but could not detect any changes in GDH activity.

Both transaminases investigated(GOT and GPT) are more active in opaque-2 endosperm from 20 to 35 days after pollination. The transamination processes in opaque-2 endosperm abruptly intensify after 15 days, reach their maximum on the 25th day(GOT) and 35th day(GPT) after pollination, respectively, and abruptly decline 45 days after pollination. In normal endosperm the same processes occur at a more uniform rate during the period studied(fig.1C,D).

Increased activities of lysine-ketoglutarate reductase coincide with the intensification of the metabolism process in the kernel for the synthesis of kernel storage proteins(fig.2). Normal maize endosperm synthesizes high amounts of zein with minimum lysine content. Considering that this protein makes up about 50% of total protein in the maize kernel, lysine is subjected to metabolism more than in opaque-2 mutant endosperm, in which zein synthesis is retarded and the amount of other protein fractions containing higher amounts of lysine is proportionally increased.

The results obtained(fig.2) show that the presence of the o_2 gene in maize endosperm leads to a decline in activity of lysine-ketoglutarate reductase, i.e., this enzyme controls the lysine level in maize endosperm.

The presence of the su_2 gene in the Oh 43 genetic background causes decreased starch and zein contents in the kernel(3) and, therefore, decreases kernel weight. The kernel undergoes the development stages faster, so protein synthesis terminates earlier. The processes investigated are, therefore, less intensive in the double mutant than in the opaque-2 mutant.

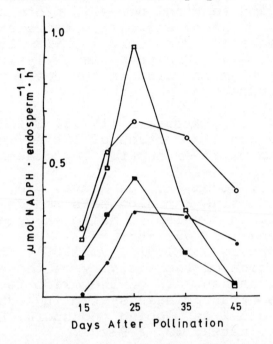

Fig.2. Lysine-ketoglutarate reductase activity in normal(o), opaque-2(●), sugary-2(◻) and opaque-2 sugary-2(■) maize endosperm.

The present results indicate that the o_2 gene affects some changes in the biosynthesis of the soluble precursors of protein synthesis in the developing maize endosperm.

REFERENCES

(1) Nelson,O.E.(1969). Genetic modification of protein quality in plants. Adv.Agron. 21, 171-194.

(2) Sodek, L.,Wilson,C.M.(1970). Incorporation
of leucine C^{14} and lysine C^{14} into protein in the developing endosperm of normal and opaque-2 corn. Arch. Biochem.
Biophys. 140, 29-38.
(3) Dalby, A.,Tsay, C.Y.(1975). Comparison of
lysine and zein and non-zein protein content in immature and mature maize endosperm mutants. Crop Sci. 15, 513-515.
(4) Sodek, L.(1976). Biosynthesis of lysine
and other amino acids in the developing
maize endosperm. Phytochemistry. 15,
1903-1906.
(5) Da Silva, W.J., Arruda,P.(1979). Evidence
for the genetic control of lysine metabolism in maize endosperm. Phytochemistry. 18, 1803-1805.
(6) Arruda, P., Sodek, L., da Silva, W.J.
(1982). Lysine-ketoglutarate reductase
activity in developing maize endosperm.
Plant Physiol. 69, 988-989.
(7) Hadži-Tašković Šukalović, V.(1983). Investigation of the activity of the more
significant enzymes of the oxido-reduc-
tase and transaminase system in normal
and opaque-2 developing endosperm. Arhiv
za polj. nauke, 43, 279-299.
(8) Hadži-Tašković Šukalović, V., Petrović, R.
(1982). The activity of some nitrogen
assimilation enzymes and synthesis of
protein fractions in the endosperm of
opaque-2 (o_2) and sugary-2 opaque-2 (su_2o_2)
maize mutants. Genetika, 14, 227-242.
(9) Misra, S., Oaks, A. (1981). Enzymes of nitrogen assimilation during seed development
in normal and high lysine mutants in
maize (Zea mays, W 64A). Can.J.Bot, 59,
2735-2743.

MOLECULAR GENETIC ANALYSIS OF NODULATION GENES IN *RHIZOBIUM MELILOTI*

ADAM KONDOROSI[1], EVA KONDOROSI[2], ISTVAN TÖRÖK[2], PETER PUTNOKY[1], ZSOFIA BANFALVI[1]
Institutes of Genetics[1] and Biochemistry[2], Biological Research Center, Hungarian Academy of Sciences, H-6701 Szeged, P.O.B. 521, HUNGARY

INTRODUCTION

The development of symbiotic nitrogen-fixing associations between rhizobia and leguminous plants is a multistage process, consisting of recognition and infection of root hairs, differentiation of root nodules, proliferation of bacteria and conversion into bacteroids within the nodules. In this paper we present a molecular genetic analysis of R.meliloti genes determining the early steps of the symbiotic development leading to the formation of nodules on *Medicago sativa* (early nodulation genes).

PLASMID CONTROL OF NODULATION

In previous studies numerous symbiotic genes coding for nodulation function (*nod* genes) or for nitrogen fixation (*fix* genes) have been identified and localized in the *R.meliloti* genome. Genetic mapping of symbiotic mutations indicated that some *fix* genes are located on the chromosome of *R.meliloti* strain 41 (1). Other *fix* genes, including the genes coding for enzyme nitrogenase (*nif* genes) and genes determining early nodulation functions are located on an extremely large plasmid (megaplasmid; 2, 3).

Proceedings of the 16th FEBS Congress
Part A, pp. 397–403
© 1985 VNU Science Press

When this megaplasmid was transferred into other
Rhizobium species or into *Agrobacterium tumefa-
ciens*, the transconjugants became able to form
nodules or nodule-like structures on alfalfa,
indicating that the early steps of nodulation
are coded by this megaplasmid (pRme41b) (4).
These nodules developed only to a certain stage,
suggesting that genes determining the later
steps of nodule development are either not on
this megaplasmid or these genes are not expressed in the new hosts (5). *R.meliloti* 41
carries two other plasmids (a 140 Md plasmid,
pRme41a, and another megaplasmid, pRme41c), but
on these plasmids no symbiotic genes have been
detected so far (6).

It was shown that *nod* and *nif* genes are
closely located to each other (2) and R-prime
plasmids carrying a section of the megaplasmid
with both *nod* and *nif* genes were isolated (8).
The physical map of a 135 kb segment containing
the *nod-nif* region was established (9) and
numerous Nod⁻ or Fix⁻ point, insertion or dele-
tion mutations were localized on it (10, 11).

CLONING OF GENES DETERMINING EARLY NODULATION
FUNCTIONS

A recombinant plasmid, made in the cosmid vehicle pLAFR1, carrying a 24 kb insert from this
megaplasmid region was identified (pPP346) which
contained all essential early nodulation genes
(14). Upon introduction of pPP346 into Nod⁻ mutants with large megaplasmid deletions, the Nod⁺
phenotype was restored. It was shown that A.*tu-
mefaciens* carrying pPP346 was able to nodulate
alfalfa, indicating that genes determining
nodulation specificity for *Medicago sativa* are
located on pPP346. When plasmid pPP346 was introduced into 5 different *Rhizobium* species of
diverse host specificity (*R.leguminosarum*,

R. trifolii, R. lupini, R. japonicum and *Rhizobium sp.* NGR234), the transconjugants were able to nodulate *Medicago*.

The mapped Nod⁻ mutations were localized on two *EcoRI* fragments which are present in pPP346. These two fragments were recloned into the broad host range vehicle, pRK290: plasmid pKSK5 contains the 8.5 kb *nod* fragment, while pEK10 carries the 6.8 kb fragment (10). It was also shown that no other *EcoRI* fragments of pPP346 contain essential *nod* genes.

ORGANIZATION AND STRUCTURE OF NODULATION GENES.

Nodulation genes were localized on the 8.5 kb fragment by the method of directed Tn5 mutagenesis (14). In this way a *nod* region of 3.0 kb and a *fix* region of about 1 kb in size were identified. The Nod⁻ mutants were defective in root hair curling (Hac⁻) which is one of the first observable steps of the infection process. The properties of these mutants are similar to those Nod⁻ derivatives of *R. meliloti* 2011 which were mapped about 20 kb away from the *nif* genes (7).

The nucleotide sequence of a 3.6 kb fragment containing the *nod* region was determined. Computer analysis of the sequence data revealed 3 large open reading frames which may code for 3 polypeptides of molecular weight of 21840, 23756, and 44125 (or 46759).

The protein-coding regions were also mapped in experiments where synthesis of proteins from this DNA segment was investigated in *E. coli* minicells and in an *in vitro* transcription/ /translation system, resulting in polypeptides of Mwt 23000, 28500 and 44000 in size (15). These proteins synthesized only when the region was placed after a strong *E. coli* promoter. In line with this observation, transcription from this DNA region was not detectable in R.*meliloti* grown *ex planta*. We suggest that 3 genes, tentatively designated as *nod*A, *nod*B and *nod*C, may code for these proteins.

A DNA region located left to the common *nod* genes on the 8.5 kb fragment is also involved in the determination of nodulation ability of R.*meliloti*, but these genes have not been analysed so far.

On the 6.8 kb *Eco*RI fragment two *nod* regions were identified by directed Tn5 mutagenesis (11). One region is only roughly defined: it is 1-2 kb in size. Mutations in this region resulted in delayed nodulation phenotype. The other *nod* region on the 6.8 kb fragment is about 1 kb. Mutants mapped in this region had a definite Nod⁻ phenotype with rather weak root hair curling ability.

Common *nod* genes

In several Nod⁻ mutants which lack the 8.5 kb fragment, the ability to nodulate alfalfa was restored (2) upon the introduction of the *sym* plasmid of R.*leguminosarum* (16), or of R.*trifolii* (obtained from Dr. B.Rolfe). Therefore, the *nod* genes carried by the 85 kb fragment were designated as "*common*" *nod* genes (11).

Hybridization of the common *nod* region with total DNA from different *Rhizobium* species demonstrated conservation of these genes also at the nucleotide sequence level. This was supported recently by comparing sequence data for the R.*meliloti nod*A,B and C genes and nucleotide sequences and the deduced amino acid sequences of 3 *nod* genes from R.*leguminosarum* obtained by the John Innes Group (A.Downie, L.Rossen and A.W.B.Johnston, personal communication). Based on these data the 3 *nod* genes of R.*leguminosarum* do correspond to the *nod*A,B and

C genes of *R.meliloti*.

Genes-controlling host specificity of nodulation

Nod⁻ mutants mapped on the 6.8 kb fragment were not complemented by the *R.leguminosarum nod* genes, and lack of interspecies homology was detected with the 1 kb *nod* region and weak homology was observed with the other region. When plasmid pEK10 was introduced into *Rhizobium sp*. NGR234 about 30% of the transconjugants induced rather sparse nodule formation on *Medicago sativa*. These results indicate that host specificity of nodulation is controlled by genes present on the 6.8 kb fragment but efficient nodulation of alfalfa requires other *R.meliloti* genes which are present on pPP346.

OTHER GENES INFLUENCING NODULATION EFFICIENCY

Preliminary results suggests that a megaplasmid region which is not present on pPP346 is also needed for efficient nodulation of alfalfa. This region was tentatively located on the right side of the *nif* structural genes about 25 kb away.

REFERENCES

1 Forrai, T., Vincze, E., Banfalvi, Z., Kiss, G.B., Randhawa, G.S., Kondorosi, A. (1983). J.Bacteriol. 153, 635-643.
2 Banfalvi, Z., Sakanyan, V., Koncz, C., Kiss, A., Dusha, I., Kondorosi, A. (1981). Mol. Gen. Genet. 184, 318-325.
3 Rosenberg, C., Boistard, P., Denarie, J.,

Casse-Delbart, F. (1981). Mol. Gen. Genet. 184, 326-333.

4   Kondorosi, A., Kondorosi, E., Pankhurst, C.E., Broughton, W.J., Banfalvi, Z. (1982). 188, 433-439.

5   Wong, C.H., Pankhurst, C.E., Kondorosi, A., Broughton, W.J. (1983). J. Cell Biol. 97, 787-794.

6   Banfalvi, Z., Kondorosi, E., Kondorosi, A. (1984). Plasmid (submitted).

7   Long, S.R., Buikema, W.J., Ausubel, F.M. (1982). Nature, 298, 485-488.

8   Banfalvi, Z., Randhawa, G.S., Kondorosi, E., Kiss, A., Kondorosi, A. (1983). Mol. Gen. Genet. 189, 129-135.

9   Kondorosi, A., Kondorosi, E., Banfalvi, Z., Broughton, W.J., Pankhurst, C.E., Randhawa, G.S., Wong, C.H., Schell, J. (1983). In: Molecular Genetics of the Bacteria-Plant Interaction, A.Pühler, (ed.), Heidelberg, Springer-Verlag, Berlin, pp. 55-63.

10   Kondorosi, E., Banfalvi, Z., Slaska-Kiss, K., Kondorosi, A. (1983). In: UCLA Symposia on Molecular and Cellular Biology 12, Plant Molecular Biology, R.Goldberg (ed.), A.R. Liss Inc., New York, pp. 259-275.

11   Kondorosi, E., Banfalvi, Z., Kondorosi, A. (1984) Mol. Gen. Genet. 193, 445-452.

12   Kondorosi,A., Kondorosi,E., Banfalvi,Z., Putnoky,P., Török,I., Schmidt,J., John,M. (1984). In: Proc. of the XIV Steenbock Symp. on Nitrogen Fixation and CO_2 Metabolism, P. W.Ludden, J.E.Burris (eds.) Elsevier Science Publ. New York, in press.

13   Kondorosi,A., Kondorosi,E., Banfalvi,Z., Dusha,I., Putnoky,P., Toth,J., Bachem,C. (1984). In: Proc. of the XV. Int. Congr. of Genetics, Oxford and IBH Publ. Co. New Delhi (in press)

14   Ruvkun,G.B.,Sundaresan, V., Ausubel, F.M. (1982) Cell 29, 551-559.

15 Schmidt, J., John, M., Kondorosi, E.,
   Kondorosi, A., Wieneke, U., Schröder, G.,
   Schröder, J., Schell, J. (1984). EMBO J.,
   3, 1705-1711.
16 Downie, J.A., Hombrecher, G., Ma, Q.-S.,
   Knight, C.D., Wells, B., Johnston, A.W.B.
   (1983). Mol. Gen. Genet. 190, 359-365.

SOME CHARACTERISTICS OF NITROGEN FIXATION BY BACTEROIDS ISOLATED FROM NODULES OF LEGUMES.

J. RIGAUD

Laboratoire de Biologie végétale, Faculté des Sciences et des Techniques, Parc Valrose, 06034 NICE Cedex, FRANCE

Rhizobia are common bacteria present in most soils and able to live in symbiosis with the roots of legumes inducing typical nodules which fix atmospheric nitrogen. As firstly evidenced in 1966 (1) the microsymbionts, called bacteroids, were responsible for nitrogen fixation activity and commonly isolated from crushed nodules for biochemical studies. To reduce molecular nitrogen to ammonia, active nitrogenase present in bacteroids requires energy and reducing power, which was essentially provided by respiration. Thus, oxygen supply appears as critical for optimal nitrogen fixation in relation to the high sensitivity of nitrogenase itself to O_2 (2). We report here some results concerning nitrogen fixation by bacteroids in relation to oxygen supply.

1. BACTEROID O_2 REQUIREMENT

Bacteroids are located in the central tissue of nodules, and the cortex constitutes a diffusion barrier for O_2 inducing near-anaerobic conditions (3). When isolated bacteroids from Phaseolus nodules were placed in the chamber of an O_2 electrode in the presence of dissolved O_2 concentrations where nitrogenase was always active (25 μM to 125 μM), no significant difference in O_2 uptake occurred by comparison with free-living bacteria. Addition of glucose (10 mM) stimulated O_2 consumption in both bacteroid and bacteria indicating a real capacity for bacteroids to utilize O_2 (4). In another way, an active manganese superoxyde dismutase (SOD) was purified from Phaseolus bacteroids (4), since a good correlation exists between the level of SOD and the O_2^- production (5), the presence of this enzyme in bacteroid was also in favour of an active respiration in vivo. This large O_2

Proceedings of the 16th FEBS Congress
Part A, pp. 405–410
© 1985 VNU Science Press

demand could also contribute to protect nitrogenase against O_2 inactivation (6).

2. OXYGEN SUPPLY TO THE BACTEROIDS

In the laboratory, dissolved O_2 can be provided to bacteroids in incubations carried out in an O_2 electrode chamber, allowing a simultaneous measurement of O_2 uptake during C_2H_2 reduction (7). In the absence of gas phase, C_2H_4 formed was determined after vacuum decompression. A more accurate system has been also used (7) (8) where O_2 was delivered to bacteroids by an O_2 carrier like leghemoglobin extracted and purified from nodules. This hemoprotein present in large quantities in the host cells exhibited a particularly high affinity for O_2 (9) and delivered an adequate O_2 flux to the bacteroids equipped with a specific system of oxidases (10). The deoxygenation of the leghemoglobin was followed spectrophotometrically, and very low O_2 concentrations (2-5 nM) were provided to the bacteroids in a range where O_2 electrode was inefficient.

3. RELATIONSHIP BETWEEN O_2 REQUIREMENT AND ENERGY-YIELDING SUBSTRATES

In the nodules, the bacteroid respiration is stimulated by organic molecules provided by the host cells. In vitro, organic acids added to bacteroid incubations exerted an efficient stimulation of respiration and were routinely used to study nitrogen fixation by bacteroids. We demonstrated the possibility for glucose or sucrose to also support C_2H_2 reduction in French-bean and soybean bacteroids, but their efficiency was in direct relation to the O_2 concentration in the medium. As shown on Fig.1, nitrogen fixation was strictly limited to a narrow range of dissolved O_2 concentration, and then declined when glucose or sucrose were present. In contrast, succinate was efficient for higher concentrations of dissolved O_2 in a wider range of O_2 values. These experiments conducted with leghemoglobin as oxygen carrier also indicated a strong stimulation of O_2 uptake exerted by succinate by comparison to carbohydrates.

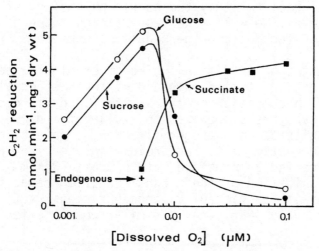

Fig. 1. C_2H_2 *reduction by soybean bacteroids in relation to O_2 concentrations provided by oxyleghemoglobin.* Trinchant et al. (8)

More information has been obtained about this bacteroid O_2 requirement related to the nature of substrates. With glucose, in the absence of nitrogenase denaturation by raising O_2 tensions providing a significant level of ATP, the responsibility for reducing power has been considered (11). Among the differences occurring between bacteria and bacteroids in the cytochrome contents, a significant increase of cyt-c has been reported in bacteroids (12). The level of cyt-c reduction, determined in whole cells by a rapid spectrometry method, always appeared very high during active C_2H_2 reduction both with glucose and succinate (11). Increasing O_2 tensions affected neither C_2H_2 reduction nor cyt-c reduction when succinate was present, but induced a rapid oxidation of cyt-c with glucose, which limited the reducing power available for nitrogenase. This effect could be in direct relation to the poor stimulation exerted by glucose on bacteroid O_2 consumption.

4. ALTERATION OF BACTEROID O_2 REQUIREMENT

Optimal conditions for nitrogen fixation by bacteroids being well defined, bacteroid preparation can appear as an original tool to study the nodule physiology at cellular level. We will take two examples : the nitrogen nutrition of legumes and the nodule senescence.

4.1. <u>Nitrogen nutrition</u> : Like other plants the legumes can also utilize combined nitrogen especially nitrate and a competition occurs with fixed nitrogen. Among the hypothesis proposed to explain the depressive effect of nitrate on nitrogen fixation, a role of nitrite has been suggested (13). Bacteroids isolated from nodules of <u>Phaseolus</u> fed 24 h before with nitrate (3.5 mM) showed a strong inhibition of their C_2H_2 reduction capacity associated with a shift of O_2 concentrations required for optimal activity (Fig. 2a). A similar double effect was

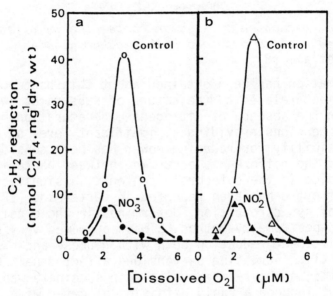

Fig. 2. *C_2H_2 reduction by French-bean bacteroids from NO_3-treated plants (a) or after addition of NO_2^- (b).* (Trinchant and Rigaud

also observed in incubations containing NO_2^- (Fig. 2b) associated with an inhibition of bacteroid respiration observed both after plant NO_3^- treatment or nitrite addition (14). In the two cases, this similarity in the bacteroid O_2 sensitivity strengthened the possibility for

NO_2^- to be involved in the nitrogen fixation inhibition due to nitrate.

4.2. Nodule senescence : Like other organs nodules senesced, and a rapid drop in their C_2H_2 reduction activity occurred after few weeks. In contrast, substantial levels of activity remained in bacteroids isolated from nodules of different age (15). However, the O_2 requirement for the oldest bacteroids was lowered as evidenced by the shift towards the lowest values of O_2 tensions required for optimal nitrogen fixation. Thus, the bacteroids were able to provide an accurate protection of their nitrogenase but largely appeared host-dependent to express this activity.

5. CONCLUSION

As in other diazotrophs, O_2 plays a major role in the nitrogen fixation by isolated bacteroids and constitutes, with the energetic substrates,an essential limiting factor. However, in spite of important progress in the bacteroid study many points concerning the electron pathways or the transfer of the reducing power to nitrogenase must be clarified for a complete comprehension of the bacteroid biochemistry.

REFERENCES

(1) KENNEDY, I.R., PARKER, C.A. and KIDBY, K.K. (1966) The probable site of nitrogen fixation in root nodules of Ornithopus sativus. Biochim. Biophys. Acta 130, 517-519
(2) BERGERSEN, F.J. (1984) Oxygen and the physiology of diazotrophic microorganisms. In : Advances in nitrogen fixation research, C. Veeger and W.E. Newton (eds) Nijhoff/Junk Pudoc, Wageningen, pp. 171-180
(3) TJEPKEMA, J.D. and YOCUM, C.S. (1974) Measurement of oxygen partial pressure within soybean nodules by oxygen micro electrodes. Planta 119, 351-360
(4) DIMITRIJEVIC, L., PUPPO, A. and RIGAUD, J. (1984) Superoxide dismutase activities in Rhizobium phaseoli bacteria and bacteroids. Arch. Microbiol. in press

(5) HASSAN, H.M. and FRIDOVICH, I. (1977) Regulation of the synthesis of superoxide dismutase in Escherichia coli. J. Biol. Chem. 252, 7667-7672

(6) GALLON, J.R. (1981) The oxygen sensitivity of nitrogenase : a problem for biochemists and micro-organisms. Trends Biochem. Sci. January, 19-23

(7) BERGERSEN, F.J. and TURNER, G.L. (1975) Leghemoglobin and the supply of O_2 to nitrogen-fixing root nodules bacteroids : studies of an experimental system with no gas phase. J. Gen. Microbiol. 89, 31-37

(8) TRINCHANT, J.C., BIROT, A.M. and RIGAUD, J. (1981) Oxygen supply and energy-yielding substrates for nitrogen fixation (C_2H_2 reduction) by bacteroid preparations. J. Gen. Microbiol. 125, 159-165

(9) WITTENBERG, J.B., APPLEBY, C.A. and WITTENBERG, B.A. (1972) The kinetics of the reactions of leghaemoglobin with oxygen and carbon monooxide. J. Biol. Chem. 247, 527-531

(10) BERGERSEN, F.J. (1982) Root nodules of legumes : structure and functions. Research Studies Press, Chichester (164 p.)

(11) TRINCHANT, J.C., BIROT, A.M., DENIS, M. and RIGAUD, J. (1983) C_2H_2 reduction, oxygen uptake and cytochrome-c reduction by bacteroids isolated from French-bean nodules. Arch. Microbiol. 134, 182-186

(12) APPLEBY, C.A. (1974) Leghemoglobin. In : The biology of nitrogen fixation, A. Quispel (ed) North-Holland, Publishing Company, Amsterdam, pp. 521-554

(13) RIGAUD, J. (1976) Effet des nitrates sur la fixation d'azote par les nodules de Haricot (Phaseolus vulgaris L.). Physiol. vég. 14, 297-308

(14) TRINCHANT, J.C. and RIGAUD, J. (1984) Nitrogen fixation in French-beans in the presence of nitrate : effect on bacteroid respiration and comparison with nitrite. J. Plant Physiol. in press

(15) BIROT, A.M., TRINCHANT, J.C. and RIGAUD, J. (1983) Nitrogen fixation in French-bean nodules in relation to ageing : role of bacteroids. Physiol. vég. 21, 715-722

NITROGEN FIXATION IN THE ANOXYGENIC PHOTOTROPHIC BACTERIA

W.G. ZUMFT, H. KÖRNER, D.J. ARP, W. KLIPP* and A. PÜHLER*

Lehrstuhl für Mikrobiologie, Universität Karlsruhe, Kaiserstr. 12, 7500 Karlsruhe 1, and *Lehrstuhl für Genetik, Universität Bielefeld, 4800 Bielefeld 1, F.R.G.

THE NITROGEN-FIXING SYSTEM

The anoxygenic phototrophic bacteria are an ecologically important group of bacteria with many members utilizing dinitrogen. Nitrogenase (EC 1.18.2.1) in the purple bacteria is subject to rapid inhibition by ammonia, termed ammonia switch-off (1). This appears to be a unique trait of this group of procaryotes and has become the basis of current efforts to explore their nitrogen-fixing system. Here we describe some pertinent properties of nitrogenase of Rhodopseudomonas palustris and the organization of nif genes in Rhodopseudomonas capsulata. Within this context, Rp1 and Rp2 refer to the MoFe protein and Fe protein of R. palustris, respectively. An analogous nomenclature is being used for other organisms.

Properties of the MoFe protein and Fe protein

MoFe proteins were recently obtained from Rhodospirillum rubrum (2,3), R. capsulata (4), and R. palustris (5). Their properties and amino acid compositions are compiled in Tables 1 and 2, respectively. Rp1 and Rp2, but not Rr1, yield two subunits of different size in detergent electrophoresis. The N-terminal sequence of Rp1 indicates that the subunits are indeed discrete polypeptides (Table 1), as was observed with other MoFe proteins for which extended sequences are available (7). The low M_r component of nitrogenase from phototrophic bacteria differs markedly

Proceedings of the 16th FEBS Congress
Part A, pp. 411–424
© 1985 VNU Science Press

TABLE I

PROPERTIES OF MoFe PROTEINS

	Rr1	Rc1 (4)	Rp1[a]
M_r (GPC)	234,000 (2) 215,000 (3)	230,000	nd[b]
M_r Subunits (SDS-PAGE)	58,500 (2) 56,000 (3)	59,500 55,000	58,000 54,000
Quarternary structure	α_4(?)	$\alpha_2\beta_2$	$\alpha_2\beta_2$
Mo (atoms/tetramer)	1.7 (2) 2 (3)	1.3	2
N-Terminal sequence	nd	nd	(S)-T/E-A-V-E/A
Fe (atoms/tetramer)	20 (2) 25-30 (3)	28	nd
S^{2-} (atoms/tetramer)	19-22 (3)	26	nd
Spec. activitity[c]	1260 (3)	1800	1100

[a] this paper   [b] not determined   [c] $nmol \cdot min^{-1} \cdot mg^{-1}$

in its chemical composition from Fe proteins of other diazotrophs. A non-proteinaceous group consisting of a phosphate residue, a pentose, and a fluorescent adenine-like
base is covalently attached to the protein (2). Whenever
the modifying group is bound to the Fe protein, the latter
is rendered inactive in nitrogenase catalyis. The group is
cleaved from the protein by heat and can be isolated in
this way (8,9). Under physiological conditions this activation process is accomplished by an activating factor
(10,11). Apparently, the entire modifying group is being
removed (9,12). At present the chemical structure of the
modifier, the linkage between the three constituents, and
the nature of the bond with the protein has not been fully
elucidated (13), but a progress report has appeared (9).

The activating enzyme

The activating factor has been recognized as a small, O_2
labile protein of M_r around 20 000 (10,13-16) that acts
catalytically on nitrogenase, and is being preferentially
referred to as activating enzyme (AE). It requires a di-
valent cation, with Mn^{2+} (apparent K_d ca. 20 µM, ref. 16)

412

being the most active one and Mg, Fe, and Co showing considerably less affinity for the protein (10,13-16). AE
acts on the Fe protein and is bound in situ to the chro-
matophore membrane. It is removed by treatment with 0.5 M
NaCl (10,11). AE has not yet been found outside R. rubrum;
however, the isolated enzyme acts on Rc2 (17-19), Rp2, and
Rhodomicrobium vannielii Fe protein (17). Unlike nitrogenase, AE synthesis is not repressed by ammonia, certain
amino acids, or by O_2. Escape from the regulation of nif
genes may indicate a role in metabolic processes not directly related to N_2 fixation (20).

Metabolic interconversion of the Fe protein

Initial observations of the effect of ammonia did not fur-
nish a coherent concept of activity regulation of nitrogenase. The elaboration of the activating system (2,10,11)
together with a renewed interest in the short-term effects
of reduced nitrogen compounds on nitrogenase (1,21) suggested that in phototrophic bacteria nitrogenase is an

TABLE II

AMINO ACID COMPOSITION OF MoFe PROTEINS AND Fe PROTEINS

| | MoFe protein | | Fe protein | |
	Rc1(4)	Rp1[a]	Rr2(6)	Rc2(4)
Asx	78	110	63	50
Thr[b]	45	59	15	28
Ser[b]	38	54	29	25
Glx	88	96	70	79
Pro	49	43	13	26
Gly	85	100	95	59
Ala	90	86	77	54
Cys	12	10	26	16
Val	64	71	32	43
Met	25	22	15	19
Ile[c]	54	70	9	43
Leu	64	77	34	45
Tyr	38	38	11	16
Phe	42	52	8	7
Lys	68	69	31	32
His	25	32	8	8
Arg	37	54	19	22
Trp	5	nd	nd	0
M_r	110,000		61,500	67,000

[a] this paper

[b] extrapolated to 0 h hydrolysis

[c] from 72 h hydrolysis

413

TABLE III

COMPARISON OF THE Fe PROTEIN FROM N_2-GROWN AND N-LIMITED CELLS OF RHODOPSEUDOMONAS PALUSTRIS

Property	Source of Fe protein	
	N_2-grown cells	N-limited cells
Requirement for activation by R. rubrum AE and Mn^{2+}	yes	no
Maximal specific activity[a]	260	730
Phosphate content[b] (mol P_i/mol protein)	1.32 ± 0.44	0.32 ± 0.19
Number of apparent subunits	2	1
M_r		33 000

[a] Fe protein from each cell type was titrated with purified Rpl_1 from N-limited cells; activity in nmol $C_2H_2 \cdot min^{-1} \cdot mg$ protein^{-1}

[b] Mean and SD of eight replicates.

[c] To remove non-covalently bound P_i, the protein (1-2 mg) was precipitated twice in 2 N HCl, resuspended in 2 ml acid, and boiled to dryness on an electric burner. The flask was then heated in a flame for 1 min, 1 ml 2 N HCl and 100 µl of 30% H_2O_2 was added. The content of the flask was again brought to dryness each time after 5 consecutive additions of 100 µl H_2O_2. The sample was dissolved in 0.5 ml H_2O and phosphate determined according to Penney (Anal. Biochem. 75: 201-210, 1976). Internal standard P_i was recovered to 85-95%. Recovery of P_i from ATP was 70-80%. All determinations were corrected for a reagent blank.

interconvertible enzyme in response to ammonia (22). Since then, evidence from several labs has supported a unifying model of Fe protein regulation. Previous proposals of two different species of nitrogenase (18,23,24) are now to be viewed in terms of Fe protein interconversion.

The donor molecule for the modifying group might be ATP, since radioactivity of uniformly labeled ^{14}C-ATP (25) and tritiated adenine (26) is incorporated into the Fe protein during inactivation. Although the modifying group is not AMP (9), it must be very similar. Cells grown under N-limitation or severe N-starvation lose sensitivity towards ammonia (17,23,24,27). This activity response is confined to cells grown on glutamate or N_2. In about 80% of experiments with R. palustris we found no nitrogenase activity in cell-free extracts of N_2-grown cells. When low activities were observed, reaction rates were nonlinear. By contrast, nitrogenase from N-limited cells always showed high activity with linear rates. The Fe proteins from both cell types were compared (Table 3). As with cell-free extracts, Rp2 from N_2-grown cells required AE, while that from N-limited cells was active without addition. Titration of the Fe proteins with Rp1 from N-limited cells yielded a nearly 3-fold higher specific activity in N-limited cells. The reason for this is unclear at present.

Loss and gain of ammonia sensitivity is a reversible process (27). N-limited cells which did not respond to ammonia, "learned" switch-off at a fairly rapid rate when sparged with N_2. Within 24 h the degree of switch-off increased from zero to 0.7 (Fig. 1). Switch-off was acquired by N_2-grown cultures at a similar rate when ammonia was added. The kinetics of loss of ammonia sensitivity of N_2-grown cells subjected to N-starvation by exchanging N_2 for Ar, is shown in Fig. 2. The loss of ammonia switch-off was slow relative to the rate at which N-limited cells gained sensitivity and was on the order of nitrogenase turnover of N_2-grown cells (5). Under those conditions there may also be a shortage of modifying group donor, as has been suggested for slow ammonia switch-off (6).

Modified Rr2 (2,12) and Rc2 (19) yield two apparent sub units of different size in detergent electrophoresis. This was also the case for Rp2 (Table 3). The chemical composition of active and inactive Fe protein is different due to the non-proteinaceous components. Prompted by results obtained with Rr2 (6), we confirmed a significantly higher level of phosphate in Rp2 from N_2-grown cells (Table 3). The amino acid composition of both proteins and their tryptic pattern, however, are identical (6). Recent evaluations of the composition of the modifying group gave slightly above one mole of phosphate and pentose per mole protein, and less than one mole of an adenine-like base (8). The modifier is attached to the apparently larger subunit of the Fe protein, as shown by radioactive labeling (8,12,19,26). Upon in vivo-inactivation with ammonia only the larger subunit becomes labeled (12,19,28). For cells grown on glutamate there is no need to add ammonia to find in vitro-inactive Fe protein. Apparently, dark

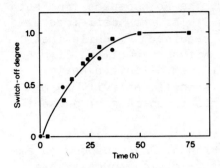 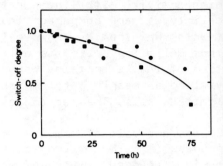

Fig. 1. Acquisition of ammonia switch-off by N-limited cells of R. palustris. A 3-day old culture with 0.5 g yeast extract as N-source was sparged at zero time with N_2. At the times indicated, the culture was sampled and assayed. The switch-off degree is expressed as the quotient of reductions rates after and before ammonia addition. Results of two independent experiments are shown.

Fig. 2. Loss of ammonia switch-off on transition from N_2 utilization to N-deficiency. A 3-day old culture of R. palustris was shifted at zero time from N_2-sparging to Ar. Data for two separate experiments are shown.

exposure of the photosynthetic cell during cell breakage and nitrogenase extraction suffices to modify the Fe protein (28).

GENETIC ANALYSIS OF nif GENES IN R. CAPSULATA

Compared to other methods of mutation, transposons have advantages that facilitate genetic analysis. Several techniques for the isolation of transposon mutants were developed for Escherichia coli. For other gram-negative bacteria modified methods have to be used. Rhizobium and Agrobacterium were successfully mutagenized with suicide plasmids, e.g. RP4::Mu. However, since these plasmids replicate stable in R. capsulata (29), a system based on in vitro constructed plasmids was used (30).

416

The Tn5 mutagenesis system and characterization of mutants

The principle of this technique is the mobilization of
plasmids that carry Tn5 but do not replicate outside E.
coli into other gram-negative bacteria. The transposition
event is selected for by the Tn5-mediated kanamycin resistance (Km^r).The special donor strain of E. coli has the
transfer functions of the broad host range plasmid RP4
chromosomally integrated. This guarantees mobilization of
plasmids with the RP4-specific origin of transfer into
other gram-negative bacteria without co-transfer of RP4.
The mobilizable plasmid was constructed in vitro by cloning the origin of transfer of RP4 into different E. coli
vectors, such as pBR325 or pACYC184 (30). The E. coli specific replication functions of these plasmids prevent a
stable establishment in most other gram-negative bacteria.
This suicide effect is used for random introduction of
Tn5 and for site-specific mutagenesis.

With this system, Tn5-carrying R. capsulata strains were
obtained with a frequency of 10^{-5} to 10^{-6} (31). The muta-
genic effect of Tn5 could be directly observed in mutants
with altered carotenoid synthesis which appeared in about
0.5% of Km^r exconjugants (ranging from greenish-white to
yellow, pink and red). Retesting of Tn5-containing R. capsulata strains for their ability to grow on N$_2$, led to
the identification of auxotrophic mutants (about 1%; among
them arg, ilv, leu, met, phe, trp, and tyr), mutants unable to grow anaerobically in the light and nif::Tn5 mutants (about 0.5%).

Mutation of nif genes can affect the structural proteins, electron transport proteins, components for activity regulation and expression of nitrogenase, and proteins involved in the processing of the enzyme or the FeMo
cofactor. Table 4 lists several assays for various nitro-
genase-related activities to which mutants were subjected.
Some tests were done with the non-regulated heterologous
proteins from Azotobacter vinelandii to circumvent the inherent regulatory mechanism of R. capsulata. These probes
catalogued mutants in distinct groups for which tentative
assignments can be made from Table 4.

TABLE IV

ANALYSIS OF THE EXPRESSION OF nif-RELATED GENE PRODUCTS IN MUTANTS OF RHODOPSEUDOMONAS CAPSULATA BY THE ACETYLENE REDUCTION ASSAY

Mutant No.	In vivo acetylene reduction	Crude extract activity	Crude extract +Mn^{2+}	DEAE-eluate +Av2 [a]	DEAE-eluate +Av1	DEAE-eluate +AE(Rr) +Rr1	Presence of Fe protein [b] (OUCHTERLONY)
1	-	-	-	-	-	-	-
12	-	-	-	-	-	-	-
13	-	-	-	-	-	-	-
3	tr[c]	+	+	+++	++	+++	+
5	tr	+	++	++	+	+++	+
8	tr	++	++	+++	+++	+++	+
9	tr	+	++	+	-	++	+
7	tr	+	++	++	tr	++	+
10	tr	tr	+	++	-	++	+
6	tr	+	+	+	tr	+++	+
18	tr	+	++	+++	++	+++	+
16	+	-	-	-	+	+++	+
15	+	+	+	+	++	+++	+
4	-	-	-	-	++	+++	+
2	-	-	-	-	-	++	+

[a] Crude extract was adsorbed onto a 1x5 cm anaerobic DEAE-Sepharose column, washed with 0.12 M NaCl in 25 mM Tris-HCl, pH 7.2, 2 mM in $Na_2S_2O_4$, and eluted with 0.5 M NaCl in the same buffer.

[b] Rabbit antibodies against Rr2 were used in the immunodiffusion assay.

[c] Non-quantifiable trace activity.

Cloning, restriction mapping, and identification of discrete nif clusters

The following strategy was applied for cloning DNA fragments with nif genes from R. capsulata into E. coli. R' plasmids carrying part of the R. capsulata chromosome, including a nif::Tn5 mutant gene, were constructed with a Km^s derivative of R68.45 (32). The R' plasmids were identified by their Tn5-mediated Km^r after conjugational transfer to an E. coli recA⁻ strain. The M_r of these plasmids was determined by agarose gel electrophoresis. R' plasmids carrying 50-100 kb of the R. capsulata chromosome flanking the nif::Tn5 region were isolated from E. coli. Restriction fragments containing the nif::Tn5 insertions were cloned into E. coli vector plasmids and further analyzed.

Cloned nif::Tn5 restriction fragments were also radioactively labeled and were used as probes for screening 500 hybrid cosmid clones by colony hybridization to identify the appropriate clone. The cosmid gene bank was obtained

by cloning partial MboI-digested total R. capsulata DNA
into the cosmid vector pHC79 (33). Restriction maps of the
corresponding cosmid were compared to cloned nif::Tn5
restriction fragments from different nif mutants.

Restriction analysis of 34 mutants showed that all of
them mapped within three regions of the chromosome which
were separated from each other. Six mutants were localized
in a cluster of about 5 kb (Fig. 3). Biochemical analysis
showed that they were affected in the structural genes of
nitrogenase. This result was supported by DNA-DNA hybridization with Klebsiella pneumoniae nifKDH DNA. The restriction analysis of this region was in good agreement with
the map of the R. capsulata region, encoding for the nitrogenase structural genes (34). No further homology of
Klebsiella nifKDH within the nif gene region of the other
Tn5 mutants was found, although copies of silent structural genes should also be present (35).

The main nif coding region harboured 24 mutants distributed over about 20 kb (Fig. 4). Mutants within this major

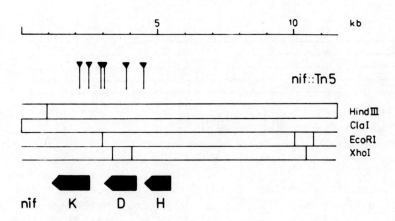

Fig. 3. Localization of the structural nif gene cluster of
R. capsulata. The site of Tn5 insertions is compared to
the restriction map of this region. The approx. site and
localization of nifKDH genes was taken from ref. 34.

nif cluster fall into likely categories of electron donor
mutants and mutants affected in the FeMo cofactor. One
mutant at the flanking region was also devoid of all ni-
trogenase-related activities. To confirm that this part of
the chromosome predominantly encodes for N_2 fixation
genes, further Tn5 mutations were introduced into that
region by site-specific mutagenesis. For that purpose different restriction fragments were cloned into mobilizable
vector plasmids and subsequently mutagenized by Tn5 in E.
coli. Different insertion sites were mapped by restriction
analysis and were introduced into the R. capsulata chromosome by homologous recombination. The restriction map of
this region (see also ref. 31), the localization of several nif::Tn5 mutants and the phenotype of mutants obtained
by site-directed mutagenesis is shown in Fig. 4.

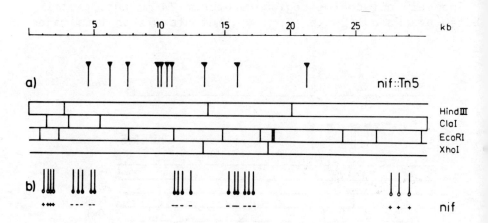

Fig. 4. Localization of nif::Tn5 mutations of R.
capsulata. Part a) shows the site of Tn5 insertion of
several nif mutants in comparison to the restriction map
of this region. The map was determined by restriction
analysis of cloned fragments and an overlapping cosmid
clone. Part b) gives the localization and the nif phenotype of Tn5 insertions by site-directed mutagenesis.

In addition, we found three nif::Tn5 mutants that mapped
close together on a 7.5 kb HindIII fragment, outside the
other two gene clusters. The fragment had four approximately equidistant recognition sites for XhoI. Mutants
within this region were negative in all biochemical tests
for nitrogenase related activities. Our results show that
contrary to Klebsiella, the nif genes of R. capsulata are
not clustered in a single region on the chromosome, but
are scattered in at least three regions, with the structural genes separated from the main nif-coding region.

ACKNOWLEDGEMENTS

We thank Dr. H. Matsubara for amino acid analyses and Dr.
P. Ludden for gifts of antibodies. The work was finan-
cially supported by the Deutsche Forschungsgemeinschaft.

REFERENCES

1. Zumft, W.G. and Castillo, F. (1978). Regulatory properties of the nitrogenase from Rhodopseudomonas
   palustris. Arch. Microbiol. 117, 53–60.
2. Ludden, P.W. and Burris, R.H. (1978). Purification and
   properties of nitrogenase from Rhodospirillum rubrum,
   and evidence for phosphate, ribose and an adenine-
   like unit covalently bound to the iron protein.
   Biochem. J. 175, 251–259.
3. Nordlund, S., Eriksson, U. and Baltscheffsky, H.
   (1978). Properties of the nitrogenase system from
   a photosynthetic bacterium, Rhodospirillum rubrum.
   Biochim. Biophys. Acta 504, 248–254.
4. Hallenbeck, P.C., Meyer, C.M. and Vignais P.M. (1982).
   Nitrogenase from the photosynthetic bacterium Rhodopseudomonas capsulata: Purification and molecular
   properties. J. Bacteriol. 149, 708–717.
5. Arp, D.J. and Zumft, W.G. (1983). Overproduction of nitrogenase by nitrogen-limited cultures of Rhodopseudomonas palustris. J. Bacteriol. 153, 1322–1330.

6. Ludden, P.W., Preston, G.G. and Dowling, T.E. (1982).
   Comparison of active and inactive forms of iron
   protein from Rhodospirillum rubrum. Biochem. J. 203,
   663-668.
7. Hase,T., Wakabayashi, S., Nakano, T., Zumft, W.G. and
   Matsubara, H. (1984). Structural homologies between
   the amino acid sequence of Clostridium pasteurianum
   MoFe protein and the DNA sequences of nifD and K
   genes of phylogenetically diverse bacteria. FEBS
   Lett. 166, 39-43.
8. Dowling, T.E., Preston, G.G. and Ludden, P.W. (1982).
   Heat activation of the Fe protein of nitrogenase
   from Rhodospirillum rubrum. J. Biol. Chem. 257,
   13987-13992.
9. Ludden, P.W., Murrell, S.A., Pope, M., Kanemoto, R.,
   Dowling, T.E., Saari, L.L. and Triplett, E. (1984).
   Regulation of nitrogen fixation in photosynthetic
   bacteria. In: Advances in Nitrogen Fixation Research, C. Veeger, W.E. Newton (eds.).Nijhoff/Junk
   Publ., The Hague, pp. 181-187.
10. Ludden, P.W. and Burris, R.H. (1976). Activating
    factor for the iron protein of nitrogenase from
    Rhodospirillum rubrum. Science 194, 424-426.
11. Nordlund, S., Eriksson, U. and Baltscheffsky, H.(1977)
    Necessity of a membrane component for nitrogenase
    activity in Rhodospirillum rubrum. Biochim. Biophys.
    Acta 462, 187-195.
12. Gotto, J.W. and Yoch, D.C. (1982). Regulation of
    Rhodospirillum rubrum nitrogenase activity. J. Biol.
    Chem. 257, 2868-2873.
13. Ludden, P.W. and Burris, R. (1979). Removal of an
    adenine-like molecule during activation of dinitro-
    genase reductase from Rhodospirillum rubrum. Proc.
    Natl. Acad. Sci. USA 76, 6201-6205.
14. Zumft, W.G. and Nordlund, S. (1981). Stabilization and
    partial characterization of the activating enzyme
    for dinitrogenase reductase (Fe protein) from Rhodo-
    spirillum rubrum. FEBS Lett. 127, 79-82.
15. Gotto, J.W. and Yoch, D.C. (1982). Purification and
    Mn^{2+} activation of Rhodospirillum rubrum nitrogen-
    ase activating enzyme. J. Bacteriol. 152, 714-721.
16. Guth, J.H. and Burris, R.H. (1983). The role of Mg^{2+}

and Mn^{2+} in the enzyme-catalysed activation of nitrogenase Fe protein from Rhodospirillum rubrum.
Biochem. J. 213, 741-749.

17. Zumft, W.G., Alef, K. and Mümmler, S. (1981). Regu-
lation of nitrogenase activity in Rhodospirillaceae.
In: Current Perspectives in Nitrogen Fixation, A.H.
Gibson and W.E. Newton (eds.). Austral. Acad.
Science, Canberra, pp. 190-193.

18. Yoch, D.C. (1980). Regulation of nitrogenase A and R
concentrations in Rhodopseudomonas capsulata by
glutamine synthetase. Biochem. J. 187, 273-276.

19. Jouanneau, Y., Meyer, C.M. and Vignais, P.M. (1983).
Regulation of nitrogenase activity through iron
protein interconversion into an active and an inactive form in Rhodopseudomonas capsulata. Biochim.
Biophys. Acta 749, 318-328.

20. Triplett, E.W., Wall, J.D. and Ludden, P.W. (1982).
Expression of the activating enzyme and Fe protein
of nitrogenase from Rhodospirillum rubrum. J.
Bacteriol. 152, 786-791.

21. Neilson, A.H. and Nordlund, S. (1975). Regulation of
nitrogenase synthesis in intact cells of Rhodospirillum rubrum: Inactivation of nitrogen fixation
by ammonia, L-glutamine and L-asparagine. J. Gen.
Microbiol. 91, 53-62.

22. Zumft, W.G. (1978). Dinitrogen reduction. Hoppe-Sey-
ler's Z. Physiol. Chemie 359, 1170-1171.

23. Carithers, R.P., Yoch, C.D. and Arnon, D.I. (1979).
Two forms of nitrogenase from the photosynthetic
bacterium Rhodospirillum rubrum. J. Bacteriol. 137,
779-789.

24. Yoch, D.C. and Cantu, M. (1980). Changes in the regulatory form of Rhodospirillum rubrum nitrogenase as
influenced by nutritional and environmental factors.
J. Bacteriol. 142, 899-907.

25. Michalski, W.P., Nicholas, D.J.D. and Vignais, P.M.
(1983). ^{14}C-Labelling of glutamine synthetase and
Fe protein of nitrogenase in toluene-treated cells
of Rhodopseudomonas capsulata. Biochim. Biophys.
Acta 743, 136-148.

26. Nordlund, S. and Ludden, P.W. (1983). Incorporation of
adenine into the modifying group of inactive iron

protein of nitrogenase from Rhodospirillum rubrum. Biochem J. 209, 881-884.

27. Alef, K., Arp, D.J. and Zumft, W.G. (1981). Nitrogenase switch-off by ammonia in Rhodopseudomonas palustris: Loss under nitrogen deficiency and independence from the adenylylation state of glutamine synthetase. Arch. Microbiol. 130, 138-142.

28. Kanemoto, R.H. and Ludden, P.W. (1984). Effect of ammonia, darkness, and phenazine methosulfate on whole-cell nitrogenase activity and Fe protein modification in Rhodospirillum rubrum. J. Bacteriol. 158, 713-720.

29. Yu, P.-L., Cullum, J. and Drews, G. (1981). Conjugational transfer systems of Rhodopseudomonas capsulata mediated by R plasmids. Arch. Microbiol 128, 390-393.

30. Simon, R., Priefer and U. Pühler, A. (1983). A broad host range mobilization system for in vivo genetic engineering: Transposon mutagenesis in gram-negative bacteria. Biotechnol. 1, 784-791.

31. Pühler, A., Aguilar, M.O., Hynes, M., Müller, P., Klipp, W., Priefer, U., Simon, R. and Weber, G. (1984). Advances in the genetics of free-living and symbiotic nitrogen fixing bacteria. In: Advances in Nitrogen Fixation Research, C. Veeger and W.E. Newton (eds.). Nijhoff/Junk Publ., The Hague, pp. 609-619.

32. Brewin, N.J., Beringer, J.E. and Johnston, A.W.B. (1980). Plasmid-mediated transfer of host-range specificity between two strains of Rhizobium leguminosarum. J. Gen. Microbiol. 120, 413-420.

33. Hohn, B. and Collins, J. (1980). A small cosmid for efficient cloning of large DNA fragments. Gene 11, 291-298.

34. Avtges, P., Scolnik, P.A. and Haselkorn, R. (1983). Genetic and physical map of the structural genes (nifH,D,K) coding for the nitrogenase complex of Rhodopseudomonas capsulata. J. Bacteriol. 156, 251-256.

35. Scolnik, P.A. and Haselkorn, R. (1984). Activation of extra copies of genes coding for nitrogenase in Rhodopseudomonas capsulata. Nature 307, 289-292.

SOME FEATURES OF THE ORGANIC ACID-INDUCED NITRATE REDUCTASE IN CUCUMBER COTYLEDONS

GÖRING, H., ULITZSCH, M., and PREUSSER, E.

Humboldt University, Section of Biology, Invalidenstrasse 43, 1040 Berlin, G.D.R.

Nitrate reductase activity (NRA) in higher plants is induced by the substrate, NO_3^-, as well as by the reaction product, NO_2^- (1, 2, 3). Enzyme activity can be induced also by other conditions: cytokinin application (4, 5), application of citric acid and some other compounds (6). Using inhibitors of nucleic acid and protein synthesis as well as antibodies directed against NR, it was shown that the increase of NRA is due to a de novo synthesis of NR (cf. 7).

It was quite unexpected that NRA in cotyledons of Cucumis sativus could be induced by all the different conditions mentioned above (6, 7). It was therefore the aim of the present work to study in more detail the properties of the extracted enzyme.

Excised cotyledons of 5-d old seedlings of Cucumis sativus L. cv. Dickfleischige Gelbe were used. Seedlings were grown at $28^\circ C$ in complete darkness. Excised cotyledones were floated on distilled water (non-inducing) or on 150 mM NH_4NO_3 (inductive conditions). Experimental conditions and enzyme extraction as well as the assay for NRA are described in detail elsewhere (7).

NR was not detectable under non-inducing conditions neither by enzymatic nor by immunological methods (7). Optimal induction was obtain-

Proceedings of the 16th FEBS Congress
Part A, pp. 425–430

ed by incubation in 100 mM KNO$_2$, 150 mM KNO$_3$ or NH$_4$NO$_3$. NH$_4$NO$_3$ was even more effective than KNO$_3$ (Fig. 1). Maximal NRA was obtained 8 to 10 h after incubation in the induction medium.

NRA (units/g FW)

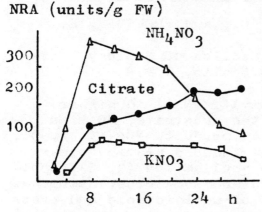

Fig. 1. Induction of NRA in excised cucumber cotyledones by KNO$_3$ (150 mM), NH4NO$_3$ (150 mM) and citric acid (100 mM, pH 2.5).

A strong induction of NRA was obtained also with citric, ascorbic and maleic acids (100 mM), especially at low pH of the medium (Fig. 1 and 2). Differently from the induction with nitrate, the organic acid-induced NRA increased continuously over the whole period investigated (Fig. 1).

NRA (units/g FW)

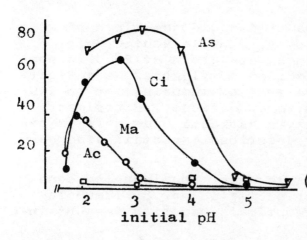

Fig. 2. NRA induction in excised cucumber cotyledones by ascorbic (As), citric (Ci), maleic (Ma) and acetic (Ac) acids in dependence on the pH of the medium (100 mM, 18 h, 28°C).

The effectiveness of the compounds was close related to their dissociation constants (PC_1 for ascorbic, citric, maleic and acetic acids are 4.17, 3.06, 1.87 and 4.76, respectively). The only exception was acetic acid which is toxic in such high concentration (100 mM) due to the high permeability of the plasmalemma for acetic acid.

Some feature of the enzyme extracted from cucumber cotyledones (7) were studied after enzyme purification. Blue-sepharose 4B was used for affinity chromatography (8). The purified NR had the same features independent of the induction way, i.e. NR induced either by nitrate or citric acid. This was true for the temperature dependency (maximal activity at 30°C), the pH dependency (maximal activity at pH 7.6) and the K_m value (about 0.5 mM). We could not find any difference between the substrate- and non-substrate-induced NR in relation to their electrophoretical or immunological behavior (not shown).

Nevertheless, there were differencies between the NR induction by nitrate or organic acids. One of the differencies was the kinetics of induction (Fig. 1).

Another difference was the NR stability of the crude enzyme extract during its storage in ice (Fig. 3). The substrate-induced NR is quite instable while the citric-acid-induced NR can be stored for a period of 2 to 3 days loosing only about 50% of its initial activity. The reason for this relatively high stability is unknown.

A further difference was detected in the induction of the nitrite reductase (NiR). NiR is usually induced by nitrate or nitrite simultaneously with NR. This was confirmed in our experiments with cucumber cotyledones (Fig. 4). The reduction of nitrite by the enzyme extract was

427

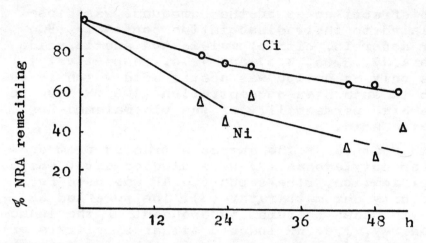

Fig. 3. Stability of NR in a crude enzyme extract. NR was induced either by 100 mM citric acid at pH 2.5 (Ci) or by 150 mM NH_4NO_3 (Ni). The crude extract was stored in ice for different time periods.

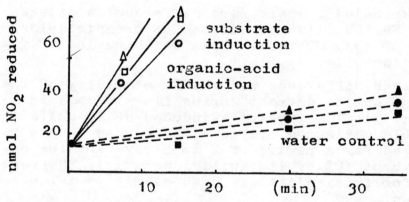

Fig. 4. Different NiR activity in enzyme extracts after induction by substrate ($\triangle$, KNO_2; $\square$, $NH4NO3$; o, KNO_3), organic acids ($\blacktriangle$, citric acid; $\bullet$, ascorbic acid) or non-inducing conditions ($\blacksquare$, water control). NiR activity is expressed as reduction of NO_2^- per enzyme assay.

428

determined after (9). In contrast to the enzyme
induction with nitrate or nitrite there was no
any significant increase in the NiR activity
after induction with citric or ascorbic acids
(Fig. 4). This is in agreement with results
obtained with embryos of Agrostemma githago
(10). In this case nitrate induced both, the NR
and the NiR, while benzylaminopurine induced
only NR.

After a joined application of nitrate and citric acid to the excised cucumber cotyledons we
found a strong synergism in the action of the
two substances (Table 1).

Table 1. Synergism of nitrate and citric acid
in induction of NR in excised cucumber cotyledons. Incubation for 18 h at 28°C in KNO_3 at
different concentrations alone or together
with citric acid (100 mM, pH 2.5).

Treatment	KNO_3 concentration (mM)				
	0	5	10	50	100
KNO_3	–	8	15	34	78
KNO_3 + citric acid	124	234	268	342	400
	±19	±24	±52	±39	±32

NRA in units/g FW, 1 units corresponds to
10^{-9} mol reduced nitrate per min.

The reason for this synergism is not understood
yet. Perhaps, nitrate can penetrate more easely
in the cotyledon tissues at low pH in citric
acid. Of course, the cotyledons are damaged at
longer incubation times in citric acid at the
very acid pH of the medium. It seems that the
synthesis of NR de novo is induced by citric
acid under conditions of gradual destruction of
the tissues. Nevertheless, the purified enzyme
is not different from the nitrate induced one.
There is rather an additional effect of nitrate,
e.g. induction of NiR and, perhaps, induction
of a NR-destabilizing factor.

Referencelist

(1) Beevers, L., and Hageman, R.H. (1969). Nitrate reduction in higher plants. Ann. Rev. Plant Physiol. 20, 495-522.

(2) Srivastava, H.S. (1980). Regulation of nitrate reductase activity in higher plants. Phytochem. 19, 725-733.

(3) Kaplan, D., Roth-Bejerano, N., and Lips, H. (1974). Nitrate reductase as a product-inducible enzyme. Eur. J. Biochem. 49, 393-398.

(4) Borriss, H. (1967). Untersuchungen über die Steuerung der Enzymaktivität in pflanzlichen Embryonen durch Cytokinine. Wiss. Z. Univ. Rostock, Math.-Naturw. Reihe 16, 629-639.

(5) Kende, H., and Shen, T.C. (1972). Nitrate reductase in Agrostemma githago - comparison of the inductive effects of nitrate and cytokinin. Biochim. Biophys. Acta 286, 118-125.

(6) Knypl, J.S., and Ferguson, A.R. (1975). pH-dependent induction of nitrate reductase in cucumber cotyledons by citric acid and other compounds. Z. Pflanzenphysiol. 74, 434 to 439.

(7) Ulitzsch, U., and Schiemann, J. (1984). Induction of NADH-dependent nitrate reductase activity in cucumber cotyledons by de novo synthesis of the enzyme. Biochem. Physiol. Pflanzen 179, 115-121.

(8) Campbell, W.H., and Smarelli, J. (1978). Purification and kinetics of higher plant NADH:nitrate reductase. Plant Physiol. 61, 611-616.

(9) Hucklesby, D.P., Dalling, M.J., and Hageman, R.H. (1972). Some properties of two froms of mitrite reductase from corn (Zea mays L.) scutellum. Planta 104, 220-233.

(10) Dilworth, M.F., and Kende, H. (1974). Control of nitrite reductase activity in excised embryos of Agrostemma githago. Plant Physiol. 54, 826-828.

PHYSIOLOGY AND MOLECULAR BIOLOGY OF PLANT GLUTAMINE SYNTHETASE

B.J. MIFLIN, M. LARA[1], R. SAARELAINEN, C. GEBHARDT and J.V. CULLIMORE[2]
Biochemistry Department, Rothamsted Experimental Station, Harpenden, Herts. U.K.
[1]Now at Centro de Investigacion sobre Fijacion de Nitrogeno, Aptdo Postal 565-A, Cuernavaca, Mexico
[2]Now at Dept. of Biological Sciences, University of Warwick, Coventry.

INTRODUCTION

The majority of nitrogen in man is derived from inorganic nitrogen that enters into organic combination in higher plants via the assimilation of ammonia. This process was originally thought to occur in all organisms via the enzyme glutamate dehydrogenase but Tempest, Meers and Brown proposed a new route in 1970 involving glutamine synthetase and a hitherto undiscovered enzyme pyridine nucleotide-linked glutamate synthase (1,2). Subsequently the existence of this route, often termed the glutamate synthase cycle, was also shown in higher plants (3,4) in which the major form of glutamate synthase uses ferredoxin as an electron donor. Evidence showing that this is the major, and probably sole route, of ammonia assimilation in higher plants will be reviewed below.

More recently it has been realized that the nitrogen assimilated into the organic form by the plant is not irrevocably locked into such molecules but is frequently released again as ammonia. This gives rise to the process of secondary assimilation which occurs most frequently during photorespiration via the photorespiratory nitrogen cycle (5) but is also important as nitrogen is transported around the plant.

Proceedings of the 16th FEBS Congress
Part A, pp. 431–439
© 1985 VNU Science Press

(For a detailed discussion of secondary ammonia assimilation consult 6,7,8). Consequently it appears that the plant must assimilate nitrogen in a number of different organs and tissues and in the course of a range of different metabolic pathways. This raises questions of how this is achieved and what are the regulatory controls that operate? To answer at least some of these questions we have begun a programme to isolate and characterise the genes for the enzyme glutamine synthetase from Phaseolus vulgaris.

EVIDENCE ON THE PATHWAY OF ASSIMILATION

This topic has been reviewed in detail many times (e.g. 7,9) but it may be useful to recall briefly the major points. There is no doubt that almost all plant tissues and organs contain both the enzymes of the glutamate synthase cycle and glutamate dehydrogenase. The occasional reported absence of the enzymes is usually due to technical difficulties or errors in assaying the enzymes. Some authors have attempted to use fluctuations in the amounts or concentrations of the different enzymes to support the operation of one or the other pathways; such evidence is at best only weakly indicative as the fluctations are rarely of great magnitude. Another much used argument of limited value is the apparently high K_m of glutamate dehydrogenase for ammonia; although the very low K_m of glutamine synthetase allows this enzyme to assimilate ammonia at low concentrations ($< 10^{-4}M$) there is evidence that the K_m of glutamate dehydrogenase may have been overestimated (Shatilov, these proceedings) at least in some organisms.

Labelling studies using ^{13}N or ^{15}N provide more valuable evidence but really require detailed analysis of the kinetics of assimilation the use of short-time experiments (only really practical with ^{13}N). Where these have been done (e.g. Meeks et al. (10), Rhodes et al (11) the results suggest that the majority of

the nitrogen is assimilated via glutamine synthetase.
Additional evidence has been obtained by the use of the
specific inhibitor methionine sulphoximine which is a
transition state inhibitor of glutamine synthetase and
azaserine and other inhibitors of glutamine-amide
transferases (i.e. glutamate synthase). Care must be
taken in interpreting results of experiments where the
incubations have taken place over a long time (because
of secondary effects of the inhibitors) or where the
investigators have failed to show that the enzymes are
fully inhibited at the time of assay. A number of
workers have published papers where these conditions
appear to have been satisfied and they show that
assimilation occurs via glutamine synthetase not
glutamate dehydrogenase in roots (12), leaves (13),
nodules (10) and whole plants (11). Using a combination
of ^{15}N kinetic analysis and the above inhibitors Rhodes
et al (11) conclude that in their experiments ammonia
assimilation took place solely by the glutamate synthase
cycle. Because the complete glutamate synthase cycle is
localized in chloroplasts and glutamate dehydrogenase in
mitochondria (14) the ability of these isolated
organelles to assimilate ammonia has been investigated.
Chloroplasts readily assimilate ammonia (4,15) which, by
use of inhibitors, has been shown to occur via the cycle
(16). In contrast, mitochondria fail to assimilate
ammonia unless it is present in relatively high
concentrations (~ 15 mM) and the mitochondria are
incubated under anaerobic conditions (17) or in the
presence of inhibitors of electron transport (18); even
under these extreme conditions the rate of assimilation
is very low.

Finally, evidence is available, from the isolation of
photorespiratory mutants that lack ferredoxin-glutamate
synthase (19,20), that all of the ammonia released in
photorespiration is reassimilated via the glutamate
synthase cycle. The fact that such mutants can
assimilate sufficient nitrogen to grow is perhaps
surprising, however, plants contain both NAD(P)H and

433

ferredoxin-dependent glutamate synthase (3,21,22) and the mutants have normal amounts of the NAD(P)H form. Presumably this enzyme is sufficient to carry out primary ammonia assimilation - a process that is quantitatively much less than that occurring during the photorespiratory nitrogen cycle.

ISOENZYMES OF GLUTAMINE SYNTHETASE

Glutamine synthetase is found in both the plastids and in the cytoplasm; in the pea leaf the activity is about equally distributed (14). Many workers (23,24,25,26,27) have shown that the activities are due to different forms of the enzyme (isoenzymes) that can be physically separated - usually by ion exchange chromatography. The proportions of the two forms in leaves differs widely according to species (25). The nature of the isoenzymes also differs between tissues; thus although the root contains both plastid and cytoplasmic glutamine synthetases (28) the cytoplasmic form is physically separable from the leaf cytoplasmic form (26). Similarly organ-specific forms of the enzyme have been reported from pea seeds that differ from the leaf forms (29). Recently we have also shown that Phaseolus vulgaris nodules produce a specific, physically separable glutamine synthetase during nodule development (30,31,32) This enzyme is probably the major route of ammonia assimilation during nitrogen fixation (see 33 for further discussion). The mature nodule contains two separable forms termed GS_{n1} and GS_{n2} whereas the uninoculated root contains only one from GS_r. Although GS_{n2} and GS_r appear identical on the basis of their chromatographic, immunological and catalytic behaviour they may differ in subunit composition (34). No enzymic form corresponding to GS_{n1} is found in the uninoculated root. However as the nodule develops GS_{n1} activity increases in concert with increases in nitrogenase and leghaemoglobin. In ineffective nodules formed using mutant strains of Rhizobium phaseoli little or no GS_{n1} is formed. One hypothesis to explain these results is that the plant contains a number of genes that specify different glutamine synthetases that are expressed in different organs. Whether or not each isoenzyme is totally distinct depends upon a knowledge of the subunit structure of the enzyme. Each enzyme is made up of 8 subunits, two dimensional electrophoresis suggests that each isoenzyme form has more than one type of subunit. Thus Lara et al. (34) have shown nodule GS (presumably GS_{n1} + $\overline{GS_{n2}}$) had two subunit forms β and γ whereas root GS had no γ subunit but only β and a third form α. This result would suggest that GS_{n2} and GS_r are not identical since GS_{n2} does not contain any α polypeptide. To test the hypothesis of differential gene expression we decided to isolate cDNA and genomic clones for the enzyme.

CLONING OF GLUTAMINE SYNTHETASE

The first step in the cloning was to demonstrate that functional mRNA could be isolated from nodule poly A^+ RNA (35). Using a reticulocyte lysate in vitro translation system and immunoprecipitation of the products we showed that about 2.4% of this RNA fraction was GS mRNA. Virtually pure glutamine synthetase mRNA was obtained by using glutamine synthetase antisera to purify polysomes containing nascent glutamine synthetase polypeptides and then releasing the poly A^+ RNA from the complex. A cDNA clone bank was then made from nodule mRNA using conventional cDNA synthesis procedures and GC tailing to insert the double stranded cDNA into the Pst1 site of the plasmid pBR322 (36). The glutamine synthetase clones were identified using a radioactive cDNA probe synthesized from the immunopurified glutamine synthetase mRNA. The identify of the clone pcGS-01 was confirmed by hybrid-select translation and DNA sequence analysis; the amino acid sequence deduced showed 85% homology, over a stretch of 20 amino acids, with a 20 amino acid peptide sequence obtained by Donn et al. (37).

pcGS-01 was hybridized to electrophoresed restriction digests of P. vulgaris DNA and to poly A⁺ RNA isolated from roots, nodules and leaves. The results showed that there were a number of genomic fragments of DNA which hybridized at moderate stringency; certain of these bands preferentially retained the probe when a higher stringency wash was used. We interpret this as showing that there are a number of glutamine synthetase genes in the P. vulgaris haploid genome and that the sequence of these copies varies. Hybridization to poly A⁺ RNA also showed that glutamine synthetase transcripts could be recognized in roots, nodules and leaves but only the RNA of nodules contained sequences that were very similar or identical to those in pcGS-01. Subsequent work (Gebhardt, C. unpublished) has led to the identification of a glutamine synthetase cDNA clone related to root glutamine synthetase which specifically hybridizes at the highest stringency to different genomic bands from pcGS-01. The clone also hybridizes at high stringency to sequences present in root and nodule RNA, implying that it is related to a polypeptide present in both root and nodule GS (probably the β polypeptide of Lara et al. (34).

CONCLUSION

The plant has a continually varied need to assimilate ammonia in a range of organs and tissues and arising in different metabolic pathways. To do this it uses a variety of different isoenzymic forms. Molecular cloning experiments confirm the hypothesis that the plant has a number of genes for glutamine synthetase which are specifically expressed in different organs and under different conditions (e.g. during nitrogen fixation). It is presumed that each of these genes will have different control sequences adjacent to the structural gene and we are currently characterizing isolated genomic clones of glutamine synthetase. This model of control contrasts with that recently described for the cyanobacterium Anabaena which has one structural gene for glutamine synthetase but two different promoter sequences 5' to that gene; one of these is used specifically under nitrogen fixing conditions (38). The existence of glutamine synthetase clones of higher plants should also enable us to investigate in more detail the number of polypeptides present in each organ and how they might be assembled into a functional enzyme.

ACKNOWLEDGEMENTS

J.V.C. gratefully acknowledges receipt of a Pickering Research Fellowship from The Royal Society. C.G. thanks the Commission of the European Communities for a training fellowship and R.S. is grateful to the Osk Huttunen Foundation, Helsinki for support.

REFERENCES

1. Tempest, D.W., Meers, J.L. and Brown, C.M. (1970) J. Gen. Microbiol. 64, 187-194.
2. Tempest, D.W., Meers, J.L. and Brown, C.M. (1970) Biochem. J. 117, 405-407.
3. Dougall, D.K. (1974) Biochem. Biophys. Res. Commun. 58, 639-646.
4. Lea, P.J. and Miflin, B.J. (1974) Nature (London) 259, 614-616.
5. Keys, A.J., Bird, I.F., Cornelius, M.J., Lea, P.J., Wallsgrove, R.M. and Miflin, B.J. (1978) Nature (London) 275, 741-743.
6. Lea, P.J. and Miflin, B.J. (1980) In: The Biochemistry of Plants, B.J. Miflin (ed.), Vol. 5, Academic Press, New York, pp. 559-607.
7. Miflin, B.J. and Lea, P.J. (1980) In: The Biochemistry of Plants, B.J. Miflin (ed.), Vol. 5, Academic Press, New York, pp. 169-202.
8. Miflin, B.J., Wallsgrove, R.M. and Lea, P.J. (1981) Current Topics in Cellular Regulation 20, 1-43.
9. Miflin, B.J. and Lea, P.J. (1977) Annu. Rev. Plant Physiol. 28, 299-329.

10. Meeks, J.C., Wolk, C.P., Schilling, N., Shaffer, P.W., Avissar, Y. and Chien, W.S. (1978) Plant Physiol. 61, 980-987.

11. Rhodes, D., Sims, A.P. and Folkes, B.F. (1980) Phytochem. 19, 357-366.

12. Probyn, T.A. and Lewis, O.A.M. (1979) J. Exp. Bot. 30, 299-305.

13. Kaiser, J.J. and Lewis, O.A.M. (1980) New Phytol. 85, 25-241.

14. Wallsgrove, R.M., Lea, P.J., and Miflin, B.J. (1979) Plant Physiol. 63, 232-236.

15. Mitchell, C.A. and Stocking, C.R. (1975) Plant Physiol. 55, 59-63.

16. Anderson, J.W. and Done, J. (1977) Plant Physiol. 60, 504-508.

17. Davies, D.D. and Teixiera, A.N. (1975) Phytochemistry 14, 647-656.

18. Wallsgrove, R.M., Keys, A.J., Bird, I.F., Cornelius, M.J., Lea, P.J. and Miflin, B.J. (1980) J. Exp. Bot. 31, 1005-1018.

19. Somerville, C.R. and Ogren, W.L. (1980) Nature (London) 286, 257-260.

20. Lea, P.J., Hall, N.P., Kendall, A.C., Keys, A.J., Miflin, B.J. and Wallsgrove, R.M. (1983) Plant Physiol. 71, 641s.

21. Matoh, T., Ida, S. and Takahashi, E. (1980) Plant and Cell Physiol. 20, 1332-1340.

22. Wallsgrove, R.M., Lea, P.J. and Miflin, B.J. (1982) Planta 154, 473-476.

23. Stasiewicz, S. and Dunham, V.L. (1979) Biochem. Biophys. Res. Commun. 87, 627-634.

24. Mann, A.F., Fentem, P.A. and Stewart, G.R. (1979) Biochem. Biophys. Res. Commun. 88, 515-521.

25. McNally, S.F., Hirel, B., Gadal, P., Mann, F. and Stewart, G.R. (1983) Plant Physiol. 72, 22-25.

26. Hirel, B. and Gadal, P. (1980) Plant Physiol. 66, 619-623.

27. Kretovich, W.L., Evstigneeva, Z.G., Pushkin, A.V. and Dzhokharidze, T.Z. (1981) Phytochemistry 20, 625-629.

28. Miflin, B.J. (1974) Plant Physiol. 54, 550-555.
29. Antonyuk, L.P., Pushkin, A.V., Vorobyeva, L.M.,
    Solvjeva, N.A., Estigneeva, Z.G. and Kretovich,
    W.L. (1982) Molecular and Cellular Biochem. 47,
    55-57.
30. Cullimore, J.V., Lara, M., Lea, P.J. and Miflin,
    B.J. (1983) Planta 157, 245-253.
31. Lara, M., Cullimore, J.V., Lea, P.J., Miflin, B.J.,
    Johnston, A.W.B. and Lamb, J.W. (1983) Planta
    157, 254-258.
32. Cullimore, J.V. and Miflin, B.J. (1984) J. Exp.
    Bot. 35, 581-587.
33. Miflin, B.J. and Cullimore, J.V. (1984) In Plant
    Gene Research ed. D.P.S. Verma and T. Hohn.
    Springer-Verlag, Vienna, pp. 129-178.
34. Lara, M., Porta, H., Padilla, J., Folch, J. and
    Sanchez, F. (1984) In: Advances in Nitrogen
    Fixation Research, C.F. Veeger and W.E.
    Newton,(eds). Nijhoff/Junk Publ. Co., The Hague,
    pp. 601.
35. Cullimore, J.V. and Miflin, B.J. (1983) FEBS
    Letts. 158, 107-112.
36. Cullimore, J.V., Gebhardt, C., Saarelainen, R.,
    Miflin, B.J., Idler, K.B. and Barker, R.F.
    (1984) J. Mol. Appl. Genet. (in press).
37. Donn, G., Tischer, E., Smith, J.A. and Goodman,
    H.M. (1984) J. Mol. Appl. Biol. (in press).
38. Tumer, N.E., Robinson, S.E. and Haselkorn, R.
    (1983) Nature 306, 337-343.

BIOSYNTHESIS OF NITROGEN TRANSPORT COMPOUNDS IN N$_2$-FIXING LEGUME AND NON-LEGUME ROOT NODULES

SVEN ERIK ROGNES
Department of Biology, Botany Division, University of
Oslo, P.O.Box 1045, Blindern, 0316 Oslo 3, Norway

INTRODUCTION: NITROGEN TRANSPORT COMPOUNDS

This paper reviews the synthesis of nitrogenous transport compounds exported from N$_2$-fixing nodules of legumes and, briefly, non-legume actinorhizal plants. Sym-
bioses involving cyanobacteria are not discussed.

The main questions are: 1) In what form is fixed N exported from nodules ? 2) What biochemical pathway opera-
tes between the initial step of assimilation of NH$_3$ generated by N$_2$ase (glutamine synthesis) and the formation
of a final export product ?

The major nitrogenous solutes known to function in export of fixed N are the amides asparagine and glutamine,
the ureido amino acid citrulline and the ureides allantoin (ALL) and allantoic acid (ALLC) (1-3). These compounds have typically low C:N ratios, 1.0-2.5, and are
translocated via the xylem to the shoot. In the nodule
they behave as sinks for the assimilated N and are end
products of N metabolism.

A second group of compounds includes N-rich non-protein
amino acids found in very high concentrations in certain
legumes. Some of them are very likely involved in N
transport; e.g. 4-methyleneglutamine (Arachis), as shown
by Fowden (4) 30 years ago, canavanine (Canavalia,Vicia),
lathyrine and 2,4-diaminobutyric acid (Lathyrus), homo-
serine (Pisum,Lathyrus) and albizziine (Albizzia,Acacia).
However, relatively little is known about their biosynthesis in general and still less about their role in
assimilation and export of N derived from N$_2$ fixation in
nodules because of the lack of ^{15}N or ^{13}N studies.

Finally, smaller amounts of amino acids like aspartate,
glutamate, 4-aminobutyrate and arginine are usually present in nodule xylem sap.

Proceedings of the 16th FEBS Congress
Part A, pp. 441–451
© 1985 VNU Science Press

AMIDE-EXPORTERS AND UREIDE-EXPORTERS

Legumes have been divided into two distinct groups according to their major nodule export product: amide-exporters and ureide-exporters (5). Within some tribes these
traits are accompanied by profound differences in nodule
structure, organization and N metabolism. Amide-exporters
are found in the Vicieae (Pisum,Vicia) and Trifolieae
(Trifolium), tribes thought to have developed in tempera-
te regions. On the other hand, tropical/subtropical members of the Phaseoleae (Glycine,Vigna,Phaseolus) have
ureide-exporting nodules. The amide-exporters utilize the
same compounds for export of fixed N from nodules as for
transport of N assimilated in the roots from combined
sources. In ureide-exporters, however,different compounds
are used for transport of fixed N and N from e.g. NO_3^-
(6,7).

The non-legume actinorhizal plants also include amide-
exporters forming asparagine or/and glutamine (Myrica,
Coriaria (1,8)) and ureide-exporters, inasmuch as citrulline (Alnus (9)) is a ureide. There seems to be no report
describing export of ALL/ALLC from such nodules.

INITIAL ASSIMILATION OF NH_3 PRODUCED BY N_2 FIXATION

Despite attempts to resurrect a role for glutamate dehydrogenase or aspartase in the primary assimilation of NH_3
generated by N_2ase in the bacteroids, there is very
strong evidence for the glutamine synthetase/glutamate
synthase (GS/GOGAT) cycle as the only pathway of significance in legume nodules (10,11). The levels of NH_3-assi-
milating enzymes in the bacteroid are too low to prevent
escape of the bulk of the NH_3 into the plant cell cytosol
with subsequent assimilation by plant GS/GOGAT. It is
thought that endophyte vesicles in non-legume nodules
also excrete NH_3 to the host cell cytosol followed by
assimilation into glutamine via GS as the first step.

AMIDE-EXPORTERS: ASPARAGINE SYNTHESIS

Nodules of Coriaria appear to export N essentially as
glutamine in unchanged form (1), but in most amide-

forming systems the bulk of the N is passed on to asparagine. A typical asparagine-exporter is Lupinus. 50-80% of
the N of lupin xylem sap is found in asparagine, usually
accompanied by aspartate (20-40% of the asparagine concentration) and smaller amounts of glutamine and glutamate (11,12).

The assimilation of NH_3 into asparagine requires operation of four enzymes: GS, GOGAT, aspartate aminotransferase and glutamine-dependent asparagine synthetase (AS).
In addition the activity of phosphoenolpyruvate carboxyl-
ase (PEPC) increases markedly during nodule development
and nodules actively fix $^{14}CO_2$ into oxaloacetate, aspartate and asparagine, indicating a role for PEPC in the
formation of oxaloacetate. Strong evidence for the involvement of these enzymes in asparagine synthesis during N_2
fixation comes from time-course studies with L.angusti-
folius (11,13) and L.luteus (14) nodules which demonstrate striking increases in their specific activities in the
plant cytoplasmic fraction concurrently with the development of N_2-fixing capacity. A steep rise in AS activity
occurred between 12 and 16 d after inoculation (11). AS
has not been detected in bacteroids (15), but there is a
report on its association with proplastids in the plant
fraction (16). The cellular and subcellular organization
of asparagine synthesis is still incompletely understood.

The biosynthetic reaction catalyzed by lupin AS is
(17-19):
Aspartate + Glutamine + ATP (Mg^{2+}, Cl^-) =
Asparagine + Glutamate + AMP + PP_i.

An attractive possibility not yet tested experimentally
is that 4-methyleneglutamine is formed in peanut plants
by an analogous reaction from 4-methyleneglutamate with
glutamine serving as amide-N donor (2,20).

Properties of asparagine synthetase

Plant AS was first isolated and purified 500-fold from
yellow lupin cotyledons (17-19). It has been partially
purified from blue lupin (11,13) and soybean (15,21,22)
nodules. The cotyledon and nodule enzymes have closely
similar properties. The specific activity of AS in lupin
nodule extracts (50-80 pkat/mg protein) is much higher

than in soybean and other ureide-exporters (3-16 pkat/mg protein) (13,15,21-23). AS is a difficult enzyme to handle as it is extremely labile in crude extracts; a low MW inhibitor has also been described (24). Cl^- ions activate the glutamine-linked reactions catalyzed by the cotyledon enzyme (19). The enzyme shows 2- to 3-fold higher reaction rates with glutamine compared to NH_4^+ as N donor and the K_m for NH_4^+ is 10- to 40-fold higher than for glutamine (2,15,17). In the absence of Cl^- and thiol protection, the glutamine site can easily be modified or destroyed so that the glutamine-dependent activity is lost although with retention of some NH_4^+-dependent activity, which may be misinterpreted as the reaction occurring in vivo. The AS activity in nodules is relatively low in comparison with the other enzymes involved (11), but for reasons given above measurements on crude extracts are likely to lead to underestimation of the in vivo activity (11,15,24).

The properties of AS strongly indicate that glutamine is the natural N donor for asparagine synthesis and that AS has no role in primary NH_3-assimilation. Additional support for this concept comes from ^{15}N and $^{14}CO_2$ incorporation studies with soybean nodules (15,25). These results indirectly confirm the role of glutamine and glutamine-dependent asparagine synthetase in nodule asparagine synthesis. That AS represents a bottleneck in the export of N as asparagine is illustrated by the presence of significant amounts of aspartate in the root xylem sap.

UREIDE-EXPORTERS: TRANSPORT OF ALLANTOIN AND ALLANTOATE

With their low C:N ratio (1.0) and apparently low energy cost of synthesis (26) the ureides ALL and ALLC are ideally suited for transport of fixed N. However, their relatively low (and highly temperature-dependent) solubility dictates a satisfactory water supply and a hot climate; ureide transport may require about 2.5 times as much water as asparagine transport (5).

The breakthrough in this field came about 1977 with the demonstration by Japanese groups that ALL + ALLC occurred in large amounts only in nodulated soybean plants actively fixing N_2 and became labelled from $^{15}N_2$ (27). The results indicated ALL synthesis in the nodules with subsequent conversion to ALLC and rapid transport into the vascular system of the root. These findings have later been extended to many tropical legumes. During the last four years very extensive studies have been carried out with cowpea (Vigna unguiculata) by a group in Australia and with soybean (Glycine max) by two groups in U.S.A.(28,29).

In N_2-dependent cowpea and soybean plants, the ureides account for 70-95% of the xylem-borne N with an emphasis on ALLC in soybean (6,26,30,31). Asparagine and other amino acids are of some significance in the early phase of nodule development before the onset of active fixation, but later on the ureides take over and dominate completely (26). In fact, the relative proportion of ureides in xylem sap is a sensitive and useful indicator of the extent of N_2 fixation (6,7,31). In NO_3^--fed plants, NO_3^- and asparagine become predominant in the xylem sap whereas nodule development and ureide synthesis are depressed; the ureide content of xylem sap drops to 5-10% of the soluble N (6,7).

Organization of ureide biosynthesis in nodules

Several models for the cellular and subcellular organization of ureide biogenesis have been proposed; these schemes have undergone rapid revisions during the last few years (16,28,29,32-34). It is now clear that the process occurs in the infected central zone of the nodule and probably involves a collaboration between bacteroid-containing and uninfected cells; further that the plant fraction of these cells catalyzes the complex and compartmented reaction sequence.

Ureide formation takes place in two stages: 1) Purine (IMP) biosynthesis de novo, and 2) Purine oxidation. These processes occur in separate compartments: the biosynthesis in proplastids, and the oxidation in the cytosol and the peroxisomes (28,29,34).

Purine biosynthesis de novo. Glycine conversion to purine nucleotides and pathway intermediates was shown with preparations of a particulate fraction which was relatively fragile, but could be purified and identified as starch-containing proplastids (16,29,35,36). These plastids apparently possess a complete pathway for IMP synthesis, although PRPP synthetase seems to be located in the cytosol (16). Serine (which would yield C_1-units via serine hydroxymethyl transferase) and CO_2 are also precursors of purines in nodules (35-37).

PRPP amido transferase (catalyzing the first committed step of purine biosynthesis) was shown to be located in the proplastids (16,35) and utilized glutamine and NH_4^+, but not asparagine. This key enzyme was purified 1500-fold from soybean nodules and there was evidence that it may be part of a large multienzyme complex including several purine biosynthetic activities (38). The enzymes implicated in purine biosynthesis show increased activities during nodule development in ureide-exporters (22, 26), but not in amide-exporters (23).

Phosphoglycerate appears to be a key compound in the formation of serine via phosphohydroxypyruvate (16). NADH is formed in the PGDH step. The action of serine hydroxymethyl transferase then gives glycine (C4,C5,N7 of the purine ring) and $N^{5,10}$-methylenetetrahydrofolate, which with generation of NADPH (36) supplies $N^{5,10}$-methenyl-tetrahydrofolate for the C8 atom in an economical way. The origin of formate (C2) is not clear. The enzymes of these associated metabolic conversions which supply glycine and C_1-tetrahydrofolate precursors are also located in the proplastids (16,29,36).

Purine oxidation. Enzymes of purine oxidation are very active in nodules of ureide-exporters, but show negligible activity in amide-exporting nodules (22,23,26). Allopurinol (4-hydroxypyrazolo(3,4-d)pyrimidine) is a very potent and specific inhibitor of xanthine oxidase and NAD^+-dependent plant xanthine dehydrogenase (XDH)(39,40). Allopurinol also inhibits hypoxanthine oxidation, a reaction catalyzed by XDH. Allopurinol-treated soybean plants contained only slight amounts of ALL and ALLC in stems and nodules, but showed a strong accumulation of xanthine in the nodules (39); similar effects were shown with cowpea (40). XDH has been purified from navy bean and soy-

bean nodules and its kinetic properties studied (41,42).
It is clearly a soluble cytosolic enzyme (16,29) and recent evidence indicates that it is located in the infected cells (32). Formation of ureides at rates commensur-
ate with those of N_2 fixation in vivo has been shown in
cell-free extracts of soybean and cowpea nodules using
various purine substrates: IMP, XMP, inosine, xanthosine,
guanine, hypoxanthine, xanthine and uric acid. ALLC formation from all compounds except urate required simultaneous addition of NAD^+ and was blocked by allopurinol
(43,44). XMP and IMP were the best mononucleotide substrates, whereas GMP and AMP were poor precursors (44).
This suggests that IMP or XMP is the key purine compound
which leaves the normal biosynthetic route (to AMP and
GMP) and becomes channelled into an oxidative pathway.

Recent work has shown that at low, physiological IMP
concentrations (10 µM), 80% of the metabolism occurs via
a pathway involving IMP dehydrogenase and leading to the
formation of XMP, xanthosine and xanthine (33). In support of the XMP/xanthosine-based pathway, a NAD^+-depen-
dent IMP dehydrogenase was demonstrated in the cytosol of
cowpea nodules (33), but was claimed to be associated
with proplastids in soybean nodules (36). Its lability
could explain the failure to detect this activity in earlier studies (28). The results from this work (33) are
consistent with the observed accumulation of xanthine
(and not hypoxanthine) following allopurinol treatment
and suggest that the in vivo pathway in the plant cell
cytosol is: IMP-XMP-xanthosine-xanthine-urate.

The uninfected cells may participate in a specific way
in the final steps of ureide synthesis (45). Urate oxidation requires a high pO_2 and a high pH (46). Urate oxidase (uricase) purified from soybean and cowpea nodules had
a fairly high K_m for O_2, about 30 µM (47,48). It was suggested that these properties could severely limit uricase
activity in infected cells, where the leghemoglobin system is believed to reduce the free dissolved O_2 concentration to 10-200 nM. Organelle fractionation studies of
soybean nodules have demonstrated that uricase is located
in the peroxisomes together with catalase (34). Electronmicroscopy further shows that peroxisomes (microbodies)

are abundant in the uninfected cells, but are virtually absent from infected cells (49). The uninfected cells are therefore probably the principal site of urate oxidation in vivo. Finally, the location of XDH in infected cells (32) indicates that urate is the compound to be transported from infected cells to uninfected cells.

Allantoinase, catalyzing the hydrolysis of ALL to ALLC, is associated with the microsomal fraction derived from the endoplasmic reticulum and is largely found in the uninfected cells (34,45).

NON-LEGUME NODULES: CITRULLINE SYNTHESIS IN ALNUS

Unfortunately, the level of sophistication attained in the research on legume N transport has no parallel in similar progress within the actinorhizal systems. Few reports on N metabolism in these nodules have appeared.

In Alnus, citrulline is the major N compound exported from nodules and becomes labelled from $^{15}N_2$ in the carbamoyl group (9). Dark fixation of CO_2 is obviously important, both via PEPC and carbamoyl phosphate synthetase. Citrulline formation will involve synthesis of ornithine from glutamate, plus carbamoyl phosphate from CO_2, ATP and glutamine amide-N. Ornithine carbamoyl transferase action then gives citrulline. The latter enzyme was found by a cytochemical staining technique to be located in the mitochondria of the host cell, but not in hyphae or vesicle stages of the endophyte nor in host cell proplastids (50). Glutamine synthetase is probably a host cell cytosolic enzyme, but the locations of the other enzymes required for citrulline biosynthesis are unknown.

REFERENCES

1. Pate,J.S. (1976) in "Encyclopedia of Plant Physiology" N.S., Vol.2 (Transport in Plants II, Part B Tissues and Organs, U.Lüttge and M.G.Pitman, eds), pp. 278-303, Springer-Verlag.
2. Lea,P.J. and B.J.Miflin (1980) in "The Biochemistry of Plants", Vol.5 (B.J.Miflin, ed), pp.569-607, Academic Press.

3. Sprent,J.I. (1981) in "The Physiology and Biochemistry of Drought Resistance in Plants" (L.G.Paleg and D.Aspinall, eds), pp. 131-143, Academic Press, Australia.
4. Fowden,L. (1954) Ann.Bot.N.S. 18, 417-440.
5. Sprent,J.I. (1980) Plant,Cell and Environment 3, 35-43.
6. McClure,P.R. and D.W.Israel (1979) Plant Physiol. 64, 411-416.
7. Pate,J.S., C.A.Atkins, S.T.White, R.M.Rainbird and K.C.Woo (1980) Plant Physiol. 65, 961-965.
8. Leaf,G., I.C.Gardner and G.Bond (1959) Biochem.J. 72, 662-667.
9. Leaf,G., I.C.Gardner and G.Bond (1958) J.Exp.Bot. 9, 320-331.
10. Robertson,J.G. and K.J.F.Farnden (1980) in "The Biochemistry of Plants", Vol.5 (B.J.Miflin, ed), pp. 65-113, Academic Press.
11. Boland,M.J., K.J.F.Farnden and J.G.Robertson (1980) in "Nitrogen Fixation" (W.E.Newton and W.H.Orme-Johnson, eds), Vol.2, pp. 33-52, University Park Press, Baltim.
12. Atkins,C.A., J.S.Pate, M.B.Peoples and K.W.Joy (1983) Plant Physiol. 71, 841-848.
13. Scott,D.B., K.J.F.Farnden and J.G.Robertson (1976) Nature 263, 703-705.
14. Radyukina,N.A., A.V.Pushkin, Z.G.Evstigneeva and V.L.Kretovich (1977) Dokl.Akad.Nauk SSSR 234, 1209-1212.
15. Huber,T.A. and J.G.Streeter (1984) Plant Physiol. 74, 605-610.
16. Boland,M.J., J.F.Hanks, P.H.S.Reynolds, D.G.Blevins, N.E.Tolbert and K.R.Schubert (1982) Planta 155, 45-51.
17. Rognes,S.E. (1970) FEBS Lett. 10, 62-66.
18. Rognes,S.E. (1975) Phytochemistry 14, 1975-1982.
19. Rognes,S.E. (1980) Phytochemistry 19, 2287-2293.
20. Winter,H.C., G.K.Powell and E.E.Dekker (1982) Plant Physiol. 69, 41-47.
21. Chan,Y.-K. and R.V.Klucas (1980) Plant Physiol. 65S, 111.
22. Reynolds,P.H.S., M.J.Boland, D.G.Blevins, K.R.Schubert and D.D.Randall (1982) Plant Physiol. 69,1334-1338.
23. Reynolds,P.H.S., D.G.Blevins, M.J.Boland, K.R.Schubert and D.D.Randall (1982) Physiol.Plant. 55, 255-260.

24. Joy,K.W., R.J.Ireland and P.J.Lea (1983) Plant Physiol. 73, 165-168.
25. Fujihara,S. and M.Yamaguchi (1980) Plant Physiol. 66, 139-141.
26. Schubert,K.R. (1981) Plant Physiol. 68, 1115-1122.
27. Matsumoto,T., M.Yatazawa and Y.Yamamoto (1977) Plant & Cell Physiol. 18, 353-359; 459-462; 613-624.
28. Reynolds,P.H.S., M.J.Boland, D.G.Blevins, D.D.Randall and K.R.Schubert (1982) TIBS 7, 366-368.
29. Shelp,B.J., C.A.Atkins, P.J.Storer and D.T.Canvin (1983) Arch.Biochem.Biophys. 224, 429-441.
30. Herridge,D.F., C.A.Atkins, J.S.Pate and R.M.Rainbird (1978) Plant Physiol. 62, 495-498.
31. McClure,P.R., D.W.Israel and R.J.Volk (1980) Plant Physiol. 66, 720-725.
32. Triplett,E.W. (1984) Plant Physiol. 75S, 8.
33. Shelp,B.J. and C.A.Atkins (1983) Plant Physiol. 72, 1029-1034.
34. Hanks,J.F., N.E.Tolbert and K.R.Schubert (1981) Plant Physiol. 68, 65-69.
35. Atkins,C.A., A.Ritchie, P.B.Rowe, E.McCairns and D.Sauer (1982) Plant Physiol. 70, 55-60.
36. Boland,M.J. and K.R.Schubert (1983) Arch.Biochem. Biophys. 220, 179-187.
37. Boland,M.J. and K.R.Schubert (1982) Arch.Biochem. Biophys. 213, 486-491.
38. Reynolds,P.H.S., D.G.Blevins and D.D.Randall (1984) Arch.Biochem.Biophys. 229, 623-631.
39. Fujihara,S. and M.Yamaguchi (1978) Plant Physiol. 62, 134-138.
40. Atkins,C.A., R.Rainbird and J.S.Pate (1980) Z.Pflanzenphysiol. 97, 249-260.
41. Triplett,E.W., D.G.Blevins and D.D.Randall (1982) Arch.Biochem.Biophys. 219, 39-46.
42. Boland,M.J., D.G.Blevins and D.D.Randall (1983) Arch. Biochem.Biophys. 222, 435-441.
43. Triplett,E.W., D.G.Blevins and D.D.Randall (1980) Plant Physiol. 65, 1203-1206.
44. Atkins,C.A. (1981) FEBS Lett. 125, 89-93.
45. Hanks,J.F., K.Schubert and N.E.Tolbert (1983) Plant Physiol. 71, 869-873.

46. Woo,K.C., C.A.Atkins and J.S.Pate (1981) Plant
    Physiol. 67, 1156-1160.
47. Lucas,K., M.J.Boland and K.R.Schubert (1983) Arch.
    Biochem.Biophys. 226, 190-197.
48. Rainbird,R.M. and C.A.Atkins (1981) Biochim.Biophys.
    Acta 659, 132-140.
49. Newcomb,E.H. and S.R.Tandon (1981) Science 212,
    1394-1396.
50. Scott,A., I.C.Gardner and S.F.McNally (1981) Plant
    Cell Reports 1, 21-22.

REGULATION OF AMMONIA ASSIMILATING ENZYMES IN PLANTS

VALERY R. SHATILOV
A. N. Bach Institute of Biochemistry, Academy of
Sciences, Leninsky Prospekt 33, Moscow 117071, USSR.

The process of nitrogen utilization by microorganisms
and plants for their growth eventually comes to assimilation of ammonium resulting in formation of α-
amino nitrogen. That is why every researcher, investigating nitrogen metabolism tries to answer the question:
in what way ammonium assimilation occur. This question
became of principle after the discovery of NAD(P)H-
dependent glutamate synthase by Tempest et al. in 1970
(1) and finding the ferre-doxin-dependent glutamate
synthase by Lea and Miflin in 1974 (2). Nowadays the
most of researchers believe that the main route of
ammonium assimilation in plant kingdom goes via glutamine synthetase (GS) and glutamate synthase (3).
However, up to the early 70's it was glutamate dehydrogenase (GDH) that had been considered as a major enzyme
to be responsible for ammonium assimilation (4). But
at present tha participation of GDH in ammonium assimilation in plants is almost denied (3).

In this paper I will present some data and arguments
on the assimilatory function of GDH at least in unicellular green algae.

We have been studying in detail GDHs as well as other
enzymes participating in ammonium assimilation in unicellular green algae (5, 6, 7). All the species investigated have the coenzyme-nonspecific GDH, which is a
constitutive enzyme, being present in cells constantly
at a high level. Members of Ankistrodesmus and Scenedesmus genera have in addition the second GDH, which
is NADP-specific. Its activity greatly increases in
nitrogen-starved cells and continuously falls down to
the original level after the addition of nitrate or
ammonium, with the latter more rapidly (6); GS behaves
in the same way (7). NADP-GDH and GS activity rise in
Ankistrodesmus and Scenedesmus cells during nitrogen

Proceedings of the 16th FEBS Congress
Part A, pp. 453–459
© 1985 VNU Science Press

starvation is blocked by the mixture of chloramphenicol and actidione (8). Separately they inhibit the process only partially. These data indicate the involvement of 70S and 80S ribosomes in the NADP-GDH and GS synthesis during nitrogen starvation. GS behaviour is in a good agreement with the data reported recently by Sumar et al. (9). They found two isoforms of GS in Chlorella kessleri. The authors assumed them to be a chloroplastic and cytosolic ones, like in higher plants.

Among the Chlorella species NADP-GDH have been found only in three thermophilic strains; its appearance is induced by ammonium (5). The induction is completely blocked by α-amanitin, actinimycin D and cycloheximide, but not by chloramphenicol (8). Thus it is clear that the inducible NADP-GDH is encoded in the nuclear genome and is formed on cytoplasmic 80S ribosomes. Unfortunately there are no data about the location of this GDH in a unicellular green algae cell, otherwise that would help to elicit its physiological role. Nevertheless some properties of NADP-GDH may be certainly considered as an evidence for its involvement in ammonium assimilation. Firstly, it is strong inhibition of deamination by 2-oxoglutarate and ammonium taken at physiological concentrations almost without L-glutamate effect on amination (5, 10). Thus in the presence of 2-oxoglutarate ammonium and NADP the enzyme appears to function in the assimilatory fashion. Secondly, NADP-GDH has a sufficient affinity for ammonium ions (10, 11). The plots, characterizing the dependence of the Chlorella pyrenoidosa 82T and Ankistrodesmus braunii NADP-GDH activity on ammonium ion concentration show that the enzyme from both algae displays a negative kinetic cooperativity in the range of low ammonium concentrations, the Hill coefficient (h) being about 0.5; for this reason the Lineweaver-Burk plots are biphsic (fig. 1). Biphasicity gives two meanings of the apparent K_m - relatively low and rather high. In the most publications devoted to kinetic properties of plant GDH rather high K_m values have been reported, and they were considered by many authors as a strong argument against an effective participation of GDH in ammonium assimilation. Unfortunately the reported values of K_m

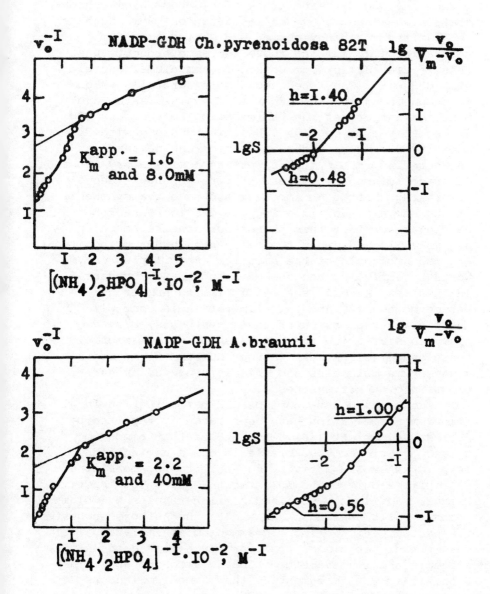

Figure 1. The Lineweaver-Burk and Hill plots characterizing the kinetic behaviour of NADP-GDH from Ch. pyrenoidosa 82T (redrawn from 11) and from A. braunii (redrawn from 10).

often correspond to the range of high ammonium concentration, near and above half-saturation. Some authors re-examined the behaviour of GDH during ammonium saturation (12, 13) and found the same property, as that we did earlier for Chlorella ammonium-inducible NADP-GDH (11). Thus one should more carefully taken into consideration the reported K_m values as an argument against or for the assimilation role of any GDH. Strong elevation of NADP-GDH activity along with GS activity during nitrogen starvation can be taken as one more indirect evidence for its assimilatory function in unicellular green algae. At first sight it seems surprising that at an ammonium shortage the synthesis of the ammonium assimilating enzymes increases. But at closer scrutiny this phenomenon appears to be reasonable. Indeed, when the cells are abundant in nitrogen each molecule of the ammonium assimilating enzyme works effectiviley because of a substrate abundance. In this case a cell requires a limited number of the enzyme molecules, and this limitation is controlled via the partial repression of their synthesis. During nitrogen starvation there is a shortage of ammonium, therefore a cell needs a alrger number of the scavenging enzyme molecules and this is achieved by derepression of their synthesis.

The convincing data on NADP-GDH participation in ammonium assimilation have been recently reported by Everest and Syrett (14). They showed that ammonium uptake by Stichococcus bacilaris cells having high level of NADP-GDH activity is inhibited by methinine sulfoximine only up to 50%, though GS was 90% inactive. Peltier and Tibault obtained similar results on Chlamydomonas cells. Based on these data the authors suggested the participation of GDH in ammonium assimilation (15).

As for higher plants there are much less data which evidence the involvement of GDH in ammonium assimilation. It is well documented, that ammonium induces de novo synthesis of a new GDH isoform in some plants and stimulates the synthesis of a certain GDH isoform originally present in some other plants (16). Besides, Schuber et al. found that the inhibition of GS by methionine sulfoximine caused an enhancement of N^{13}-

456

ammonium flow into glutamate in alder nodules (17).
Based on this fact they suggested the important role
of GDH in ammonium assimilation. Then Singh and Srivastava came to the same conclusion about the role of
GDH in maize plants (18). There is one paper which
should be especially mentioned in this context. It is
the paper by Sommerville and Ogren (19), who showed
that the Arabidopsis mutant with extremely low, if any,
the ferredoxin-dependent glutamate synthase activity
could not survive under conditions favouring photorespiration, but the mutant plants could normally grow
and develop utilizing nitrate at suppressed photorespiration. Then, a reasonable question arises - by what
pathway was ammonium derived from nitrate reduction
assimilated in the latter case? The authors did not
give the answer. They only wrote: "More surprising,
perhaps, is the normal growth of the mutants in non-
-photorespiratory conditions. This implies that the
plant does not require leaf GOGAT activity for NH_3 assimilation from primary nitrate reduction. Rather the
sole requisite function of leaf GOGAT seems to be
reassimilation of photorespiratory NH_3". In my opinion
the most probable candidate for ammonium assimilation
in mutant plants is GDH, though NAD(P)H-dependent
glutamate synthase, if it is present, can not be excluded, however its activity may be very low (3).

Two more definite conclusions can be drawn from
this paper. The first one is two pathways fo ammonium
assimilation are functioning in Arabidopsis plants,
both of them are of vital importance; one pathway is
assigned for assimilation of photorespiratory ammonium
by means of GS and the ferredoxin-dependent glutamate
synthase; another pathway, probably GDH reaction,
exists to assimilate ammonium, which comes directly
from nitrate reduction. The second conclusion is ammonium pools, chanelling through two pathways, are separated in space so, that the pool derived from photorespiration is inaccessible to GDH. If to accept the
existance of two separate ammonium pools then becomes
clear why an enhancement of ammonium flow through GDH
reaction when GS had been blocked by methionine sulfoximine was not observed in many reported experiments.

REFERENCES

1. Tempest, D. W., Meers, J. L. and Brown, C. M.
   (1970). Synthesis of glutamate in <u>Aerobacter</u>
   <u>aerogenes</u> by hitherto unknown route. Biochem. J.
   117, 405-407.
2. Lea, P. J. and Miflin, B. J. (1974). An alternative route for nitrogen assimilation in higher
   plants. Nature 251, 614-616.
3. Miflin, B. J. and Lea, P. J. (1982). Ammonia
   assimilation and amino acid metabolism. In: Encyclopedia of Plant Physiology, New Series, vol. 14A,
   Nucleic Acids and Proteins in Plants. I Structure,
   Biochemistry and Physiology of Proteins, D. Boulter
   and B. Parthier (Eds), springer-Verlag Berlin
   Heidelberg New York, pp. 5-64.
4. Kretovich, W. L. (1965). The most important aspects
   of amino acid and amide biosynthesis in plants.
   Izvestiya Academii Nauk SSSR 5, 647-665.
5. Shatilov, V. R. and Kretovich, W. L. (1977).
   Glutamate dehydrogenases from <u>Chlorella</u>: forms,
   regulation and properties. Mol. and Cell. Biochem.
   15, 201-212.
6. Shatilov, V. R., Sof'in, A. V., Kasatkina, T. I.,
   Zabrodina, T. M., Vladimirova, M. G., Semenenko,
   V. E. and Kretovich, W. L. (1978). Glutamate
   dehydrogenases of unicellular green algae: effect
   of nitrate and ammonium in vivo. Plant Sci. Lett.
   11, 105-114.
7. Sof'in, A. V., Shatilov, V. R., Zabrodina, T. M.,
   Pushkin, A. V., Evstigneeva, Z. G. and Kretovich,
   W. (1981). Control of ammonium assimilating enzymes
   in unicellular green algae. Plant Physiol. (USSR)
   28, 398-403.
8. Shatilov, V. R., Sof'in, A. V., Zabrodina, T. M.
   and Kretovich, W. L. (1982). The role of chloro-
   plast and cytoplasm in the NADP-glutamate dehydrogenase and glutamine synthetase synthesis in
   <u>Ankistrodesmus</u> cells. Mol. and Cell. biochem. 47,
   77-79.
9. Sumar, N., Casselton, P. J., Mc Nally, Sh. F. and
   Stewart, G. R. (1984). occurrence of isoenzymes

of glutamine synthetase in the algae Chlorella kessleri. Plant Physiol. 74, 204-207.

10. Sof'in, A. V., Shatilov, V. R. and Kretovich, W. L. (1984). glutamate dehydrogenases of unicellular green algae Ankistrodesmus braunii. Kinetic properties. biochimiya 49, 334-343.

11. Shatilov, V. R., Ambartsumjan, W. G. and Kretovich, W. L. (1974). properties of the Chlorella ammonium ion-inducible NADP-specific glutamate dehydrogenase. Biochimiya 39, 571-576.

12. Wootton, J. C. (1983). re-assessment of ammonium ion affinities of NADP-specific glutamate dehydrogenases. activation of the Neurospora crassa enzyme by ammonium and rubidium ions. Biochem. J. 209, 527-531.

13. Palich, E. and Gerlitz, C. (1980). Deviation from Michaelis-Menten behaviour of plant glutamate dehydrogenase with ammonium as variable substrate. Phytochemistry 19, 11-13.

14. Everest, S. A. and Syrett, P. J. (1983). Evidence for the participation of glutamate dehydrogenase in ammonium assimilation by Stichococcus bacillaris. New Phytol. 93, 581-589.

15. Peltier, G. and Thibault, P. (1983). Ammonia exchange and photorespiration in Chlamydomonas. Plant Physiol. 71, 888-892.

16. Shatilov, V. R. (1982). Glutamate dehydrogenases of microorganisms and plants. Uspekhi Biologhicheskoj Chimii 23, 185-209.

17. Schubert, K. R. and Coker III, G. T. (1981). Ammonia assimilation in Alnus glutinosa and Glycine max. Short-term studies using N^{13}-ammonium. Plant Physiol. 67, 662-665.

18. Singh, R. P. and Srivastava, H. S. (1982). Glutamate dehydrogenase activity and assimilation of inorganic nitrogen in maize seedlings. biochem. Physiol. Pflanzen B177, 633-642.

19. Sommerville, C. R. and Ogren, W. L. (1980). Inhibition of photosynthesis in Arabidopsis mutants lacking leaf glutamate synthase activity. Nature 286, 257-259.

Symposium VII

EVOLUTIONARY BIOCHEMISTRY

ON THE ORIGIN OF TYPICALLY BIOLOGICAL PROPERTIES IN THE EVOLUTION OF AUTOCATALYTIC SYSTEMS.

R. BUVET Université Paris Val de Marne - CRETEIL, France
J.M. DELARBRE Ecole Nationale Supérieure Universitaire
de Technologie - DAKAR, Sénégal
C. GRAVET Université de LIEGE, Belgique

THE PRODUCTS OF PRIMITIVE EARTH CHEMISTRY

From the first proposal of the theory of primitive chemical evolution, presented sixty years ago by Oparin (1), and from the numerous experiments which have been carried on in all countries as soon as proper analytical tools were available at the beginning of fifties (2) it is now well established on experimental grounds that the supply of any kind of energy, which can be absorbed by electronic excitation of carbonaceous components, in any simple mixture of reduced compounds of carbon, oxygen, nitrogen and sulfur, in the presence of condensed water, results, after only some hours, in the production in solution of relatively large amounts of many chemicals and even of structures which are now currently used by living organisms.
These include small molecules such as aminoacids and other simple acids, sugars, pyrimidic and puric bases and other heterocyclic compounds, but also oligomers and polymers of these compounds such as peptidic ones and proteïnoïds, and polynucleotidic polymers in the presence of phosphate. In the same way, globular precipitates involving hydrophobic properties have been formed in different conditions and peripheric membrane structures roughly comparable to cell membranes have been put into evidence (3)

THE PRIMITIVE REACTIONS AT EARTH PERIPHERY AND THE BIOCHEMICAL METABOLISM

However, such structural resemblances could be of no real biological significance if functional parallels

Proceedings of the 16th FEBS Congress
Part A, pp. 463–473
© 1985 VNU Science Press

between the primitive chemistry of earth periphery and
the contemporary biochemistry could not also be cleared
of experiments.
First, this concerns the principle of the mechanisms of
reactions set in place in both cases.
I have shown previously, e.g. in the book published in
honor of Marcel Florkin (4), that starting from the
first overview of metabolic steps which is given by the
classification of enzymes, it is possible to reduce even
more the number of classes of elementary processes from
which the metabolism is built, by dissociating some
metabolic steps, said coupled ones, in two elementary
processes, in general respectively energy coupling and
energy coupled, as it is usually done more restrictive-
ly, e.g. for the primary productions of energy-rich
condensed bonds from redox reactions.
In this classification of biochemical elementary processes, more meaningful as it concerns the properties of
substrates than the enzyme classification, seven classes
of processes do suffice to read the metabolism, and
three classes only are sufficient to read 90 % of it :
- condensations leading to condensed group such as ester, amide, osidic ... etc groups according to :

$$
\left.\begin{array}{c} \gtrdot C- \\ \\ \gtrdot P- \\ \; \end{array}\right\}-OH \; + \; H-\left\{\begin{array}{c} -O- \\ -S- \\ -N\lessgtr \end{array}\right. \; \rightleftharpoons \; \gtrdot C- \atop \gtrdot P- \Big\}\Big\{ \begin{array}{c} -O- \\ -S- \\ -N\lessgtr \end{array} \; + \; H_2O
$$

and, reciprocally hydrolyses of such groups.
- syntheses and reciprocally degradations of C-C bonds
according to additions of polarized C-H bonds to C=O

$$
\begin{array}{c} \gtrdot C = O \\ \gtrdot C - H \end{array} \; \rightleftharpoons \; \begin{array}{c} \gtrdot C - OH \\ \gtrdot C \end{array}
$$

- and redox reactions involving at most a transfer of
two electrons, between two redox couples defined by :

$$
1 \; or \; 2 \; Ox \; + \; 1 \; or \; 2 \; e^- \; + \; p \; H^+ \; \rightleftharpoons \; 1 \; or \; 2 \; Red \; + \; q \; H_2O
$$

Refering to theses three main kinds of elementary processes involved in the biochemical metabolism, the stoechiometries and the mechanisms of reactions which should have produced the first carboxylated and phosphorylated condensed bond or formed the first C-C bonds in the primitive aqueous media on the earth were experimentally studied by many authors, mainly in connection with the problem of the formation of primitive polymers (5). And it was evidently shown that these stoechiometries and mechanisms are identical as it concerns the involved substrates reactivities to those stoechiometries and mechanisms implicated in contemporary enzymic processes.

Less experimental studies were devoted up to now to the identification and mechanisms of redox reactions on the primitive earth, but I have shown at the sixth conference on the origin of life held in Jerusalem (6) that the choice of biochemical redox processes, although worked enzymically in contemporary organisms, is also determined by simple principles relating to the energetics and kinetics of substrates properties. Moreover, Krasnovskii's works on the photoactivation of redox processes (7) associated with results obtained by F.Stoetzel and I (8) on the ultraviolet absorption of solutions obtained in the course of experiments simulating the primitive earth chemistry, have shown that the bases of the photosynthetic absorption of solar energy in aqueous media were gathered as soon as some evolution of these aqueous media was achieved at the primitive earth periphery.

In conclusion of this comparison of reactions which lead to biochemicals in contemporary organisms and in experiments simulating the conditions which must have prevailed on primitive earth, it clearly appears now that products formed in both cases, are roughly the same because the reactions which produce them are also the same as it concerns the substrates reactivities implicated in both cases, simply because both groups of processes occur in aqueous media. The metabolism of living beings is as it is because it entirely exploites the only set of reactions possible in aqueous media from carbonaceous compounds and for this reason it could not be different of what it is.

CATALYTIC EFFECTS, ADAPTATION
AND DISSYMETRY IN BIOCHEMISTRY

Nevertheless, we have still to be faced with two groups of essential differences between both sets of reactions.

First, the biochemical metabolism is acted by catalysts which are products of this metabolism itself and we have to define how this "egg and chicken" situation could evolve.

Secondly, perfectly functional coenzymes, peptidic sequences qualified for having proper catalytic properties, polynucleotidic catalysts able to improove the production of these sequences, perfectly adapted membrane structures and these even more admirably adapted structures which are organisms in their whole, are so omnipresent in biology that they should have led Voltaire, if he could have known these molecular bases of biological adaptation, to emphasize even more his famous "I cannot believe that this clock does exist, and has no watchmaker".

To which we must add that some apparent watchmaker's whim made him choose L aminoacids and D sugars, when it was less painful in terrestrial surrounding to produce racemic aminoacids and sugars.

Let us look at the first problem, and see if its solution does not allow to clarify the other ones.

AUTOCATALYTIC EFFECTS IN THE PRIMITIVE CHEMISTRY
OF EARTH PERIPHERY

As a matter of fact, many experimental data also show that some products of the very first reactions on the primitive earth were able to modify, and particularly to catalyze the course of reactions which produced these compounds themselves.

From Jencks (9) and Benkovic's (10) works on Bronstedt and nucleophilic catalyses of transacylation processes implicated in the formation of carboxylated condensed groups and in C-C bond syntheses, we can on this respect deduce that all acidic and basic compounds formed from

the begining, and particularly amino and imidazolic derivatives were able to catalyse at least some of the
reactions which led initially to their formation.
More directly, a series of works from Fox, Dose and
co-workers (11) showed that polypeptidic polymers simply
obtained by thermal copolymerisation of aminoacids mixtu-
res present always, at least at some extent, catalytic
properties relating to the main group of enzymes defined
by the enzyme classification.
In Bach Institute, Oparin and co-workers showed (12)
that the globular precipitation of coacervates including
some less hydrosoluble catalysts shall lead to some kind
of primordial nutrition-excretion cycle which makes chemical energy available in the coacervates surrounding
usable for the development of these coacervates.
These experimental facts, related to the role of autocatalytic effects of products of primitive reactions on
the rate of these reactions, although needing a lot of
further demonstrations and precisions, do suffice in my
opinion to show that such autocatalytic processes and
any possible subsequent evolution were at least most
probable on the primitive earth.
Let us now look more closely at the consequences of such
evolutions.

THE EVOLUTION OF AUTOCATALYTIC REACTION NETWORKS

More than thirty years ago, a theory was proposed by
F.C. Frank (13) to justify the origin of the optical
activity of biological compounds. This theory was developed as a mathemetical treatment of the kinetics of a
reaction network :

- supplied in a reagent A

- able to be competitively transformed in two products
C_1, and C_2, by reactions presenting an autocatalytic
effect by their own product and a mutual inhibition by
the other product.
Many mathematical treatments were furtherly developed
(14) with the aid of computers from this basis, and have
shown that such systems are unstable if C_1 and C_2 have
quantitatively the same properties, and that this un-

467

stability shall result in the final selection of only one of these products, let us say, enantiomers.

I personnally consider that such developments are beautiful introductions to the potentialities of studies based on the evolution of autocatalytic systems. And this is even more the case if we take also into account all studies more or less derivated from the Lotka-Volterra problem which have shown that autocatalytic processes placed in series may lead to oscillatory phenomena.

However, as up to now we have no precise ideas about the exact mathematical expression of autocatalytic properties set in place in the primitive evolution, we shall firstly try to define what are the minimal requirements which a reaction network occurring in an open system must quantitatively present for being able to deliver by evolution states and properties of this open systems having some biological relevance.

In addition of this, for many didactic, psychological and philosophical reasons we are also faced with the need to insure the acquisition of the conciousness of the importance of the results of such studies as easily as possible to as many as possible scientists and, as far as possible, other men and women.

To stay here on scientific grounds, let us simply start, with some oversimplification of autocatalytic effects set in place from the beginning of earth evolution, by considering :

- an open system steadily supplied out of equilibrium with reagent A at a constant flux ϕ ;
- which can be transformed by two autocatalytic processes in two different products, C_1 and C_2 ;
- which are eliminated from the system without any discrimination between both, i.e. in proportion of their respective quantities and, e.g. to keep the system mass constant, at the same total flux ϕ than A is supplied.

In the simplest case, we can assume that the autocatalytic effects for both reactions can be described by the first order degeneracy of Michaelis equation, as :

$$\dot{\xi}_i = - \frac{dA}{dt}_i = \frac{dc_i}{dt} = k_i . A . C_i$$

with k_1 and k_2 different, but as little different as decided, one from the other, or even identical.

Under these conditions, the evolution of the system follows the differential equations :

$$\frac{dA}{dt} = - (k_1 C_1 + k_2 C_2) \, A$$

$$\frac{dC_1}{dt} = k_1 C_1 A - \frac{C_1}{C_1 + C_2} \, \phi$$

$$\frac{dC_2}{dt} = k_2 C_2 A - \frac{C_2}{C_1 + C_2} \, \phi$$

Although naïvely simple, this differential system cannot be explicitly solved, and our scientifically trained mind is unable to visualize at first sight the evolutionary properties of the physical model that it mathematically represents.

However, two simple general properties can be extracted from these equations with the use of a single pencil. The first one emphazises the selective character of the evolution of this physical model. For this purpose, let us simply divide the second and third equations respectively by C_1 and C_2 and substract them.

It comes :

$$\frac{1}{C_1} \frac{dC_1}{dt} - \frac{1}{C_2} \frac{dC_2}{dt} = \frac{d \, \text{Log} \, C_1/C_2}{dt} = (k_1 - k_2) \, A$$

The last equality, which I usually name the Malandain's theorem, in honor of the friend of mine who proposed it to my attention, shows that since A is necessarily positive, the logarithm of the ratio of C_1 to C_2, is necessarily of the same sign that the difference $(k_1 - k_2)$. This means that, in any circumstance such as defined by other parameters, the evolution of the system tends to increase the proportion of the very product which is the best autocatalytic tool.

But, let us now look more closely at what state of completion shall come this tendency. In the stationary state, the differential systems gives :

$$0 = k_1 C_1 A - \frac{C_1}{C_1 + C_2} \phi$$

$$0 = k_2 C_2 A - \frac{C_2}{C_1 + C_2} \phi$$

We can again try to divide these equations by C_1 and C_2, respectively. It should give :

$$k_1 A = \frac{\phi}{C_1 + C_2} = k_2 A$$

which should imply, A being different from zero since continuously supplied in the system at the flux ϕ different from zero, :

$$k_1 = k_2$$

even when :

$$k_1 \neq k_2$$

This is evidently impossible and prooves that we were in fact not allowed to divide the stationary equations by C_1 and C_2 because one of these concentrations was necessarily zero. From the Malandain's theorem, this could concern only the less efficient catalyst, corresponding to the lower kinetic constant k. Finally, if we ask a computer the step to step solution of this differential system, its answer, e.g. corresponding to the initial state $A(0) = 0$ and $C_1(0) = C_2(0)$ and k_1 k_2 presents the shape given by the figure 2.

This establishes that the excellency of the very exclusive choices made by evolution which led to Life, can be explained in a quite deterministic viewpoint, such as described by any set of differential equations against time, as well as, but perhaps not better than, it is usually done with the help of a great architect of the universe, by some of these which are not used to manipulate physics.

470

If both kinetic constants k_1 and k_2 are strictly identical as it should be for two enantiomers in any properly symetrical surrounding, it can be easily seen from Malandain's equation that starting from $C_1 \neq C_2$ as well as from $C_1 = C_2$ no shift at all could be observed. It means that any fluctuation of C_1/C_2 e.g. imposed by any externally applied accident, is simply conservative, i.e. that any set of fluctuations around an average value of this ratio results statistically in no shift at all from this average value.

Things are completely different if the rates of catalysed reactions are more than proportional to the catalysts concentration, i.e. if :

$$\left(\frac{\partial^2 \dot{\xi_i}}{\partial c_i^2} \right)_{c_i = 0} > 0$$

Here, it can be easily seen that even if both catalysts have exactly the same properties, e.g. as enantiomers in a symetrical surrounding, and if they are initially present at the same concentrations, any fluctuation around this state inevitably results in a shift of the system which proceeds until one of the catalyst is entirely swept out.

This allows us to understand that the selection of only one kind of enantiomer of aminoacids and sugars which was made by life should result either from the existence of any kind of very small convenient dissymetry at earth periphery amplified by linear autocatalytic retroaction or, even, of no dissymetry at all under the influence of non-linear autocatalytic retroactions acting from unavoidable fluctuations of local conditions or even at the molecular level.

In conclusion, my willing is giving this talk as I did it, was to show that some of the most physically strange properties of living systems, which were not yet accounted for by experimental studies of chemical evolution because the duration of such experiments was too short, are probably simple cumulative results of the auto-catalytic character of this evolution occurring on a

471

time long enough on the earth periphery under the flux of solar energy.

I am deeply grateful to the organizers of this conference, and particularly to Professor E.M.Kreps, chairman of this symposium on Evolutionary Biochemistry for having invited me to review some of our recent works in the field of the origin and evolution of life at this 16th FEEBS meeting in Moscow.
My feelings of honour and pleasure are strengthened when I consider that this meeting is held in the town which saw during so many years the development of the activity of Alexandre Ivanovich Oparin and Nina Petrovna Oparina. I am deeply honoured for having been one of their very close friends, and I would like to dedicate to their memory the content of this talk which was directly inspired by some of our conversations.

REFERENCES

(1) Oparin A.I. (1924) Proiskhozhdenie zhizni. Izd. Moskovskii Rabochi
(2) see e.g. Buvet R. (1974) L'Origine des Etres Vivants et des Processus Biologiques. Masson ed. Paris
(3) Fox S.W. (1967) in Biogenèse, Masson ed. Paris
(4) Buvet R. (1980) Comp.Biochem.Physiol. 67 B, 381-387
(5) (1971) Chemical Evolution and the Origin of Life. Buvet R., Ponnamperuma C. (eds). North Holland publ., Amsterdam
(6) Buvet R. (1981) Origin of Life. Y.Wolman (ed) D.Reidel Publ. 589-599
(7) Krasnovsky A.A. (1971) Chemical Evolution and the Origin of Life. Buvet R. and Ponnamperuma C. (eds) North Holland publ. Amsterdam, 279-287
(8) Buvet R., Le Port L. and Stoetzel F. (1976) Cosmochemical Evolution and the Origins of Life. Oro J., Miller S.L., Ponnamperuma C., Young R.S. (eds) D.Reidel publ., 253-262
(9) Jencks W.P. (1969) Catalysis in Chemistry and Enzymology. Mc Graw-Hill publ.
(10) Bruice T.C., Benkovic S. (1966) Bioorganic Mechanisms. Benjamin W.A. publ.

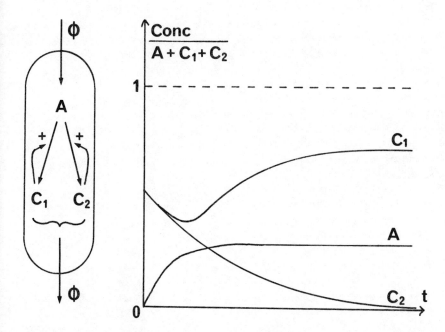

Figure 1 - Schematic re-
presentation of a bi-di-
rectional   autocatalytic
system.

Figure 2 - Shape of the
computed evolution again-
st time of the composi-
tion of a bidirectional
linear autocatalytic sys-
tem $(A(0) = 0, \quad C_1(0) = C_2(0), \quad K_1 > K_2)$

(11) Dose K. (1974) Cosmochemical Evolution and the
    Origins of Life. Oro J., Miller S.L., Ponnamperuma C.,
    Young R.S (eds) D.Reidel publ. 239-252
(12) Oparin A.I. (1958) see e.g. The Origin of Life on
    Earth. Oliver and Boyd.
(13) Franck F.C. (1953) Bioch.Biophys.Acta 11, 459
(14) see e.g. Seelig F.F, Ziclke R. (1975) J.Mol.Evol.
    6, 117

EVOLUTION OF NEUROPEPTIDES : THE NEUROHYPO-PHYSIAL HORMONE-NEUROPHYSIN MODEL

R. ACHER

Lab. of Biological Chemistry, University of Paris VI
96, Bd Raspail   75006 Paris   (France)

Neurohypophysial hormones and neurophysins are mainly biosynthesized in the supraoptic and paraventricular nuclei of hypothalamus as common macromolecular precursors split during the transport until neurohypophysis (1-3).

We have shown in 1955 that they can be extracted from the neurohypophysis associated in non-covalent and reversible complexes (4, 5). The stoichiometry of the complex components suggested that a neurohypophysial hormone and a neurophysin could be fragments of a common precursor. This view has been substantiated first by Sachs(6) and later by Gainer, Brownstein and their coworkers (7) who have purified proteins immunologically reactive with both anti-vasopressin and anti-neurophysin. Richter and associates have deduced the amino acid sequences of vasopressin/MSEL-neurophysin and oxytocin/VLDV-neurophysin precursors from bovine cDNA studies (8, 9) and more recently their genes have been characterized in both the rat and the ox (9, 10, 11). Vasopressin and oxytocin genes are organized in a similar way, both comprising three exons and two introns (10, 12). Because the variabilities of these exons and their peptide products greatly differ when several mammalian species are compared, it seems that each exon has its own evolution and that the dogma "one gene - one protein" should now be converted into "one exon - one domain". We will examine successively the evolution of the hormones, the neurophysins and the copeptins (C-terminal domain).

Proceedings of the 16th FEBS Congress
Part A, pp. 475–484
© 1985 VNU Science Press

I - EVOLUTION OF NEUROHYPOPHYSIAL HORMONES

a) Structures of neurohypophysial hormones.

Although neurohypophysial peptide-like material has been detected by immunochemistry in invertebrates, namely in insects (13) and coelenterates (14), chemical identification has, up to now, been carried out only in vertebrates. About 50 species have been investigated to date, and 10 peptides have been characterized. The general conclusion can be drawn that on the one hand each species usually has two neurohypophysial peptides, on the other, that the neurohypophysial hormones are evolutionary very stable. All of them have the same nonapeptide pattern, the same hormones being generally found in species belonging to the same class and substitution dealing usually with one or two residues out of nine.

Five main groups can clearly be distinguished in vertebrate species. These groups are :
1. The mammals. They are clearly distinct in having one or two vasopressin(s) instead of vasotocin found in all other vertebrates. In Prototheria (egg-laying mammals) and Eutheria (placental mammals), oxytocin and virtually always arginine vasopressin have been identified (15). In Metatheria the evolution appears more complex and differ in Australian and American species. As oxytocic principle, Australian marsupials have mesotocin ([Ile ^{8}]-oxytocin)(16, 17), a peptide found in nonmammalian tetrapods ; South-American species have oxytocin (18, 19) and the North-American opossum has both. As vasopressor principle(s), the brush-tailed possum, belonging to the Australian family Phalangeridae, has arginine vasopressin (16), whereas 5 species belonging to the Australian family Macropodidae have both lysine vasopressin ([Lys ^{8}]-vasopressin) and phenypressin ([Phe ^{2}]-vasopressin (17) ; South and North-American opossums have both lysine vasopressin and arginine vasopressin

(18, 19). Because all the individuals examined up to now have two vasopressins, it seems that there is a duplication of the vasopressin gene rather than heterozygocity.

2. The nonmammalian tetrapods, namely birds, reptiles, amphibians, and lungfishes, in which two peptides, mesotocin ([Ile^8]-oxytocin) and vasotocin ([Ile^3]-vasopressin), have been characterized (15).

3. The bony fishes, including primitive bony fishes such as Polypterus, in which isotocin ([Ser^4, Ile^8]-oxytocin) and vasotocin have been identified (15).

4. The cartilaginous fishes, which show a rather great heterogeneity in contrast to the other classes. Two peptides are again usually found. However, if cartilaginous fishes have vasotocin, like all the other nonmammalian vertebrates, the amount is here remarkably small ; the second hormone differs in each subgroup, namely rays, sharks, and chimaeras. In four species of rays, glumitocin ([Ser^4, Gln^8]-oxytocin) has been characterized. In the spiny dogfish, Squalus acanthias, two oxytocin-like hormones, valitocin ([Val^8]-oxytocin) and aspargtocin ([Asn^4]-oxytocin), have been found and it remains to be determined whether both peptides are produced by a single gland or not (15). In the chimaeras, the ratfish Hydrolagus colliei has been examined, and a peptide having the amino acid composition of oxytocin has been isolated (20). The presence of oxytocin in a fish is rather puzzling.

5. The Cyclostomes, the most ancient living vertebrates, in which a single hormone, vasotocin, has been disclosed (15).

b) Phylogeny of neurohypophysial hormones.
Up to now, six oxytocin-like hormones and four vasopressin-like hormones have been identified. All these peptides have nine amino acid residues, five of which are invariant. They can be arranged in two lineages corresponding to the oxytocin-like and vasopressin-like hormo-

nes. The peculiar duplication of the vasopressin-like gene in Marsupials suggests the existence of a multi-gene family for the pressor peptide.

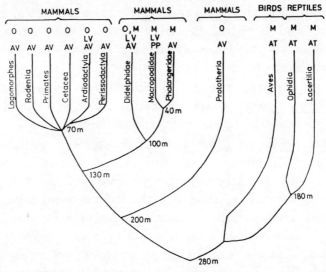

Fig.1. Neurohypophysial hormones and tetrapods evolution according to paleontological data. The letters indicate hormone identified in modern representatives of the groups: O, oxytocin; AV, arginine vasopressin; LV, lysine vaso-pressin; M, mesotocin; PP, phenypressin; AT, arginine vasotocin. The numbers give the time in millions of years (m) since the divergence.

The number of vasopressin-like genes in placental mammals is a matter of discussion (17). In the foetus of sheep and seal, a mixture of vasotocin and arginine vasopressin has been detected at mid-gestation, vaso-pressin remaining alone at the birth (21). Because the rat vasopressin gene contains a single hormonal peptide moiety and not repeated sequences, a duplication of the whole gene is necessary to explain the simultaneous pre-sence of vasotocin and vasopressin. If it is so, a family of vasopressin-like genes could exist with an ordered schedule of expression during development as found, for instance, for hemoglobins (22).

478

II - EVOLUTION OF NEUROPHYSINS

Neurophysins are small (93-95 residues) acidic proteins found associated with neurohypophysial hormones in non-covalent complexes. The association is specific and reversible; it probably exists between the corresponding domains of the precursors before processing.

a) The two types of neurophysins

Investigations carried out on eight placental mammals led to the conclusion that despite the number of components detected by electrophoresis varies from one species to another, only two distinct neurophysins exist in each species (15). We have proposed to call these two types MSEL- and VLDV-neurophysins according to the nature of the amino acids in positions 2, 3, 6 and 7. In fact the two neurophysins differ by the N-terminal sequences (residues 1 to 9) and the C-terminal sequences (residues 75 to 93/95), the central parts being nearly identical.

MSEL-neurophysins. MSEL-neurophysins of eight species, namely ox, sheep, pig, horse, whale, rat, guinea pig and man, have been completely sequenced (23). These neurophysins have 93/95 residues. Variations virtually occurred only in the last seven positions. Within the family the number of substitutions varies from 1 to 10 when the ox is taken as reference.

VLDV-neurophysins. Amino acid sequences of the VLDV-neurophysins from five species, namely ox, pig, horse, rat and man, have been determined (23). VLDV-neurophysins have 93 residues. The number of substitutions varies from 6 to 13 when the ox is taken as reference.

b) Comparison between the two types of neurophysins

Comparison between the two families is shown in Fig. 2. In a given species, there are about 20 substitutions between the two types of neurophysins. Because these

479

substitutions are concentrated in N- and C-terminal sequences, these regions act as specific antigens and the two types of neurophysins can be distinguished by monospecific antibodies (24). Half-cystines residues are in the same positions in the two types so that it can be assumed that the 7 disulfide bridges are identical. Because of the strong homology in the sequences (80 %), the general conformations are likely very similar.

The striking feature is the central part (residues 10-74), nearly invariant between the two neurophysins of a given species and between the species. This central part is encoded by a particular exon. The nearly identity within the species has been explained by a recent gene conversion (10,12). The invariance from species to species, however, must be explained by another reason, perhaps a hormone-binding function subjected to selective pressure.

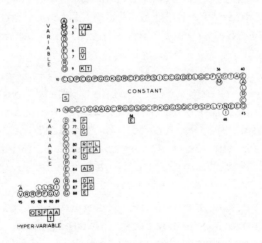

Fig.2. Comparison between MSEL- and VLDV neurophysin families. Bovine MSEL-neurophysin amino acid sequence is indicated by circles and substitutions in other MSEL-neurophysins by adjacent circles. Positions substituted in VLDV-neurophysins are indicated by squares. The N-terminal part (1-9) is variable between the two types of neurophysins but the C-terminal part (76-95) is also variable within the families; the central region (10-75) is virtually constant.

III - EVOLUTION OF COPEPTINS

The third domain of the vasopressin precursor, copeptin, is a 39-residue glycopeptide that has been characterized in ox, sheep, pig (25), man (26), rat (27) and guinea-pig (28). The polysaccharide is postranslationally attached to asparagine in position 6. It may account for 50% of the molecular weight that is around 10.000 daltons. The possible function of copeptin is unknown.

It is interesting to note that the C-terminal part of MSEL-neurophysin (residues 77-95) and copeptin are encoded by the same third exon (8), and that the percentages of substitutions, when man and rat are compared, are 58% and 62%, respectively (27). Clearly the three exons of the vasopressin gene have different rates of evolution and because MSEL-neurophysin depends upon the three, these different rates reflect in the three parts of its sequence.

IV - EVOLUTION OF MULTIPRECURSORS

Although neurophysins of lower vertebrates are not yet characterized, their presence has been demonstrated by radioimmunoassays and immunocytochemistry. Furthermore neurohypophysial hormone-like and neurophysin-like polypeptides have been detected in some invertebrates by using the same techniques (13, 14). It can be assumed that a protogene has been formed before the invertebrate-vertebrate divergence although the function of its protein product can not be guessed. This protein could have been a precursor for both a hormone-like peptide and a neurophysin-like protein or could have been a multifunctional protein with several domains. Processing appeared, at the latest, in early vertebrates. Because Cyclostomes seem to have a single neurohypophysial hormone, namely vasotocin, whereas fishes have two, a duplication likely occurred before the emergence

of fishes. We can postulate in bony fishes the presence
of two macromolecular precursors, one for isotocin
and one for vasotocin. Parallel evolutions could have
led to the eutherian hormones, oxytocin and vasopressin, with their respective VLDV- and MSEL-neurophysins.

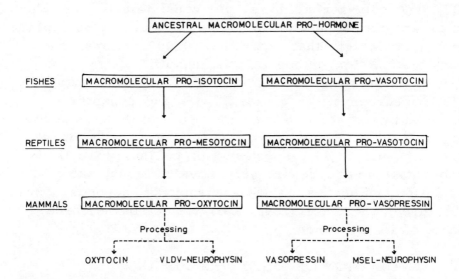

Fig. 3. Hypothetic evolution of common neurohypophysial
hormone-neurophysin precursors.A duplication between
Cyclostomes and bony fishes gave two distinct macromolecular precursors; subsequent mutations led to two evolutionary lines, an oxytocin-like/VLDV-neurophysin line
and a vasopressin-like/MSEL-neurophysin line. A similar
processing in each vertebrate   class made the nonapeptide hormones and the corresponding neurophysins.

Because all the neurohypophysial hormones have nine
residues with a C-terminal glycinamide, the processing
of the precursors, which could involve a three-enzyme
system (29), remained remarkably precise and invariant
during vertebrate evolution. It will be of interest to examine marsupial neurophysins in order to see whether the
additional vasopressor peptide is accompanied with an additional MSEL-neurophysin and, if it is so, how much the
two proteins have diverged.

REFERENCES

1. Acher, R. (1980)
   Proc. R. Soc. Lond. B 210, 21-43.
2. Acher, R. (1981)
   Trends in Neurosci. 4, 226-230.
3. Acher, R. (1984)
   In:"Evolution and Tumor Pathology of the Neuroendo-
   crine System", S. Falkmer, R. Håkanson and
   F. Sundler (eds) Elsevier, Amsterdam, in press.
4. Acher, R., Chauvet, J. and Olivry, G. (1956)
   Biochim. et Biophys. Acta 22, 421-427.
5. Chauvet, J., Lenci, M.T. and Acher, R. (1960)
   Biochim. Biophys. Acta 38, 266-272.
6. Sachs, H., Fawcett, P., Takabatake, Y. and
   Portanova, R. (1969)
   Rec. Prog. Horm. Res. 25, 447-492.
7. Brownstein, M.J., Russell, J.T. and Gainer, H (1980)
   Science 207, 373-378.
8. Land, H., Schütz, G., Schmale, H and Richter, D. (1982)
   Nature 295, 299-303.
9. Land, H., Grez, M., Ruppert, S., Schmale, H.,
   Rehbein, M., Richter, D. and Schütz, G. (1983)
   Nature 302, 342-344.
10. Ruppert, S., Scherer, G. and Schütz, G. (1984)
    Nature 308, 354-358.
11. Schmale, H., Heinsohn, S. and Richter, D. (1983)
    The EMBO J. 2., 763-767.
12. Ivell, R. and Richter, D. (1984)
    Proc. Natl. Acad. Sci. USA, in press.
13. Remy, C. (1984)
    In: "Evolution of the Hormonal System", M. Gersh, and
    P. Karlson (eds) Nova acta Leopoldina, in press.
14. Grimmelikhuijzen, C.J.P. (1983)
    Neuroscience 9, 837-845.

15. Acher, R., Chauvet, J. and Chauvet, M.T. (1981)
In : "Medicinal Chemistry Advances", F.G. de las
Heras and S. Vega (eds) Pergamon Press, Oxford
and New York, pp. 473-485.

16. Hurpet, D., Chauvet, M.T., Chauvet, J. and
Acher, R. (1982)
Int. J. Peptide Prot. Res. 19, 366-371.

17. Chauvet, M.T., Colne, T., Hurpet, D., Chauvet, J.,
and Acher, R. (1983)
Biochem. Biophys. Res. Commun. 116, 258-263.

18. Chauvet, J., Hurpet, D., Chauvet, M.T. and
Acher, R. (1984)
Bioscience Rep. 4, 245-252.

19. Chauvet, J., Hurpet, D., Colne, T., Michel, G.,
Chauvet, M.T. and Acher, R. (1984)
Gen. Comp. Endocrinol. in press.

20. Pickering, B.T. and Heller, H. (1969)
J. Endocrinol. 45, 597-606.

21. Vizsolyi, E. and Perks, A.M. (1969)
Nature 223, 1169-1171.

22. Foldi,J., Cohen-Solal, M., Valentin, C., Blouquit, Y.,
Hollan, S.R. and Rosa, J. (1980)
Europ. J. Biochem. 109, 463-471.

23. Chauvet, M.T., Hurpet, D, Chauvet, J. and Acher, R.
(1960) Proc. Natl. Acad. Sci. USA 80, 2839-2843.

24. Chauvet, M.T, Chauvet, J., Acher, R. and Robinson,
A.G. (1979) FEBS Lett. 101, 391-394.

25. Smyth, D.G. and Massey, D.E. (1979)
Biochem. Biophys. Res. Commun. 87, 1006-1010.

26. Seidah, N.G., Benjannet, S.,and Chrétien, M. (1981)
Biochem. Biophys. Res. Commun. 100, 901-907.

27. Chauvet, M.T., Chauvet, J. and Acher, R. (1983)
FEBS Lett. 163, 257-260.

28. Chauvet, M.T., Chauvet, J. and Acher, R. (1984)
7th Int. Congr.Endocrinology, Abstract n°187.

29. Bradbury, A.F., Finnie, M.D.A. and Smyth, D.G. (1982)
Nature 298, 686-688.

EVOLUTIONARY APPROACH TO THE ANALYSIS OF STRUCTURE AND FUNCTION OF GANGLIOSIDES

N.F. AVROVA
Sechenov Institute of Evolutionary Physiology and
Biochemistry USSR, Academy of Science, Leningrad
194223, USSR.

INTRODUCTION

A rapid progress is characteristic for the modern
studies in glycolipid biochemistry. The structural
variety of gangliosides, their role in cell-cell interaction, in regulation of immune response, their participation in the reception processes have been elucidated to a greater extent in the recent years than
before. These achievements are mainly due to the development and application of new methods of chemical
analysis, of different immunochemical methods and of
tissue culture method. The good choice of the modern
methods is necessary, but not enough for the success
of the studies. The choice of the right line of investigation is indispensable as well. One of the effective
approaches to the understanding of the functional role
of the compounds is an evolutionary approach. In biochemistry a great contribution in this field was made
by works of Florkin, Hochachka, Oparin, Kreps and
other scientists.

The aim of the present communication is to describe
the importance of comparative studies of gangliosides
for understanding of their structural variety and
function in animals, including mammals, to try to elucidate the main trends of such studies, perspectives.

NEW FORMS OF GANGLIOSIDES

Many novel gangliosides were found in the recent years,
studying extraneuronal organs of mammals. Among the
fractions identified some are of special interest as
tumour-associated antigens expressed in early onto-

Proceedings of the 16th FEBS Congress
Part A, pp. 485–493
© 1985 VNU Science Press

genesis (1).

A number of new gangliosides was revealed, studying lower vertebrate brain. Thus in sixties Tettamanti and co-workers and our group found large amounts of tetra- and pentasialogangliosides in amphibia and fish brain (2, 3). Their presence in mammalian brain was established later on, thus pentasialoganglioside was revealed only in 1980 (4). polysialogangliosides appear to play special role in the differentiation of nervous cells, especially in synaptogenesis (4, 5).

Trisialogangliosides with short carbohydrate chain (G_{T3} and G_{T2}) were at first found in the cartilagenous and bony fish brain (6, 7). Then they were revealed as minor components in mammalian brain. Their discovery provides additional evidences for the existence of one of the pathways of ganglioside biosynthesis, postulated in recent years, these gangliosides being the intermediate products in this pathway.

Gangliosides with high per cent of poluunsaturated fatty acids were revealed by us in cold-water fishes, but they were not described previously (8). Their functional role in the processes of adaptation will be discussed later on.

It has been shown that gangliosides partially exist in the forms of O-acyl derivatives. The study of gangliosides from lower vertebrate brain appear to be very helpful in revealing the structural variety of these forms of gangliosides. O-acyl derivatives of gangliosides seem to be much more abundant in lower vertebrates as compared to mammals. Thus according to our data at least 90 % of lamprey brain gangliosides are susceptible to alkaline hydrolysis, this treatment dramatically diminishing their migration rates (9). Large per cent of gangliosides from fish brain, especially from bony fish brain, is alkali-labile as well, while in mammalian brain alkali-stable gangliosides predominate (10). The data obtained in our common work with Dr. Ghidoni, Dr. Nalyvaeva and Dr. Karpova, suggest that in cyclostomia, in contrast to other vertebrates, gangliosides with substituted carboxylic group predominate.

GANGLIOSIDE ROLE IN ADAPTATION OF ANIMALS TO THEIR ENVIRONMENT

Comparative studies are helpful for elucidation of new aspects of ganglioside function. After the creation of the evolutionary theory the efforts of the biologists were focussed on the study of the strategy of adaptation of the organisms to their environment. The changes of chemical organization of biological membranes were found to be of great importance for adaptation of animals to varying ecological factors. It has been shown that cell membrane phospholipids of nervous and other tissues of ectothermic "cold--blooded" animals, living at low temperature of habitat, are as a rule more unsaturated than phospholipids of animals, living at higher temperature. However, rather unexpected data were obtained when glycolipids were studied. Thus, no statistically significant differences in fatty acid composition and degree of unsaturation of cerebrosides and sufocerebrosides from brain of cold- and warm-water fishes were revealed according to the data of Levitina and co-workers (11).

The role of ceramide portion of gangliosides in adaptation to different environmental factors has not been investigated yet. While studying the natural adaptations of fishes our most important tasks were to answer the following questions: whether the adaptive function is characteristic of gangliosides, what components of their complex molecule reveal the adaptive changes of composition due to the varying environmental factors and whether the compensatory changes of ganglioside molecule make considerable contribution to the adaptive changes of biochemical organization of cell membranes.

Fatty acid composition of fish brain gangliosides was found to correlate with the environmental temperature, when 42 species of cartilagenous and bony fishes were studied. The data on brain lipid fatty acid composition of 7 most cold and deep-water and 7 most warm-water species studied have been compared. Brain gangliosides of cold-water species contain two times higher relative content of monoenoic fatty acids as

compared to those of the warm-water species. They
contain 15 % of polyenoic fatty acids which are practically absent in gangliosides from warm-water species.
The degree of unsaturation is thus much higher in brain
gangliosides from cold-water species than in those
from warm-water species. All these differences are
statistically significant ($p < 0.01$). The lowering of
the temperature of the habitat and the increase of the
depth of living appear to have synergetic effect.
It appears that the differences in fatty acid composition of gangliosides are much more pronounced than
those of other lipids. The data on phospholipid fatty
acid composition were obtained by Kreps, Pomazanskaya
and co-authors (12, 13), studying the same fish species.
In search of some quantitative criteria unsaturation
indexes were calculated and compared. It was shown
that gangliosides from brain of cold-water species
of fishes contained 92 double bonds more per 100 of
fatty acid residues than gangliosides of warm-water
species, for phosphatidylcholine this value was found
to be 38-43, for phosphatidylserine 52-56, for phos-
phatidylethanolamine and sphingomyelin the differences
in number of double bonds constituted only 9 and 19
respectively (14, 15).
   In the process of phylogenetic development of vertebrates the pronounced increase in the degree of saturation of brain ganglioside fatty acids took place,
reaching more than 95 % in mammals (14). These changes
appear to be adaptive in their nature as the membranes
of highly developed vertebrates (birds and mammals)
function at much higher temperature than the membranes
of lower vertebrates studied.
   A priori one could expect that the adaptive changes
of composition are characteristic of the second ganglioside hydrocarbon chain, belonging to sphingosine
bases, as well. Thus in phospholipids such changes were
shown both for fatty acids and aldehydes (12, 13).
However, no statistically significant differences in
the degree of saturation of brain ganglioside long
chain bases were found when cold and warm-water fishes
or representatives of different vertebrate classes
were compared (8, 14).

The data obtained provide evidences that the adaptive functions are characteristic of gangliosides. The changes of ganglioside fatty acid composition of nerve cells membranes under the influence of the environmental factors are directed to the maintainance of optimal phase condition and the degree of fluidity of biological membranes.

Gangliosides may play an adaptive role in extraneuronal membranes as well, in which their concentration is much lower. Thus it seems probable that the fluidity of the receptor sites in the membranes depends on ganglioside fatty acid composition. Its changes may cause the changes in the receptor properties of the membranes. There are certain possibilities to check this suggestion. Thus it is of interest to study the influence of ganglioside composition on the processes of interaction between cells of immune system and target cells. it seems that exogenous gangliosides may change the fluidity of the receptor sites and the susceptibility of the target cells (for example malignant cells) to the effectors.

THE ROLE OF GANGLIOSIDES IN THE FUNCTION OF NERVOUS CELLS

In the process of phylogenetic development of vertebrates ganglioside concentration in brain increases (15). It is several times higher in brain of birds and mammals, than in lower vertebrate brain. Reptiles occupy intermediate position when these values are compared. Somewhat higher content of gangliosides in lamprey brain than in fish and amphibia brain is most probably due to the absence of myelin in lampreys, myelin having low ganglioside concentration. In the nervous system of lower chordates (ascidia) ganglioside content was found to be approximately 10 times lower than in fishes and amphibia. These data confirm the general rule. In all vertebrates from lamprey to mammals ganglioside content in the nervous tissue is one - two orders higher than in other tissues and organs, being most high in the neuronal plasma membranes. These data suggest the specific role of the gangliosides in the function of the nervous cells of vertebrates. It is confirmed by model experiments, by studies of pathological cases and other data.

In animal kingdom gangliosides appear to be characteristic only for the two types of animals - chordates and echinoderms, both belonging to the branch of Deuterostomia. Previously the investigators failed to show the presence of gangliosides in lower chordates. However, in our studies, made together with Dr. Karpova and Dr. Nalyvayeva, gangliosides were revealed in nervous and other tissues of ascidia, sialic acid was identified as N-acetylneuraminic acid. Even in lower chordates ganglioside content is much lower in extraneuronal tissues as compared to the nervous tissue.

it is of interest to note that in echinoderms ganglioside distribution is quite different from that in chordates, most high ganglioside concentration being found in the tissue of gonads (16).

Gangliosides are polyfunctional compounds. The increase in brain ganglioside concentration during phylo- and ontogenetic development of vertebrates appear to be due to their role in the propagation of nerve impulse and to their role in nerve cell differentiation and synaptogenesis as well. It is of interest to note that in higher vertebrates most polar gangliosides, including tetrasialogangliosides, contain almost exclusively chains, consisting of two sialic acids. On the contrary, in lower vertebrates the chains, consisting of three successively attached sialic acids predominate in tri-, tetra- and pentasialogangliosides.

Comparative studies of gangliosides made with the aid of tissue culture method seem to be of great interest for understanding of the role of these lipids in the processes of cell-cell interaction, in the formation of complex assemblies of neurons, characteristic of vertebrates, especially of higher ones.

IMMUNOCHEMICAL STUDIES OF THE FUNCTIONAL ROLE OF GANGLIOSIDES AND OF THEIR DISTRIBUTION

Comparative immunochemical studies appear to be of even greater importance. Thus ontogenetic and evolutionary approaches are widely used in the investigation of cell surface antigens. There is a number of antigens, which are characteristic both for the malignant tumours, and for early stages of embyonic development. Thus sialylated Lewis[a] and a ganglioside, containing sialic acid, bound to 6 atom of external galactose ($6'-L_{M1}$) are abundant on early stages of embryonic development of mammals, while in adult animals they are either absent, or present in a very low concentration. At the same time they were shown to be tumour-associated antigens, being found in different types of carcinomas (1, 17). The search in various tumours of the compounds, for example gangliosides, expressed on early stages of embryonic and, probably, evolutionary development of vertebrates seems to be a fruitful approach to revealing of the tumour-associated antigens.

Gangliosides were found to be specific antigens of the nervous cells. They were shown to be present on the surface of glial cells as well. During ontogenetic development of vertebrates the composition of cell surface antigens, including gangliosides, reveals certain changes (18). Thus the increase of main brain monosialoganglioside and the disappearence of tetrasialoganglioside from cell surface was described to be characteristic of the process of maturation of some types of glial cells.

Gangliosides appear to be cell surface markers of different types of neurons. Thus an antigen, specific for cholinergic neurons, appears to be a ganglioside. it is of interest to note that an evolutionary approach was used to reveal this antigen, which was found to be present in different vertebrates - from fishes to mammals. as a source of antigen, used for immunization of animals, plasma membranes of nerve cell endings from electrical organ of a ray were used (19).

Thus, comparative biochemical studies appear to be an interesting and effective approach to understanding of structural variety and functional role of gangliosides.

REFERENCES

1. Hakomori, S. I. (1981). Glycosphingolipids in cellular interaction, differentiation and onco-genesis. A. Rev. Biochem. 50, 733-764.
2. Tettamanti, G., Bertona, L., Gualandi, V. and Zambotti, V. (1965). Sulla distribuzione dei gangliosidi de sistema nervoso in varie specie animali II. Contenuto percentuale dei signoli gangliosidi. Lombardo Acad. di Scienz. Lettere. Rendiconti 99, 173-188.
3. Avrova, N. F. (1968). Comparative studies of gang-liosides from brain of various vertebrates. J. Evol. Biochem. Physiol. 4, 128-136. (In Russian).
4. Svennerholm, L. (1980). Gangliosides and synaptic transmission. Adv. Exp. Med. Biol. 125, 533-544.
5. Mandel, P., Dreyfus, H., Yusufi, A. N. K., Sarlieve, L., Robert, J., Nescovic, N., Harth, H. and Rebel, G. (1980). Neuronal and glial cell cultures, a tool for investigation of ganglioside function. Adv. Exp. Med. Biol., 125, 515-532.
6. Avrova, N. F., Li, Y. T. and Obukhova, E. L. (1979). On the composition and structure of individual gangliosides from the brain of elasmobranches. J. Neurochem. 32, 1807-1815.
7. Yu, R. K. and Ando, S. (1980). Structure of some new complex gangliosides in fish brain. Adv. exp. Med. Biol. 125, 33-45.
8. Avrova, N. F. (1980). Gangliosides in fish brain. Adv. Exp. Med. Biol. 125, 177-186.
9. Avrova, N. F. (1979). Composition and structure of main gangliosides of lamprey brain. J. Evol. Physiol. Biochem. 15, 280-285. (Translated from Russian).
10. Chogorno, V., Sonnino, S., Ghidoni, R. and Tettamanti, G. (1982). Densitometric quantification of brain gangliosides separated by two-dimensional thin-layer chromatography. Neurochem. Internat. 4, 397-403.
11. Levitina, M. V., Abramova, L. N. and Kreps, E. M. (1979). Cerebrosides and sulfatides in brain of fishes and representattives of other vertebrate

classes. In: Physiology and Biochemistry of marine
and fresh-water animals, E. M. Kreps (Ed), Nauka,
Leningrad, pp. 89-129. (In Russian).

12. Kreps, E. M. (1981). Lipids of biological membranes.
Nauka, Leningrad, pp. 1-339.

13. Pomazanskaya, L. F., Chirkovskaya, E. V., Pravdina,
N. I., Kruglova, E. E., Chebotareva, M. A. and
Kreps, E. M. (1979). Phospholipids in brain of
fishes and representatives of other vertebrate
classes. In: Physiology and biochemistry of marine
and fresh-water animals, E. M. Kreps (Ed), Nauka,
Leningrad,, pp. 22-88. (In Russian).

14. Avrova, N. F. and Zabelinskiĭ, S. A. (1971).
Fatty acids and long chain bases of vertebrate
brain gangliosides. J. Neurochem. 18, 675-681.

15. Avrova, N. F., Obukhova, E. L. and Kreps, E. M.
(1979). Gangliosides in brain of fishes and representatives of other vertebrate classes. In: Physiology and biochemistry of marine and fresh-water
animals, E. Kreps (Ed), Nauka, Leningrad, pp. 130-
-155. (In Russian).

16. Avrova, N. F., Karpova, O. B. and Nalyvayeva, N. N.
(1983). Content and composition of gangliosides
from nervous tissue of a sea urchin Strongylo-
centrotus intermedius. J. Evol. Biochem. and
Physiol. 19, 127-132. (In Russian).

17. Lindholm, L., Holmgren, J., Svennerholm, L.,
Fredman, P., Nilsson, O., Persson, B., Marvold,
H. and Lagergard, T. (1983). Monoclonal antibodies
against gastrointestinal tumour-associated antigens
isolates as monosialogangliosides. Int. Arch.
Allergy Appl. Immunol. 71, 178-181.

18. Schachner, M. (1982). Cell type specific surface
antigens in mammalian nervous system.
J. Neurochem. 39, 1-8.

19. Richardson, P. J., Walker, J. H., Jones, R. Th.
and Whittaker, V. P. (1982). Identification of a
cholinergic specific antigen Chol-1 as a ganglioside. J. neurochem. 38, 1605-1614.

EVOLUTIONARY ADAPTABILITY OF BIOCHEMICAL SYSTEMS
(CONCEPT OF THE SUPERINFLAMMATORY RESPONSE)

MICHAEL CONRAD
Departments of Computer Science and Biological Sciences
Wayne State University
Detroit, Michigan 48202 USA

ABSTRACT

Adaptability theory suggests that biological organization
is subject to a number of important tradeoffs. The first
tradeoff is among evolutionary adaptability, information
processing efficiency, and programmability. The second
involves compensating changes in different forms of biological adaptability (genetic, developmental, immunologic,
behavioral, populational,...). These tradeoffs present
biological systems with problems of control and defense
which are logically intractable, though manageable in an
approximate sense. Defense mechanisms are discussed as
an example. Correction of an overly strong or an overly
weak defense (or inflammatory) response is called a superinflammatory response. If the superinflammatory response
is overly effective the organism will be resistant to
allergy and to autoimmune disease, but will be susceptible
to neoplasms. All these tradeoffs should be considered
by the biotechnologist embarking on the enterprise of
"genetic programming".

1. INTRODUCTION

I wish to look at the organization of biochemical systems
in the light of adaptability theory. By adaptability I
mean the ability to continue to function in the face of
an uncertain environment. The formal structure of adaptability theory and applications to a variety of systems
at different levels of biological organization has been
thoroughly described in a recent monograph [1]. It
would be redundant to redescribe the formalism here.
Instead I will focus on three principles which emerge

Proceedings of the 16th FEBS Congress
Part A, pp. 495–509
© 1985 VNU Science Press

from the theory. These three principles are the ones
most relevant to the relationship between biochemical organization and evolution.

2. THE TRADEOFF PRINCIPLE

The first principle is that of tradeoff. A system
(whether natural or artificial) cannot at the same time
be evolutionarily adaptable, process information in an
efficient manner, and be structurally programmable. By
evolutionary adaptability I mean the capacity to learn
through the evolutionary mechanism of variation and natural selection. By information processing I mean the
ability to transform patterns of input to patterns of output. An information processing system is efficient to
the extent that it can solve a particular input-output
problem with economical usage of its space and time resources (space resources might be components such as atoms
or molecules). This corresponds to one notion of computational efficiency. A system is called structurally programmable if the rule (program, or more generally, map in
the mathematical sense) which generates its behavior is
encoded in the states and connectivity of its components
in a manner which is completely defined by a finite pro-
grammer's manual. All present day digital computers are
structurally programmable. But in general systems in
nature are not structurally programmable.

Without going into details we can argue thus. If a
system is structurally programmable it is universal in
the sense that it can simulate any other system. The relation between its structure and its behavior is arbi-
trary. As a consequence it is unlikely to use its physical resources efficiently for information processing.
Furthermore, slight changes in the structure of a structurally programmable system are equivalent to slight
changes in the rule which generates its behavior. But
in general slight changes in a rule of the computer program type leads to radical changes in behavior. (For the
details of this argument see [2].)

Man made computers are programmable. According to the
tradeoff principle this limits their adaptability and

496

computational efficiency, features which correspond to
realities of present day computing. Biological systems
are the products of evolution. Hence they must be evolutionarily adaptable. If they are to be efficient information processors they cannot at the same time be programmable. It is evident that systems such as the brain and
the immune system are fantastic information processing
devices. So it is hardly surprising that we cannot prescribe the rules they are to follow in the same all controlling sense that we can prescribe the rules which a
digital computer follows. We may speak of genetic programming. This makes sense to the extent that we can now
manipulate genes with some degree of precision. But this
does not mean that we can design and prescribe the behavior of biochemical systems in a manner which is similar
to that which we have gained from our experience with
machines. According to the tradeoff principle it would
be very dangerous to design plants and animals in a manner
which would allow them to be programmed in the digital
computer sense. Such plants and animals could no longer
be evolutionarily adaptable; and in fact they would not
be very efficient processors.

3. THE BOOTSTRAPPING PRINCIPLE

What makes biological organizations suitable for evolution? The fundamental control elements in biology are enzymes and other macromolecules. The important changes
which underlie evolution involve either sequences of
amino acides or regulatory elements which control the expression of DNA. Amino acid sequences fold up to form
the tertiary structures of proteins. This process of
folding is a continuous dynamic process. When the sequence is altered a bit it is often (though not always)
the case that the three dimensional structure and function is altered in a gradual manner. When the regulatory
genes are altered a bit it is often (but not always) the
case that the structure and function of the phenotype as
a whole is altered in a gradual manner. This type of
dynamic gradualism is absent in formal systems such as
computer programs. This is why computers are not well

suited to evolution by variation and selection. On the other hand, the number of possible control elements in a biological system is almost arbitrarily large. For example, there are 20^{300} possible proteins of length 300. This is why biological systems are not suited for effective programming. Of course it is in principle possible to use digital computers to simulate the dynamic features of biological systems which make evolution possible. But this is a computational cost. This is why the tradeoff principle must include efficiency as well as evolutionary adaptability and programmability.

The dynamic features which facilitate evolution are in general thermodynamic costs to an individual organism. One can imagine two forms of a protein, A and A', which perform the same mechanistic function. Protein A might consist of a smaller number of types of amino acids altogether. But however more efficient A is than A' from the thermodynamic point of view it would never be able to come into being through the process of evolution unless it could be discovered through a reasonably probable sequence of genetic changes—in other words, unless it has the gradualism property. Those proteins which have the gradualism property—which are well constructed for evolution—will always predominate in the course of evolution. Furthermore, suppose that by adding some redundant types of amino acids or some extra amino acids to A we produce an A' which is capable of undergoing an evolutionary advance. Then these redundant features will hitchhike along with the evolutionary advance which they facilitate. In this way protein structures can become more suited to evolutionary search through the process of evolution.

I call this principle of self-facilitation the bootstrap principle because of the fable about the man who picks himself up by his own bootstraps. Evolution picks up evolutionary adaptability through the process of evolution [3].

The bootstrap principle also applies to levels of biological organization above that of the protein. Examples are genetic regulatory processes, the metabolic organizations proposed by Sel'kov [4], hormonal and second messenger systems [5[, the immune system, and nervous

systems [6]. How the principle manifests itself at these
different levels of organization is reviewed in [1].

4. THE PRINCIPLE OF COMPENSATION

Now I want to consider a third principle of adaptability
theory, that of compensation among different forms of
adaptability. A biological system might utilize a variety of different forms of adaptability: for example,
genetic, developmental, immunologic, behavioral, populational. Each of these involves some thermodynamic cost.
High genetic adaptability entails the occurrence of variant organisms which are not optimally suited to a particular environment; high developmental adaptability requires
machinery for alternative patterns of growth; populational adaptability might involve culturing of organisms,
therefore rapid changes in population size. It is reasonable to assume that organisms will tend to dispense with
adaptabilities which are never required by their environment. It is also reasonable to assume that the costs of
different forms of adaptability depend on the morphological character of an organism. For a plant genetic and
developmental modes of adaptability are inexpensive--
many different variant structures are possible. For a
vertebrate the variety of morphological structures is more
limited. Genetic and developmental modes of adaptability
become relatively more expensive. Culturability is also
expensive since the lifespan is long and the cost of producing an offspring is high. To live in an uncertain environment a vertebrate must develop compensating modes of
adaptability. Physiological adaptabilities such as those
provided by the immune system and brain compensate for
the reduction in genetic and developmental adaptability.
    Several other factors enter into adaptability. Variab-
ility contributes to adaptability only if it is coupled
to anticipation of the environment. Information processing plays a role here. Protective mechanisms which reduce
the organism's sensitivity to features of the environment
also play a role. According to the principle of compensation a restriction on one mode of adaptability must
either be compensated by the enhancement of another mode

or by a narrowing of the environment (or niche) in which
the organism lives.

5. DEFENSE SYSTEM AS EXAMPLE

Plants, owing to their open growth systems, have a much
simpler defense problem than vertebrates. Physical damage to a plant or a root is largely localized. Diseases
of the xylem or phloem are the most serious since these
can have global ramifications. Higher plants thus become
more sensitive to disease processes. Unfortunately this
fact is now being manifested by some of the forests of
the world, such as those of Central Europe.
   Some specific defense mechanisms are probably present
in plants. But I think the most important one, possibly
of importance even for animals, is largely overlooked.
Both plants and animals are ecosystems with rich microbial
flora. Some of these microorganisms are symbionts which
contribute to nutrition. Others are parasites, still
others are generally thought to be neutral residents.
   However, even these mechanistically neutral residents
may contribute to a defense function. Suppose that the
plant or animal provides a niche which is occupied by a
minimally harmful microbial species. Suppose this species
becomes locally extinct, due to changes in external conditions or perhaps to the application of a drug. The
niche is then freed for occupancy by some other species,
one which might be harmful to the host organism. Of
course if this second species were competitively superior
to the original occupant it would probably eventually re-
place it in any case. But one can reasonably suppose
that the original species coevolved with the host organism and is therefore an evolutionarily stable occupant.
Furthermore, it might be a link in a very complex sequence
of material transformations involving other microbial
residents and the host organism itself. It might, for
example, detoxify the toxic products of other residents.
Such resident flora provide the first line of defense
against infectious disease whether or not they contribute
to any process which is otherwise physiologically necessary for the health of the host organism.

Vertebrates, because of their morphological complexity and the closed character of their growth system, are much more sensitive to infectious disease. Their external membranes (skin, alimentary and urogenital tract, conjunctiva,...) are all occupied by a rich resident flora. Many viruses appear to reside in individual cells. It is true that germ free organisms can be raised which suffer only nutritional deficiencies. However, as soon as these are exposed to a normal environment they are occupied by microbial forms. The extent to which they are subject to invasion by undesirable forms is not known. But ecological theory suggests that a coevolved resident flora should provide a first line of defense even if many components of this flora have no obvious physiological function.

Because of the sensitivity of vertebrates to infection it is essential to eliminate certain microorganisms altogether and at least to prevent significant numbers from invading internal tissues. There are a variety of defense mechanisms, such as outflowing mucus, antiseptic properties of body fluids, and antiviral mechanisms involving interferon. But the best known defense mechanism is that of antibody-based immunity. Each antibody species (or each lymphocyte clone) can be thought of as blocking a niche which could otherwise be occupied by some microbial form. As animals become phylogenetically more complex this second line of defense becomes more important and more elaborate.

The immune system, along with the central nervous system, is one of the great organ systems of compensating adaptability. The microbial forms can largely adapt to changing circumstances through evolutionary mechanisms. Physiological mechanisms are also available to them, but their simple structure and short generation times allow for evolutionary adaptation on a fairly short time scale. The vertebrates are the opposite extreme. The clonal selection mechanism of immunity [7] is in effect an internalized mechanism of evolutionary adaptation which compensates for the constraints on phylogenetic evolution imposed by the morphological complexity and lifespan of vertebrates.

The tradeoff principle applies to the immune system in

501

a particularly clear way. The large number of graded antibody specificities which are possible allows for high evolutionary adaptability, important both for phylogenetic evolution and ontogenetic learning. The immune system is also a powerful and highly efficient information processing system. The most fundamental level of information processing is recognition of antigen by antibody. From the computational point of view this is a difficult pattern recognition task. It is quick and effective in nature due to the tactile matching of antibody and antigen conformation and due to the fact that the antibody molecules are small enough to explore the antigen through Brownian motion. Higher levels of information processing are also important in the immune system. The lymphocyte must decide when to proliferate and when to export antibody into the blood. The decision is influenced by the pattern of antibodies which accumulate on the cell membrane as well as by signals from other cells and by mediators which carry information from other parts of the body. There are many higher levels of control which are inadequately understood. The key point is that the evolutionary adaptability and information processing efficiency of the system is based on the large number of control elements (the antibodies) and on dynamical information processes of a special purpose nature at the cellular level. These features exclude structural programmability of the type present in digital computers.

The bootstrap principle is also illustrated. Antibodies contain looped regions whose amino acid structure can vary. It is these looped regions which make the great variety of specificities possible. In principle it would be possible to design antibodies without loops which could perform the mechanistic task of pattern recognition more efficiently. But evolutionary adaptation would be much slower. The antibody molecule must have evolved to facilitate effective evolutionary adaptation. The same type of consideration could be applied to the higher levels of cellular and hormonal information processing in this system.

The idea that the resident microbial flora provides a first line of defense against infectious disease has an interesting and perhaps disturbing implication. The classical infectious diseases (measles, tuberculosis, syphilus,...) are caused by specific microorganisms which can be shown to have a unique connection to the disease. Many of the bacterial infections may be treated by antibiotics or other drugs. These drugs inevitably reduce or eliminate normal bacterial species. The diversity of the microbial flora on some of the body surfaces may be decreased, on others increased due to the elimination of control inherent in the normal competition among different species. To the extent that surfaces are sterilized by drugs the first line of defense is weakened. Niches are opened up which can be occupied by undesirable forms, especially when they come into communication with tissues which are overgrown with unusual forms. Even if these tissues are repopulated by species which were originally present the overall ecological balance will be initially disturbed, or may remain disturbed until a sufficient number of species can immigrate in, perhaps from body reservoirs. One can expect inflammatory reactions under these circumstances, in some cases initially aggravating the imbalance. A number of subtle infectious diseases which have become more prominent in recent times are probably due to this sequential process of stabilization, which in all respects is an ecological succession process.

6. THE SUPERINFLAMMATORY RESPONSE

Now I want to look a little more carefully at the adaptability structure of the immune system. When an animal is invaded by an outside agent it exhibits the well known inflammatory response. Roughly speaking, chemotactic stimuli are released from the wound, in some cases the area is blocked off by structural changes, antibodies are either released by memory cells or new lymphocyte lines are activated, antibodies catch on to antigenic sites of the invading agent, neutrophil leukocytes migrate in to ingest and destroy antibody coated bacteria, macrophages enter to ingest the neutrophils and other debris... The process is much more complicated than this [8]. The main point is that by and large it is a fairly purposeful

sequence of events which lead from a perturbed state of
the organism back to its stable state.

There are a number of circumstances in which the inflammatory response is either too strong or too weak for the
health of the organism. Allergy and autoimmunity are
cases in which it is too strong. Diseases in which the
insult is directed against the mechanisms of the inflammatory response result in a weakened defense. These diseases include various acquired deficiencies in leukocyte
lines or in various other components of the inflammatory
response, or exhaustion of these components by the disease process. The possibilities are too varied to be enu-
merated here [9]. In all these cases one can view the
organism as being moved to an unusual perturbed state. If
it returns to a stable state of organization the return
would appear to have a purposeful aspect, just as the return to a stable state after a normal insult which does
not affect the inflammatory mechanisms appears to have a
purposeful aspect. The difference is that the sequence
of states through which the organism passes will be much
more variable due to the fact that it is starting from
highly atypical regions of its phase space. More simply
stated, the organism is returning to a normal inflammatory
response from either an overly strong or overly weak inflammatory response. I will call this return the superinflammatory response.

There are a number of known mechanisms of superinflammatory response. One is Burnet's mechanism of acquired immunological tolerance [7]. Lymphocytes which recognize
antigens present in low numbers for a long period of time
recognize this fact and essentially commit suicide. A
second mechanism is provided by the idiotype-anti-idiotype
concept of Jerne [10]. Antibodies present in large quantities serve as antigens for other antibodies. Eventually
a network of antigens and antibodies are formed which
serves to control the growth dynamics of different antibody species. This control is superimposed on more direct mechanisms of feedback inhibition. If too many free
antibodies of a certain species are present the production of that species will be reduced. Undoubtedly there
are many other control processes operating in the immune

system and in the defense system overall [11].

The most obvious function of the immune system is to distinguish non-self from self. Another function is to recognize and control abnormal self. An idea which is often alluded to is that immunity helps to control neoplasms [12]. Errors in replication in a large metazoan organism are bound to produce abnormal, "neoplastic" cell lines. In plants these remain relatively localized. Plant galls and tumors are not too serious. But in vertebrates an abnormal growth or dissemination of neoplastic lines can have devastating systemic effects. If the cells of these lines have unusual surface structures, they can be controlled by the organism's own immune system. In effect, the inflammatory response can be used to control "subversive" tissue as well as foreign invaders.

Now I want to look at this whole system of inflammation and superinflammation in the light of the principle of compensation. Recall that the high development of the immune system compensates for restrictions on genetic evolution in morphologically complex animals. The immune system allows the rate of internal evolution to match the rate of viral and bacterial evolution. The morphological complexity which makes such an internal system of evolutionary adaptation necessary in the vertebrates also makes them particularly sensitive to neoplastic disease. A strong inflammatory response is thus necessary for the morphological integrity of the organism. As a consequence allergies and autoimmune diseases become inevitable. To mitigate these a strong superinflammatory response is necessary. But if the superinflammatory response is too effective, control of neoplasms will be weakened. For example, allergies may be corrected through the mechanism of acquired immunological tolerance. But if the mechanism of acquired immunological tolerance is too effective the organism will too easily tolerate neoplastic cell lines. Allergies and autoimmune diseases may also be corrected through the idiotype-anti-idiotype network. Any antibody which remains in the body too long will eventually be controlled by antibodies which respond to its idiotype. But if this mechanism is too effective antibodies to neoplastic cell lines may not be able to grow as fast

505

as these lines.

Adaptability theory thus suggests tradeoffs among a number of different types of diseases. There are the inherited (or genetic) diseases, the infectious diseases, the autoimmune and allergic diseases, and the neoplastic diseases. The genetic diseases are expressions of evolutionary adaptation. Genetic variation inevitably leads to organisms which are unsuited to the environment and in some cases unsuited to any environment (due to a serious organizational defect). As the morphological form of the species becomes more complex the liklihood of such genetic diseases increases, therefore the cost of evolutionary adaptability increases. Genetic variability is reduced. In vertebrates this is compensated by special organ systems of behavior and defense. If the defense mechanisms are too strong (if the inflammatory response is strong) the organism is resistant to infectious disease and to neoplastic disorders. But then it is susceptible to allergy and autoimmune disease. If the defense mechanisms are weak the susceptibility to neoplasms and to infectious disease or other outside insults increases. Mechanisms of superinflammation exist which can allow the organism to have a strong inflammatory response, but nevertheless weaken it when it leads to allergy or self-destruction due to immunity. But when the superinflammatory response is overly effective the defense against neoplasms will fail. Similarly the defense against persistent infectious disease and control over the resident flora will fail.

These remarks are of course very general. Not much is yet known about the theory of the superinflammatory response. In fact, not much is known about its phenomenology or about how the symptoms of various diseases are modified in different superinflammatory states. Undoubtedly new mechanisms of superinflammation will be discovered. After all, organisms continue to live and reproduce despite being faced by the logically intractable problem of eliminating all forms of disease. Hopefully in the future a better appreciation of the tradeoffs between these different disease mechanisms will be obtained. In the meantime it is important to recognize that treatments which are directed against one class of disease--say the

use of antiinflammatory or anticancer drugs--are likely to
arouse diseases of other classes.

7. PROBLEMS OF BIOTECHNOLOGY

The principles which I have listed are, I believe, highly
relevant in the upcoming age of biotechnology. The biochemists and molecular biologists have succeeded in developing powerful methods of specifically altering genes and
potentially of producing a large variety of specific proteins in commercial quantities. The effect on agricul-
ture, chemical technology, and medicine will probably be
revolutionary. It is likely that some great human bene-
fits will accrue; undoubtedly it will be impossible to
avoid painful mistakes.

One mistake would be to try to build biology-based technologies which are controllable in the same precise sense
that programmable computers are controllable. Such systems will not be evolutionarily adaptable. They will be
catastrophe prone and any society which relies on them
will be catastrophe prone. Another mistake would be to
try to achieve efficiency--say agricultural efficiency--
at the expense of evolutionary adaptability. A third mistake would be to ignore the principle of compensation. If
one part of a system becomes too complex to be adaptable
this should be compensated by adaptability in some other
part. Our present day digital computers have the potential to enhance adaptability by enhancing information
processing. But they are not evolutionarily adaptable.
Attempting to automate functions which require evolutionary adaptability and computational efficiency comparable
to that found in biological systems will inevitably lead
to a catastrophe prone civilization.

When gene technology based systems are developed it must
be recognized that they will be subject to the same types
of diseases as naturally evolved biological systems. They
will be subject to infection, to neoplastic disorders,
and to undesired genetic variation. Defense mechanisms
(fault tolerance) will have to be built into such systems.
If these defense mechanisms are too strong, counterpro-
ductive defensive reactions will occur. If they are too

507

weak undesirable internal disorders will be inevitable. Adaptability theory implies that these tradeoffs are inherent in both natural and artificial systems. Living with them is possible, though sometimes discomforting and sometimes even impossible for the individual. But trying to eliminate them completely is logically impossible and in practice dangerous.

Acknowledgments. This work was supported by NSF Grant MCS-82-05423. I acknowledge stimulating discussion with Professors O. and R. Rössler.

REFERENCES

1. Conrad, M. (1983). Adaptability: the Significance of Variability from Molecule to Ecosystem. Plenum Press, New York.
2. Conrad, M. (1983). Design principles for a molecular computer, Technical Report CSC-83-011. Also see reference [1] above.
3. Conrad, M. (1979). Bootstrapping on the adaptive landscape. BioSystems 11, 167-182. For a discussion of the connection of the bootstrap principle to informational value see Conrad, M. and Volkenstein, M.V. (1981). Replaceability of amino acids and the self-facilitation of evolution. J. theor. Biol. 92, 293-299.
4. Sel'kov, E.E. (1975). Stabilization of energy charge, generation of oscillations and multiple steady states in energy metabolism as a result of purely stoichiometric regulation. Eur. J. Biochem. 59, 151-157.
5. Liberman, E.A., Minina, S.V., and Golubtsov, K.V. (1975). The study of the metabolic synapse. I. Effect of intracellular microinjection of 3'5'-AMP. Biofizika 20, 451-456.
6. Conrad, M. (1984). Microscopic-macroscopic interface in biological information processing. BioSystems 16, 345-363.
7. Burnet, F.M. (1959). The Clonal Selection Theory of Acquired Immunity. Vanderbilt University Press, Nashville, Tennessee.
8. For example see A.W. Ham and T.S. Leeson (1961). Histology, ch. 8. J.B. Lippincott Co, Philadelphia.

9. See Wintrobe, M.M. (1981). Clinical Hematology. Lea and Febiger, Philadelphia.
10. Jerne, N.K. (1974). Towards a network theory of the immune system. Ann. Immunol. Inst. Pasteur 125C, 373-385.
11. For interesting suggestions see Rössler, O.E. and Lutz, R.A. (1979). A decomposable continuous immune network. BioSystems 11, 281-285.
12. For example see Frei, E. and Bodey, G.P. (1974). Principles of neoplasia. In: Harrison's Principles of Internal Medicine. McGraw-Hill, New York.

THERMOGENESIS OF BROWN ADIPOSE TISSUE (BAT) DURING DEVELOPMENT

Z.DRAHOTA, J.HOUŠTĚK, P.JEŽEK, J.KOPECKÝ, H.RAUCHOVÁ, and Z.RYCHTER

Institute of Physiology, Czechoslovak Academy of Sciences, Vídeňská 1083, 142 20 Prague 4, Czechoslovakia

INTRODUCTION

Heat production of BAT represents an important site of nonshivering thermogenesis in mammals. The thermogenic capacity of BAT depends (for ref. see 1) on developmental status, thermal environment and possibly also on dietary intake. Therefore, BAT is very dynamic tissue with respect to its amount, composition and metabolism.

Heat production in BAT results from physiological incoupling of oxidative phosphorylation (1). The energy of respiration-generated gradient of protons across the inner mitochondrial membrane is dissipated via a specific, regulatable conductance for protons, independent of H^+-ATPase function. The thermogenic pathway is represented by an abundant membrane protein with Mr of 32,000 called uncoupling protein (UP). This protein binds various purine nucleotides, including GDP (also GDP-binding protein), and is strictly specific for BAT. Besides H^+-conductivity, UP is also involved in the typical high permeability of BAT mitochondria for Cl^- and some other anions. Purine nucleotides inhibit both H^+- and Cl^--conductance. The second important regulatory ligand of UP free fatty acids (FFA) which activate specifically only H^+-conductance due to a direct interaction with UP. They most probably serve as an acute regulator of the rate of energy dissipation in BAT.

Proceedings of the 16th FEBS Congress
Part A, pp. 511–518
© 1985 VNU Science Press

RESULTS AND DISCUSSION

Embryogenesis of UP

The amount of UP correlates well with thermogenic
function of BAT during postnatal development and
during adaptive changes. To assess the embryonic
development of UP, its occurence was investigated
during the embryogenesis of rat. An immunodetection technique was used. UP was isolated from
cold adapted hamsters and antibodies were raised
in rabbits. Samples of rat embryonal BAT were
subjected to SDS-polyacrylamide gel electrophoresis, the separated proteins were transferred
to sheet of nitrocellulose and the reaction with
anti-UP serum was detected using a second antibody (swine) labeled with peroxidase (Sw Ar/Px).
As apparent from Fig. 1, homogenates of BAT of
21-d old (embryonal age) and older rats (after
the birth) exhibit high reactivity of the protein
band of 32,000-Mr which corresponds in mobility
to UP. This band is also clearly the most reactive one of all bands detected by this technique.

Fig. 1.   Fig. 2.

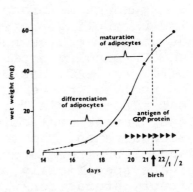

Immunodetection of UP   Organogenesis in rat
during prenatal deve-   of BAT.
lopment in rat.

512

Similarly, high reactivity of the 32 000-Mr band
is found at the day 20, but not at the day 19
(only traces) and before. The UP antigen thus
occurs rather suddenly at the day 20 of embryonal
life, which corresponds (Fig. 2) to the stage of
maturation of brown adipocytes (formation of
lipid droplets, smooth endoplasmic reticullum
etc.). Interestingly, the well differentiated
structure of mitochondria can be detected by
electronmicroscopy already at the day 18 (not
shown).

H^+- and Cl^--conductivity of BAT mitochondria

While the high H^+-conductivity plays apparently
a role in the thermogenic function, the physiological significance of the high Cl^--conductivity
is unclear. It has been previously concluded (1)
that Cl^- competes with transport of H^+-indicating
that both ions are translocated via the common
pathway. The most frequent method used to measure
Cl^- transport in BAT mitochondria was the induction of K^+-diffusion potential by suspending BAT

Fig. 3.

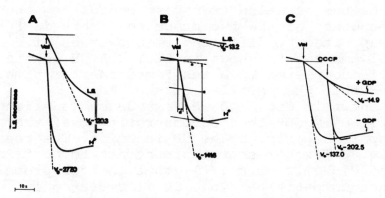

Val-induced H^+-extrusion (H^+) and Cl^--uptake
(L.S.) in hamster BAT mitochondria suspended in
KCl (A) or K_2SO_4 (B,C) media. In C only
H^+-extrusion induced by val is shown.

mitochondria in an isotonic KCl medium containing the ionophor valinomycin (val). In these conditions it was assumed (1) that K^+-movement across the mitochondrial membrane is compensated for only by Cl^- uptake. However, in submitochondrial particles or in liposomes identical conditions resulted in H^+-movements via another H^+-channel - F_0 of H^+-ATPase (2). Therefore, we have analysed (3) simultaneously H^+- and Cl^--conductance of BAT-mitochondria suspensed in isotonic K^+-media (+ val). As apparent from Fig. 3 A, in 150 mM KCl swelling (light scattering decrease; Cl^--uptake) and also extrusion of protons pH change were observed. Both Vo and the extent of these processes were several times higher than in rat liver mitochondria, thus confirming that the measured processes are specific for BAT. It is evident that in BAT the val-induced K^+-diffusion potential is compensated for not only by Cl^--uptake but also by H^+-extrusion. As shown in Fig. 3 B, also in isotonic K_2SO_4 an intensive H^+-extrusion is observed, no matter that no swelling, i.e. no anion uptake is found. Therefore, the BAT specific H^+-transport is induced both in the presence and absence of anion transport indicating the independence of the two processes. This is further supported by different time courses of H^+- and Cl^--movements shown in Fig. 3 A. H^+-extrusion is completed in a ten times shorter time period than the parallel Cl^--uptake.

As shown in Fig. 3 C, H^+-extrusion is strongly inhibited by GDP thus demonstrating that the transport depends on the UP function. The results of Fig. 3 further show, in contrast to conclusions of Nicholls et al. (1) that the two processes are not competitive. This is illustrated in Table 1 by Vo values of H^+-extrusion. In the presence of a parallel anion transport (Cl^--uptake - KCl) the H^+-conductance is rather higher than lower with respect to K_2SO_4 value, equivalent to the sole H^+-transport. As also

514

Tab. 1.

Experimental conditions	V_O (nmol H^+.min^{-1}.mg protein^{-1})	(%)	n
150 mM KCl	305.0 + 70.0	100	8
+ 200 μM GDP	33.8 + 5.2	11	4
+ 2 mg BSA/ml	86.9 + 3.7	28	4
110 mM K_2SO_4	141.0 + 12.0	100	10
+ 200 μM GDP	20.0 + 11.0	14	4
+ 2 mg BSA/ml	35.5 + 4.1	25	5

Initial rates of val-induced H^+-extrusion from BAT mitochondria in the KCl and K_2SO_4 media.

indicated in Tab. 1, the H^+-extrusion is equally sensitive to GDP and also to bovine serum albumin in both types of media (BSA; removal of FFA), again in contrast to a previous proposal (1) of a higher sensitivity to BSA when both ions are transported. That the two transport activities are independent and represented by two different pathways is also inferred by the lower sensitivity of H^+-transport (Ki = 6 μM) versus Cl^--transport (Ki = 2 μM). The movement of H^+ under the conditions used is opposite to the physiological situation, where protons extruded by respiratory chain reenter the mito-chondria via UP. However, as shown in Fig. 4, the loading of BAT-mitochondria by KCl and their subsequent suspension in sucrose + val results in exactly opposite movements of ions - similar-ly to the situation in vivo; H^+ is taken up by mitochondria and Cl^- is extruded. The relevance of the method presented to the physiological role of BAT is demonstrated in Fig. 5. It is evident, that during the postnatal development of BAT in the rat Vo values of H^+ and Cl^--transport correlate very well the amount of UP determined by estimation of GDP binding sites(4).

Fig. 4.   Fig. 5

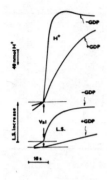

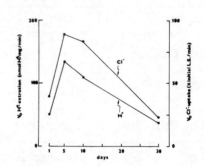

(H^+) and (L.S.)- see
Fig.3,in KCl loaded
mitochondria.

Val-induced Cl^--uptake
and H^+-extrusion in rat BAT
mitochondria during post-
natal development (measu-
red as in Fig. 3.A).

Nucleotide binding site (NBS) of UP, modification by diazobenzene sulfonate (DABS)

Each dimer of UP contains one NBS, which is localized on the cytosolic surface of the membrane.
The properties of these sites can be investigated by means of a chemical modification technique
which generally helps to recognize functionally
important amino acid residues. DABS acting in
intact mitochondria only on cytosolic surface
of the inner membrane was used as a modifying
agent. As shown in Fig. 6, (+GDP; lower trace),
50 nmol DABS added per mg of BAT-mitochondria,
prevents 10 μM nucleotide to inhibit H^+-trans-
location and similarly also Cl^--transpolation
(not shown). This treatment, however, has no

effect on the transport proper of any of the two
ions. As further shown in Fig. 6 (+GDP; upper
trace), the most of the DABS effect can be prevented when GDP is added before DABS. This
indicates that the two ligands can compete for
the identical site. The type of DABS-NBS (5)
interaction is illustrated by Scatchard plot
analysis (5) of ^{3}H-GDP binding in Fig. 7. As a
result of DABS treatment the binding of GDP is
clearly altered. When increasing the concentration of DABS from 10-75 nmol/mg prot, the
affinity of the binding decreases and Kd changes
from 2.6 to 15.0 μM. The amount of NBS, however,
does not significantly change. Therefore, even
after the DABS treatment the nucleotide can
reach the NBS when higher concentrations of the
nucleotide were used.

Fig. 6.   Fig. 7.

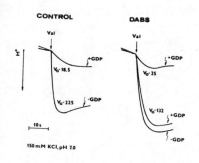 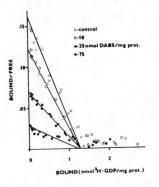

Effect of DABS on val-   Effect of DABS on ^{3}H-
induced H$^+$-extrusion in GDP binding to hamster
hamster BAT mitochond-   BAT mitochondria. Per-
ria (measured as in   formed as in ref. 5.
Fig. 3. B).

REFERENCES

1. Nicholls,D.G., and Locke,R.M. (1984). Thermogenic mechanisms in brown fat. Physiol.Rev.
   64, 1-64.
2. Kopecký,J., Houštěk,J., and Drahota,Z.(1984).
   Molecular aspects of structure-function relationship in mitochondrial H$^+$-ATPase. In:Struc-
   ture and properties of cell membranes, Benga,
   G., ed. CRC Press (in press).
3. Kopecký,J., Guerrieri,F., Ježek,P., Drahota,
   Z., and Houštěk,J. (1984). Molecular mechanism
   of uncoupling in brown adipose tissue mitochondria. FEBS Lett. 170, 186-190.
4. Sundin,U., and Cannon,B. (1980). GDP-binding
   to brown fat mitochondria of developing and
   cold-adapted rat. Comp.Biochem.Physiol. 65B,
   463-471.
5. Rial.E., and Nicholls,D.G. (1983). The regulation of proton conductivity of brown adipose
   tissue mitochondria. Identification of functional nucleotide binding sites. FEBS Lett. 161,
   184-288.